HORMONE REPLACEMENT THERAPY AND BREAST CANCER RISK

HORMONE REPLACEMENT THERAPY AND BREAST CANCER RISK

Edited by R. D. Mann

The Parthenon Publishing Group
International Publishers in Medicine, Science & Technology

Casterton Hall, Carnforth,
Lancs, LA6 2LA, UK

120 Mill Road, Park Ridge,
New Jersey 07656, USA

This volume is the Proceedings of a special symposium held at the Royal Society of Medicine, London, in September 1991

Published in the UK by
The Parthenon Publishing Group Limited
Casterton Hall, Carnforth,
Lancs, LA6 2LA, England

Published in the USA by
The Parthenon Publishing Group Inc.
120 Mill Road,
Park Ridge,
New Jersey 07656, USA

British Library Cataloguing in Publication Data
Hormone Replacement Therapy and Breast Cancer Risk
I. Mann, R. D.
618.1

ISBN 1-85070-399-x

Library of Congress Cataloging-in-Publication Data
Hormone replacement therapy and breast cancer risk / edited by R. D. Mann.
p. cm.
Includes bibliographical references and index.
ISBN 1-85070-399-X
1. Breast–Cancer–Risk factors. 2. Estrogen–Therapeutic use–Side effects.
3. Menopause–Hormone therapy–Side effects.
[1. Breast Neoplasms–chemically induced. 2. Estrogen Replacement Therapy–adverse effects.] I. Mann, Ronald D. (Ronald David), 1928–
[DNLM: 1. Risk Factors.]
RC280.B8H64 1992
616.99′449071–dc20
DNLM/DLC
for Library of Congress 92–14083
CIP

First published 1992

Phototypesetting by Lasertext Ltd., Manchester
Printed and bound in Great Britain by
Butler & Tanner Ltd., Frome and London, Great Britain

Contents

List of principal contributors

H.-O. Adami
Cancer Epidemiology Unit
University Hospital
S-751 85 Uppsala
Sweden

L.A. Brinton
Environmental Epidemiology Branch
National Cancer Institute
Executive Plaza North
Bethesda
Maryland 20892
USA

I. Burn
King Edward VII Hospital
Midhurst
West Sussex
UK

C.E.D. Chilvers
Department of Public Health Medicine and Epidemiology
Queen's Medical Centre
University of Nottingham
Nottingham NG7 2UH
UK

G.A. Colditz
Nurses' Health Study
180 Longwood Avenue
Boston
Massachusetts 02115
USA

E. Daly
Department of Public Health and Primary Care
University of Oxford
Gibson Building
Radcliffe Infirmary
Oxford OX2 6HE
UK

W.D. Dupont
Vanderbilt University School of Medicine
Department of Preventive Medicine
A-1124 Medical Center North
Nashville
Tennessee 37232-2637
USA

M.C. Ellerington
King's College Menopause Clinic
King's College Hospital
Denmark Hill
London SE5 9RS
UK

R.D. Gambrell, Jr
Department of Physiology and Endocrinology
Medical College of Georgia
Augusta
Georgia 30912
USA

B.S. Hulka
Department of Epidemiology
University of North Carolina
Chapel Hill
North Carolina 27599
USA

H.S. Jacobs
Division of Endocrinology
Medical Unit
University College and Middlesex School of Medicine
The Middlesex Hospital
Mortimer Street
London W1N 8AA
UK

D.W. Kaufman
Slone Epidemiology Unit
Boston University School of Medicine
1371 Beacon Street
Brookline
Massachusetts 02146
USA

R.D. Mann
The Royal Society of Medicine
1 Wimpole Street
London W1M 8AE
UK

M. Roche
Oxford Regional Health Authority
Old Road
Headington
Oxford OX3 7LF
UK

T.E. Rohan
NCIC Epidemiology Unit
Faculty of Medicine
University of Toronto
Toronto M5S 1A8
Canada

L. Rosenberg
Slone Epidemiology Unit
Boston University School of Medicine
1371 Beacon Street
Brookline
Massachusetts 02146
USA

R.K. Ross
USC School of Medicine
Norris Cancer Hospital and Research Institute
1441 Eastlake Avenue
Los Angeles
California 90033-0804
USA

M.A. Smith
Leeds Bone Mineralisation Unit
Department of Medical Physics and Department of Obstetrics
University of Leeds
Leeds General Infirmary
Leeds LS1 3EX
UK

M.A. Upsdell
Weaver Vale Practice
Hallwood Health Centre
Runcorn
Cheshire WA7 2UT
UK

C. La Vecchia
Istituto di Richerche Farmacologiche 'Mario Negri'
Via Eritrea 62
20157 Milan
Italy

M.P. Vessey
Department of Public Health and Primary Care
University of Oxford
Gibson Building
Radcliffe Infirmary
Oxford OX2 6HE
UK

N.S. Weiss
School of Public Health and Community Medicine
Department of Epidemiology
University of Washington
Seattle
Washington 98195
USA

Sir David Innes Williams
The Royal Society of Medicine
1 Wimpole Street
London W1M 8AE
UK

P.A. Wingo
Women's Health and Fertility Branch
Division of Reproductive Health
Center for Chronic Disease Prevention and Health Promotion
Atlanta
Georgia 30333
USA

Foreword

The Royal Society of Medicine, of which I have the honour to be the current President, embraces a wide range of specialist sections; it also provides a forum at which the non-medical professions and the health conscious laity can confront doctors and surgeons and discuss the issues of the day. There could, therefore, be no more appropriate venue than this Society for the symposium of which this volume provides the Proceedings, because the subject of hormone replacement therapy (HRT) and breast cancer risk not only involves a lot of specialists, but is also of very great public concern – a concern which is not infrequently whipped up by articles in the lay press.

These days, there is an element of autonomy amongst patients and a need for them to make their own choices but, as we all know, the assessment of risk and benefit is seldom achieved on any reasonable ground. Decisions are apt to be made emotionally and to be based upon over-optimistic hopes and unjustified fears. Thus, however much patients are autonomous, it remains the business of the doctors to advise them properly on the meanings and implications of the best available data, and this volume – based on a 3-day symposium to which many of the world's experts contributed – will, I am sure, help the doctors to fulfil their responsibilities to the greatest extent currently possible.

The choice which patients make regarding HRT will have very large implications, both for the pharmaceutical industry and for those who frame and implement health policy. The financial consequences of a large-scale move to long-term HRT would be enormous. Perhaps there are benefits, perhaps there are not – this is what those who attended this meeting or who study these Proceedings will need to decide.

Thus, I welcome this book which will, I believe, help women make informed choices regarding this important subject. I am glad to record my thanks from the Society to those who contributed to these Proceedings and I wish this volume success in the hands of those physicians and surgeons to whom it is addressed.

Sir David Innes Williams
President, The Royal Society of Medicine
London

Acknowledgements

It is a pleasure to acknowledge the expert help of Dr Mary Firth with the transcription and of Dr Andrew Cowling, of Parthenon Publishing, with the editing of this volume. The editor also wishes to thank Dr Helen Townsend for her invaluable help with proofreading, Miss Fiona Morris for help in organizing the symposium and Miss Tracey Greenhough for her very valuable assistance with wordprocessing. Warmest thanks are also due to those who gave presentations in this meeting and participated in the discussion which, at several points, indicates the way forward towards achieving an increased understanding of this difficult and important subject.

1

Hormone replacement therapy and breast cancer risk: studies of the last fifteen years

R.D. Mann

The need to strike a proper balance between the benefits and risks of the long-term use of hormone replacement therapy is obvious, but difficult and challenging. This book records the proceedings of an important symposium, held in London in September 1991, which attempted this task but with special reference to the possibility that hormone replacement therapy might increase the risk of breast cancer. Thus, the meeting gathered together many representatives of those groups that have conducted epidemiological and other studies on hormone replacement therapy and breast cancer risk; it went on to consider many of the broader issues that need to be kept in mind in evaluating the overall benefits and risks of such therapy. The focus of the meeting was, nevertheless, on cancer risk – and for the good reason that most general practitioners and patients are likely to demand a high standard of safety in respect of such risks when taking, for long periods of time, a prophylactic agent.

It is perhaps not unreasonable to look upon hormone replacement therapy as having two rather different places in therapeutics. On the one hand, it is used as a therapeutic agent in the management of the symptoms of the menopause. It is also used, for very much longer periods, for prophylactic purposes by those who believe that it offers a clinically useful degree of cardiovascular protection, and that it limits postmenopausal bone loss. If these benefits carry forward into the late decades of life and reduce the number of women dying from myocardial infarction and osteoporotic fractures, the place of long-term hormone replacement therapy seems likely to become increasingly important – unless the risks of cancer of the breast outweigh these benefits in the minds of women making their own choices from these alternatives.

There is already a very considerable and complex literature on the subject of hormone replacement therapy and breast cancer risk. It is reasonably well established that the results of animal studies suggest that exogenous oestrogens can induce breast cancer and that, in women, endogenous sex hormones seem to exert some such effect. A late onset of the menopause increases the risk of breast cancer and an early or surgical menopause reduces it; early menarche also increases the risk. Early childbirth is reported to be protective against breast cancer, but the risk increases with late age at first birth and with nulliparity. A positive family history of the disease elevates breast cancer risk but the effect of a history of benign breast disease is more controversial. These subjects will recur, from time to time, in considering this subject because the issues mentioned can act as confounders in epidemiological studies; they are, therefore, directly relevant to the subject of this symposium. The place of smoking, alcohol, and obesity in relation to breast cancer risk is well defined but each of these subjects already has its own well-known and extensive literature.

The specific studies on hormone replacement therapy and breast cancer risk go back to the very early 1970s – some of them having arisen from the work on the oral contraceptive and thromboembolism. This present introduction, however, will be limited to an initial consideration of the main studies of the last 15 years. These studies are of the case–control and cohort type and some show the effect of prolonged therapy.

Table 1 gives the overall relative risks reported from 21 case–control studies[1–21]. The first 13 of these reports suggest that hormone replacement therapy produces increased risks in specific groups, such as women receiving a higher total dose[2,3,5], those experiencing a natural menopause[1,2], those with a history of benign breast disease[7,9], nulliparous women[11], and those given injectable oestrogens[5]. In two of these studies[1,8], the relative risk is raised two- or threefold and the lower limit of the confidence intervals

Table 1 Case–control studies: ever-use of hormone replacement therapy vs. never-use

Reference	*Relative risk*	*95% confidence intervals*	*Type of controls*
Jick *et al.* 1980[1]	3.4	2.1–5.6*	Hospital
Ross *et al.* 1980[2]	1.1	0.8–1.9	Community
Hoover *et al.* 1981[3]	1.4	1.0–2.0	Community
Brinton *et al.* 1981[4]	1.24	1.0–1.5	Community
Hulka *et al.* 1982[5]	1.3	NS	Community
Hiatt *et al.* 1984[6]	0.7	0.3–1.6	Community
Brinton *et al.* 1986[7]	1.03	0.9–1.2	Community
La Vecchia *et al.* 1986[8]	1.93	1.35–2.75	Hospital
Nomura *et al.* 1986[9]	0.9	0.5–1.3	Community
Wingo *et al.* 1987[10]	1.0	0.9–1.2	Community
Rohan and McMichael 1988[11]	1.03	0.62–1.69	Community
Ewertz 1988[12]	1.28	0.96–1.71	Community
Bergkvist *et al.* 1989[13]	1.1	1.0–1.3	Community
Casagrande *et al.* 1976[14]	1.2	($p = 0.40$)	Community
Sartwell *et al.* 1977[15]	0.82	0.6–1.2	Hospital
Kelsey *et al.* 1981[16]	0.9	0.6–1.2	Hospital
Sherman *et al.* 1983[17]	0.71	0.34–1.11	Hospital
Horwitz and Stewart 1984[18]	0.9	0.5–1.7	Hospital
Kaufman *et al.* 1984[19]	0.9	0.7–1.1	Community
Talamini *et al.* 1985[20]	0.9	0.5–1.3	Hospital
McDonald *et al.* 1986[21]	0.74	0.51–1.08	Community

*90% confidence interval

exceeds unity; the remaining 19 studies have confidence intervals which include unity – none of the studies has an upper confidence limit below unity. Both studies with raised relative risks[1,8] have hospital controls; the rest of the studies have relative risks which cluster around unity in such a way to suggest that the overall risk of breast cancer is little affected by the use of hormone replacement therapy.

Table 2 summarizes the overall results of the ten cohort studies[22–31] which have been reported in the last 15 years and which have received most attention. Some of these studies[22–29] suggest specific groups that are at increased risk in relation to the use of hormone replacement therapy; these risks include women with benign breast disease[22,25], women using unopposed ethinyloestradiol[24] and current (as distinct from past) hormone replacement therapy use[25,28]. Several studies show that those receiving high-dose or prolonged therapy are at risk, but these two factors clearly confound one another and can, with advantage, be considered in examining the specific effects of prolonged therapy. Of these ten cohort studies, three[24,25,30] indicate raised relative risks with confidence intervals which exceed unity and one additional study[28] shows this in respect of current users of hormone replacement therapy. One study[31] appears to be an exception, but the rest have relative risks exceeding unity by what is perhaps a slightly greater margin than was seen in the case–control studies.

A number of these different studies show the effect of prolonged therapy and the relevant 14 case–control studies[3–13,15,19,21] are summarized in Table 3. Six of these studies[3,4,7,8,12,13] show a significant linear trend, in relation to duration of hormone replacement therapy administration, or show an increased relative risk with confidence intervals which exclude unity. The remaining studies show no such clear-cut effect, but it is notable that all seven studies[4,5,7,10,12,13,19] which report periods of administration exceeding 9–10 years show slightly raised relative risks associated with long durations of administration.

Table 2 Cohort studies

Reference	*Relative risk*	*95% confidence intervals*	*Types of control*
Hoover *et al.* 1976[22]	1.3	($p = 0.06$)	2nd and 3rd National Cancer Surveys
Buring *et al.* 1987[23]	1.1	0.8–1.4	Internal: ever-users vs. never-users
Hunt *et al.* 1987[24]	1.59	1.18–2.10	Cancer registry rates
Mills *et al.* 1989[25]	1.67	1.17–2.39	Internal
Dupont *et al.* 1989[26]	0.98	0.73–1.3	Internal: biopsy specimens
Bergkvist *et al.* 1989[27]	0.68	0.52–0.87	Community
Colditz *et al.* 1990[28]	0.98* 1.36†	0.81–1.18 1.11–1.67	Internal: ever-users vs. never-users
Hunt *et al.* 1990[29]	1.00	0.55–1.45	Cancer registry rates
Thomas *et al.* 1982[30]	1.80	1.04–3.10	Internal
Gambrell *et al.* 1983[31]	0.7	0.5–1.1	Internal/NCI-SEER 3rd National Cancer Survey

*Past users; †current users

Table 3 Studies showing the effect of prolonged therapy: case–control studies

Reference	*Duration of HRT* (years)	*Relative risk*	*95% confidence intervals*
Hoover *et al.* 1981[3]	≤ 4	1.4	
	≥ 5	1.7	
		(trend: $p = 0.022$)	
Brinton *et al.* 1981[4]	≤ 5	1.19	
	5–9	1.29	
	10+	1.21	
		(trend: $p = 0.03$)	
Hulka *et al.* 1982[5]			
community controls	0.5–3	2.1	($p < 0.05$)
	4–9	1.5	
	10+	1.7	
hospital controls	0.5–3	2.6	($p < 0.05$)
	4–9	1.6	
	10+	0.7	
Hiatt *et al.* 1984[6]	< 3	1.0	
	3–5	2.2	
	5+	0.8	
		(trend: $p = 0.41$)	
Brinton *et al.* 1986[7]	< 5	0.89	0.8–1.0
	5–9	1.09	0.9–1.3
	10–14	1.28	0.9–1.6
	15–19	1.24	0.9–1.8
	20+	1.47	0.9–2.3
		(trend: $p < 0.01$)	
La Vecchia *et al.* 1986[8]	≤ 2	1.66	1.06–2.58
	> 2	2.04	1.01–4.10
		(trend: $p = 0.001$)	
Nomura *et al.* 1986[9]			
Caucasian group:			
community controls	< 1	0.9	0.4–2.0
	1–6	0.7	0.4–1.5
	6+	1.3	0.7–2.6
hospital controls	< 1	0.5	0.2–1.0
	1–6	1.4	0.6–2.9
	6+	0.8	0.4–1.6
Japanese group:			
community controls	< 1	2.4	1.3–2.7
	1–6	0.7	0.3–1.5
	6+	1.9	0.8–4.4
hospital controls	< 1	1.0	0.6–1.8
	1–6	0.6	0.3–1.2
	6+	1.2	0.6–2.4
Wingo *et al.* 1987[10]	< 1	1.0	0.7–1.3
	1–4	1.1	0.8–1.3
	5–9	1.1	0.8–1.5
	10–14	0.8	0.5–1.3
	15–19	1.3	0.6–2.6
	≥ 20	1.8	0.6–5.8
		(trend: $p = 0.7$)	

continued

Table 3 (*continued*)

Reference	*Duration of HRT* (years)	*Relative risk*	*95% confidence intervals*
Rohan and McMichael 1988[11]	< 2	0.99	0.56–1.76
	≥ 2	0.94	0.40–2.21
Ewertz 1988[12]			
postmenopausal*	< 3	0.89	0.56–1.41
	3–	0.93	0.52–1.68
	6–	1.82	0.98–3.37
	9–	1.34	0.70–2.54
	12+	2.32	1.31–4.12
		(trend: $p = 0.002$)	
Bergkvist *et al.* 1989[13]	≤ 0.5	0.7	0.4–1.0
	0.5–3	1.1	0.9–1.4
	3–6	1.0	0.8–1.4
	6–9	1.3	0.9–1.9
	≥ 9	1.7	1.1–2.7
		(trend: $p = 0.002$)	
Sartwell *et al.* 1977[15]	< 0.5	0.87	
	0.5–< 1	0.61	
	1–1.9	1.40	
	2–4.9	0.70	
	≥ 5	0.62	
Kaufman *et al.* 1984[19]			
Postmenopausal (natural menopause)	< 1	0.9	0.5–1.5
	1–4	0.9	0.5–1.5
	5–9	0.7	0.4–1.5
	≥ 10	1.3	0.6–2.8
McDonald *et al.* 1986[21]	1–5	0.83	
	≥ 6	0.68	
		(trend: $p = 0.06$)	

*Ewertz gives comparable figures for premenopausal women (analysis for linear trend, $p = 0.29$), menopausal women (trend: $p = 0.44$) and women following artificial menopause (trend: $p > 0.5$)

The five cohort studies showing the effects of prolonged periods of treatment are summarized in Table 4. Two of these reports[24,25] show either a significant linear trend in relation to duration of treatment or raised relative risks with confidence intervals which exclude unity (at least until the effect of small numbers in the relevant cells of the analyses becomes evident).

In general, it may be said that very few of this large total of 31 reports suggest a protective effect. Five of the reports suggest a slightly increased risk in terms of overall results, but most of them have confidence intervals which straddle unity in a way that might suggest either that there is no increased risk, or that many of the studies lack the power to detect any drug-related effect that may be present. Eight of the 19 reports showing the effects of prolonged therapy show rather convincing evidence of a slightly increased risk at the longest periods of administration, but the remaining studies show no such effect. The final impression might be that a very limited increased risk is present – and it is the purpose of this volume to explore that possibility and consider its implications.

Table 4 Studies showing the effect of prolonged therapy: cohort studies

Reference	*Duration of HRT* (years)	*Relative risks*	*95% confidence intervals*
Buring *et al.* 1987[23]	< 1	1.0	0.6–1.7
	1–< 3	1.0	0.7–1.6
	3–< 5	1.0	0.6–1.6
	5+	1.3	0.9–2.1
	5–< 10	1.5	1.0–2.2
	10+	0.9	0.4–1.6
Hunt *et al.* 1987[24]	1–2.5	1.0	
	2.5+–4	4.8	1.5–15.6
	4+–6	5.3	1.4–20.2
	6+	3.6	0.9–15.0
Mills *et al.* 1989[25]	< 1	2.28	1.38–3.79
	1–5	1.56	0.95–2.56
	6–10	2.75	1.64–4.64
	10+	1.53	0.92–2.54
		(trend: $p = 0.01$)	
Bergkvist *et al.* 1989[27]	1–3	0.86	0.60–1.22
	3+	0.66	0.44–1.00
	continuous	0.997	0.992–1.001
Colditz *et al.* 1990[28]			
current users of HRT	< 1	1.28	0.8–2.1
	1–< 2	1.32	0.8–2.2
	2–< 3	1.44	0.9–2.2
	3–< 5	1.26	0.9–1.9
	5–< 10	1.62	1.2–2.1
	10–< 15	1.28	0.8–2.0
	15+	1.19	0.6–2.2
		(trend: $p = 0.61$)	
past users of HRT	< 1	1.0	0.7–1.4
	1–< 2	1.05	0.7–1.5
	2–< 3	0.65	0.4–1.1
	3–< 5	1.02	0.7–1.5
	5–< 10	1.05	0.7–1.5
	10–< 15	0.92	0.5–1.7
	15+	0.79	0.3–2.5
		(trend: $p = 0.90$)	

This process will be facilitated by the fact that a small number of meta-analyses have been reported. Two of these have received particular attention. Dupont and Page (1991)[32] reported an overall relative risk of 1.07, and commented that with 0.625 mg/d of conjugated oestrogen, the relative risk was 1.08 (confidence intervals (CI), 0.96–1.2); these authors found that in women with benign breast disease the relative risk was 1.16 (CI, 0.89–1.5). This analysis produces, therefore, results which are reassuring.

Steinberg and colleagues (1991)[33], in a meta-analysis based on a very critical and systematic assessment of the individual studies, produced rather different results; they found that there was no increased risk with up to 5 years of use, but that after 15 years the relative risk would be 1.3 (CI, 1.2–1.6). With a positive history of breast cancer, a relative risk of 3.4 (CI,

2.0–6.0) was reported. These authors commented that in the United States of America a 30% increase in risk following 15 years of hormone replacement therapy use would equal 4708 attributable breast cancer cases with 1468 attributable deaths a year.

It is clear that the implications for public health of even a small increase in the breast cancer risk are considerable, simply because this is a common killing cancer of women. This volume must then set out to tackle a number of important questions. Is there an increased risk of long-term therapy and, if so, how big or small is it? If there is an increased risk, is it causal or consequential, or an artefact due to the experimental error (chance, bias, confounding, etc.) of epidemiological methods? Do other benefits (to the heart and bone etc.) outweigh these risks and, if they do, how do we handle the ethics of the community taking the most cost-effective decision regarding benefit and risk for the community, whilst the woman, as an individual, may be much more troubled about breast cancer than cardiovascular disease and osteoporosis? How do we sort out the obvious questions concerned with dose, duration of medication, route of administration, and the differences between the various chemical agents used in hormone replacement therapy? Finally, although there are really many more questions, how do we design and execute the definitive study that will quantify the risks of contemporary formulations of hormone replacement therapy, if all of today's expensively collected data merely serve to leave us puzzled?

REFERENCES

1. Jick, H., Walker, A.M., Watkins, R.M., D'Ewart, C.C., Hunter, J.R., Danford, A., Masden, S., Dinan, B.J. and Rothman, K.J. (1980). Replacement estrogens and breast cancer. *Am. J. Epidemiol.*, **112**, 586–94
2. Ross, R.K., Paganini-Hill, A., Gerkins, V.R., Mack, T.M., Pfeffer, R., Arthur, M. and Henderson, B.E. (1980). A case–control study of menopausal estrogen therapy and breast cancer. *J. Am. Med. Assoc.*, **243**, 1635–9
3. Hoover, R., Glass, A., Finkle, W.D., Azevedo, D. and Milne, K. (1981). Conjugated estrogens and breast cancer risk in women. *J. Natl. Cancer Inst.*, **67**, 815–20
4. Brinton, L.A., Hoover, R.N., Szklo, M. and Fraumeni, J.F. (1981). Menopausal estrogen use and risk of breast cancer. *Cancer*, **47**, 2517–22
5. Hulka, B.S., Chambless, L.E., Deubner, D.C. and Wilkinson, W.E. (1982). Breast cancer and estrogen replacement therapy. *Am. J. Obstet. Gynecol.*, **143**, 638–44
6. Hiatt, R.A., Bawol, R., Friedman, G.D. and Hoover, R. (1984). Exogenous estrogen and breast cancer after bilateral oophorectomy. *Cancer*, **54**, 139–44
7. Brinton, L.A., Hoover, R. and Fraumeni, J.F. (1986). Menopausal estrogens and breast cancer risk: an expanded case–control study. *Br. J. Cancer*, **54**, 825–32
8. La Vecchia, C., Decarli, A., Parazzini, F., Gentile, A., Liberati, C. and Franceschi, S. (1986). Non-contraceptive oestrogens and the risk of breast cancer in women. *Int. J. Cancer*, **38**, 853–8
9. Nomura, A.M.Y., Kolonel, L.N., Hirohata, T. and Lee, J. (1986). The association of replacement estrogens with breast cancer. *Int. J. Cancer*, **37**, 49–53
10. Wingo, P.A., Layde, P.M., Lee, N.C., Rubin, G. and Ory, H.W. (1987). The risk of breast cancer in postmenopausal women who have used oestrogen replacement therapy. *J. Am. Med. Assoc.*, **257**, 209–15
11. Rohan, T.E. and McMichael, A.J. (1988). Non-contraceptive exogenous oestrogen therapy and breast cancer. *Med. J. Australia*, **148**, 217–20

12. Ewertz, M. (1988). Influence of non-contraceptive exogenous and endogenous sex hormones on breast cancer risk in Denmark. *Int. J. Cancer*, **42**, 832–8
13. Bergkvist, L., Adami, H.-O., Persson, I., Hoover, R. and Schairer, C. (1989). The risk of breast cancer after estrogen and estrogen–progestin replacement. *N. Engl. J. Med.*, **321**, 293–7
14. Casagrande, J., Gerkins, V., Henderson, B.E., Mack, T. and Pike, M.C. (1976). Brief communication: exogenous estrogens and breast cancer in women with natural menopause. *J. Nat. Cancer Inst.*, **56**, 839–41
15. Sartwell, P.E., Arthes, F.G. and Tonascia, J.A. (1977). Exogenous hormones, reproductive history, and breast cancer. *J. Natl. Cancer Inst.*, **59**, 1589–92
16. Kelsey, J.L., Fischer, D.B., Holford, T.R., Livolsi, V.A., Mostow, E.D., Goldenberg, I.S. and White, C. (1981). *J. Natl. Cancer Inst.*, **67**, 327–33
17. Sherman, B., Wallace, R. and Bean, J. (1983). Estrogen use and breast cancer. *Cancer*, **51**, 1527–31
18. Horwitz, R.I. and Stewart, K.R. (1984). Effect of clinical features on the association of estrogens and breast cancer. *Am. J. Med.*, **76**, 192–8
19. Kaufman, D.W., Miller, D.R., Rosenberg, L., Helmrich, S.P., Stolley, P., Schottenfeld, D. and Shapiro, S. (1984). Noncontraceptive estrogen use and the risk of breast cancer. *J. Am. Med. Assoc.*, **252**, 63–7
20. Talamini, R., La Vecchia, C., Franceschi, S., Colombo, F., Decarli, A., Grattoni, E., Grigoletto, E. and Tognoni, G. (1985). Reproductive and hormonal factors and breast cancer in a Northern Italian population. *Int. J. Epidemiol.*, **14**, 70–4
21. McDonald, J.A., Weiss, N.S., Daling, J.R., Francis, A.M. and Polissar, L. (1986). Menopausal oestrogen use and the risk of breast cancer. *Breast Cancer Research and Treatment*, **7**, 193–9
22. Hoover, R., Gray, L.A., Cole, P. and MacMahon, B. (1976). Menopausal estrogens and breast cancer. *N. Engl. J. Med.*, **295**, 401–5
23. Buring, J.E., Hennekens, C.H., Lipnick, R.J., Willett, W., Stampfer, M.J., Rosner, B., Peto, R. and Speizer, F.E. (1987). A prospective cohort study of postmenopausal hormone use and risk of breast cancer in US women. *Am. J. Epidemiol.*, **125**, 939–47
24. Hunt, K., Vessey, M., McPherson, K. and Coleman, M. (1987). Long-term surveillance of mortality and cancer incidence in women receiving hormone replacement therapy. *Br. J. Obstet. Gynaecol.*, **94**, 620–35
25. Mills, P.K., Beeson, W.L., Phillips, R.L. and Fraser, G.E. (1989). Prospective study of exogenous hormone use and breast cancer in Seventh-day Adventists. *Cancer*, **64**, 591–7
26. Dupont, W.D., Page, D.L., Rogers, L.W. and Parl, F.F. (1989). Influence of exogenous estrogens, proliferative breast disease, and other variables on breast cancer risk. *Cancer*, **63**, 948–57
27. Bergkvist, L., Adami, H.-O., Persson, I., Bergstrom, R. and Krusemo, U.B. (1989). Prognosis after breast cancer diagnosis in women exposed to estrogen and estrogen–progestogen replacement therapy. *Am. J. Epidemiol.*, **130**, 221–8
28. Colditz, G.A., Stampfer, M.J., Willett, W.C., Hennekens, C.H., Rosner, B. and Speizer, F.E. (1990). Prospective study of estrogen replacement therapy and risk of breast cancer in postmenopausal women. *J. Am. Med. Assoc.*, **264**, 2648–53
29. Hunt, K., Vessey, M. and McPherson, K. (1990). Mortality in a cohort of long-term users of hormone replacement therapy: an updated analysis. *Br. J. Obstet. Gynaecol.*, **97**, 1080–6
30. Thomas, D.B., Persing, J.P. and Hutchinson, W.B. (1982). Exogenous estrogens and other risk factors for breast cancer in women with benign breast diseases. *J. Natl. Cancer Inst.*, **69**, 1017–25
31. Gambrell, R.D., Maier, R.C. and Sanders, B.I. (1983). Decreased incidence of breast cancer in postmenopausal estrogen–progestogen users. *Obstet. Gynecol.*, **62**, 435–43
32. Dupont, W.D. and Page, D.L. (1991). Menopausal estrogen replacement therapy and breast cancer. *Arch. Int. Med.*, **151**, 67–72
33. Steinberg, K.K., Thacker, S.B., Smith, S.J., Stroup, D.F., Zack, M.W., Flanders, W.D. and Berkelman, R.L. (1991). A meta-analysis of the effect of estrogen replacement therapy on the risk of breast cancer. *J. Am. Med. Assoc.*, **265**, 1985–90

2

Physiology of the menopause

H.S. Jacobs

The proximate cause of the menopause is depletion of the ovaries' store of oocytes and follicles. Given that the supply of oocytes is finite (about 7 million germ cells can be found in the ovaries of the human fetus at the 5th month of intrauterine life) and that these cells do not thereafter divide, it is clear that some mechanism is needed to protect the species from relying on transmission of genetic information by DNA that might be over 50 years old. The protection is provided by spontaneous atresia of oocytes, a process whose rate is determined by genetic factors. For example, in individuals with a 45XO constitution, the rate of atresia is so fast that oocyte depletion is usually complete before puberty and so the patient presents with primary amenorrhoea and sexual infantilism.

Treatments with agents that destroy genetic material, such as ionizing irradiation or anticancer chemotherapy, are associated with a premature menopause; the mechanism is presumably similar to that which causes women who smoke to have their menopause at an earlier age than women who do not[1]. Certainly one can detect cotinine, a constituent of tobacco smoke, in follicular fluid obtained from the ovaries of smokers[2], so presumably ootoxic compounds in cigarette smoke, and in other pollutants, can penetrate to the oocyte's microenvironment.

From compilation of the results of several studies, it seems that the rate of disappearance of follicles from the ovary accelerates after the age of 35[3], an observation that resonates with our knowledge of the increase after this age in the rate of birth of babies with certain congenital disturbances. It also resonates with the results of longitudinal studies of bone mineralization, which indicate a fall-off of bone mineralization after this age. Premenopausal onset of complications usually attributed to the menopause (the last menstrual period a woman experiences) will clearly need to be considered when detailed strategies of public health are developed.

Complications of the menopause are the immediate symptoms of acute oestrogen deficiency and the long term problems of osteoporosis and coronary heart disease. Whilst it is widely appreciated that flushing and sweating attacks follow ovariectomy and can be prevented by treatment with oestrogen, it is curious that even with detailed assessment it is not possible to detect a difference in endogenous oestrogen levels between postmenopausal women who do and do not have these symptoms[4]. In contrast, women with symptoms that arise from atrophy of the genital tract have serum oestradiol concentrations that are about half those in women without such symptoms. I think postmenopausal women with symptoms of organ atrophy declare themselves as candidates for long-term preventative treatment with oestrogen, firstly for the obvious medical reason of the relief of symptoms but also because, in the case of osteoporosis at least, there is evidence of a dose–response relationship, in that the more severe the oestrogen deficiency, the more severe the bone rarefaction.

It is now widely recognized that postmenopausal osteoporosis represents a major hazard for postmenopausal women. By osteoporosis I mean the combination of bone rarefaction with fracture. The reason it is important to reiterate the clinical definition is that bone decalcification, and changes in calcification induced by treatment, are increasingly used as surrogates for the medical condition and treatment of osteoporosis. This use of bone density as a surrogate for osteoporosis has been facilitated by advances in the methodology of assessment of bone calcification[5]. It is important to bear in mind, however, that one part of the clinical definition, that is the occurrence of fractures, is dependent upon the association of trauma with brittle bones. The trauma may be trivial and cause fracture if the bones are in very poor shape; bones in relatively good shape may also fracture if the trauma is sufficiently severe. It seems that skeletal strength is determined in part by changes that are oestrogen-mediated and in part by effects of ageing that are independent of gender.

The overriding importance of oestrogen deficiency in causing osteoporosis was shown in a recent study of 200 young women (average age 27.8 years) who had presented to the reproductive endocrinology clinics at the Middlesex Hospital[6]. We found that women with amenorrhoea had a mean reduction in their bone mineral density, as assessed by the dual energy X-ray technique, of about 15%. The reduction was directly related to the duration of amenorrhoea and the degree of oestrogen deficiency. To our surprise, as many as 57 of the 200 amenorrhoeic women we studied gave a history of fracture. In these women the mean bone density was lower than in those without such a history. Usually the fracture had been caused by an easily-remembered event, such as falling off a bicycle or horse, or off skis, but ten of the women had no recollection of trauma and in these cases bone density was lower still. Presumably, the more severe the bone lesion, the milder the trauma required to cause fracture. Recently we have studied the changes in bone mineralization in these women after they had been placed on appropriate therapy (Guleckli, Davies and Jacobs, in preparation). While we have been able to detect an improvement over the 1st year of therapy, the size of the change has been very small (about a 2% return of bone mineral density per year). The results emphasize the importance of early reversal of oestrogen deficiency to preserve the integrity of the bones.

The model that emerges from study of the skeleton is of oestrogen deficiency causing osteoporosis and of early correction of oestrogen deficiency preventing it. The relationship to the menopause occurs because that is the time when most women become oestrogen-deficient. The effect of age is relatively minor. The position in relation to coronary heart disease is, however, not so straightforward.

Perhaps it is best to start with the size of the problem. Bush points out that coronary disease is the commonest cause of death in postmenopausal women, accounting for more than twice as many deaths as the next commonest cause[7]. It is therefore here that the potential for influencing the health of postmenopausal women must be greatest. Yet the connection to the endocrine events of the menopause is still somewhat problematic. For example, some years ago Dr Richard Heller and I analysed crude death rates from coronary heart disease in relation to age in men and women[8]. We found that the well-known change with age of the ratio of heart attacks in men and women could not be explained by an increase in the rate of heart attacks in women after the age of 50; rather, it was associated with a fall in the rate in men. These data, which have been replicated in the United States, show an uninterrupted increase in the numbers of women dying of coronary disease, with no inflection at the age of the menopause. Of course, it may be argued that national vital statistics are too crude to be used in this way; clearly, they are likely to be influenced by other factors that do not form part of the study under review (differences attributable to different types of life experience, e.g. types of employment), to differences in the rate of tobacco consumption, etc.). None the less, the inconvenience of these data has been replicated in the study of Colditz and colleagues[9]. They found that the apparent increase in the risk of heart attack after the menopause disappeared when the data were reanalysed after the age intervals of study were reduced from 5 years to 1 year and allowance was made for the effect of smoking. Colditz and colleagues did find, however, that surgical ovariectomy was associated with a doubling of the risk of a heart attack, which increase was eliminated by oestrogen replacement therapy. While it must be accepted that differences exist between women undergoing natural menopause and those having an ovariectomy (for example age, illness resulting in the need for the operation), the study did have the advantage that, with ovariectomy, at least the age of onset of oestrogen deprival was precisely known.

Perhaps the most persuasive argument for an important relationship between the oestrogen deficiency of the menopause and the risk of a heart attack comes from analyses of the protective effect of oestrogen replacement therapy. The authors of several important studies[10,11], having assessed their own data and those in the literature, conclude that treatment of postmenopausal women with oestrogens reduces the risk of a heart attack by between 30 and 50%. The data and arguments are summarized very clearly in the original articles so I will not reiterate them here, rather I will draw attention to the importance at this stage of what notion one has of the mechanism of the association.

Bush argues strongly for the mechanism to involve oestrogen-mediated effects on lipoprotein metabolism[12]. She cites the Donolo–Tel Aviv study[13] which related the risk of a heart attack in 1481 women followed for 20 years to the serum concentration of total and high-density lipoprotein (HDL) cholesterol. The study suggested that, in women, a low serum HDL cholesterol concentration was more closely associated with the risk of a heart attack than was a modestly elevated total cholesterol.

The importance of the above argument lies in the fact that in order to make decisions on optimizing oestrogen replacement therapy, one needs to have a view on whether such therapy does have prophylactic potential with respect to coronary disease and, if that is one's view, on which surrogate markers to use to assess particular regimens of therapy. The point has been made very forcibly in a recent survey of 43 trials of oestrogen replacement therapy published since 1984[14]. In essence, the authors concluded that oestrogen replacement with natural steroids lowers total serum cholesterol and raises serum HDL cholesterol, although treatment with conjugated oestrogens (Premarin®) was associated with an increase of serum triglyceride concentrations. These mainly beneficial effects on the surrogate measurements are, as mentioned above, reflected in the clinical outcome of postmenopausal hormone replacement therapy. The problem comes when the authors analysed the results of treatment with oestrogen together with progestogen. Addition of norgestrel to treatment with oestrogen completely negates the putative benefit of the oestrogen on circulating HDL concentrations.

It is instructive to reflect at this stage that in the UK at least, oestrogen replacement therapy of normal postmenopausal women (rather than of hysterectomized women) is usually administered with a combination of oestrogen with progestogen. Most schedules of therapy involve a monthly course of progestogen. Moreover, the market leaders in the field (Prempak-C® and Cyclo-Progynova®) both contain norgestrel – that is to say, the only gestagen that reliably affects HDL adversely. It is clear that we urgently need more information in this area; equally it is clear that postmenopausal women urgently need the pharmaceutical industry to produce combination therapies which incorporate the newer 'third generation' progestogens. It seems hardly credible that new combinations of ethinyloestradiol with compounds like norethisterone and norgestrel are still being developed for postmenopausal hormone replacement therapy. From their survey, Rijpkema, van der Sanden and Ruijs[14] deduced that the combination of oestradiol valerate with cyproterone acetate should produce the most favourable effects on the surrogate markers of heart disease. Perhaps this is so, but clinical benefit has yet to be demonstrated rather than deduced. One can only ally oneself with those who call for these issues to be the subjects of controlled trials of clinical outcome[15], particularly because the area becomes clouded rather than clarified by the inevitable development of new surrogate markers of the risk of coronary heart disease[16].

REFERENCES

1. Stampfer, M.J., Colditz, G.A. and Willett, W.C. (1990). Menopause and heart disease: a review. *Ann. N.Y. Acad. Sci.*, **592**, 193–203
2. Weiss, T. and Eckart, A. (1989). Cotinine levels in follicular fluid and serum of IVF patients: effect on granulosa–luteal cell function *in vitro*. *Hum. Reprod.*, **4**, 482–5
3. Richardson, S.J., Senikas, V. and Nelson, J.F. (1987). Follicular depletion during the menopausal transition: evidence for accelerated loss and ultimate exhaustion. *J. Clin. Endocrinol. Metab.*, **65**, 1231–7

4. Hutton, J.D., Jacobs, H.S., Murray, M.A.F. and James, V.H.T. (1978). Relation between plasma oestrone and oestradiol and climacteric symptoms. *Lancet*, **1**, 678–81
5. Cullum, I.D., Ell, P.J. and Ryder, J.P. (1989). X-ray dual photon absorptiometry; a new method of measurement of bone density. *Br. J. Radiol.*, **592**, 13–20
6. Davies, M.C., Hall, M.L. and Jacobs, H.S. (1990). Bone mineral loss in young women with amenorrhoea. *Br. Med. J.*, **301**, 790–3
7. Bush, T.L. (1990). The epidemiology of cardiovascular disease in postmenopausal women. *Ann. N.Y. Acad. Sci.*, **592**, 263–71
8. Heller, R.F. and Jacobs, H.S. (1978). Coronary heart disease in relation to age, sex, and the menopause. *Br. Med. J.*, **1**, 472–4
9. Colditz, G.A., Willett, W.C.., Stampfer, M.J., Rosner, B., Speizer, F.E. and Hennekens, C.H. (1987). Menopause and the risk of coronary heart disease in women. *N. Engl. J. Med.*, **316**, 1105–10
10. Stampfer, M.J., Colditz, G.A., Willett, W.C., Manson, J.E., Rosner, B., Speizer, F.E. and Hennekens, C.H. (1991). Postmenopausal estrogen therapy and cardiovascular disease – ten year follow-up from the Nurses' Health Study. *N. Engl. J. Med.*, **325**, 756–62
11. Bush, T.L., Barrett-Connor, E. and Cowan, L.D. (1987). Cardiovascular mortality and non-contraceptive use of estrogen in women: results from the Lipid Research Clinics Program follow-up study. *Circulation*, **75**, 1102–9
12. Bush, T.L., Fried, L.P. and Barrett-Connor, E. (1988). Cholesterol, lipoproteins and coronary heart disease in women. *Clin. Chem.*, **34**, 60–70
13. Brunner, D., Weisbort, J., Meshulam, N., Schwartz, S., Gross, J., Saltz-Rennert, H., Altman, S. and Loebl, K. (1987). Relation of serum total cholesterol and high-density lipoprotein cholesterol percentage to the incidence of definite coronary events: twenty-year follow-up of the Donolo–Tel Aviv prospective coronary artery disease study. *Am. J. Cardiol.*, **59**, 1271–6
14. Rijpkema, A.H.M., van der Sanden, A.A. and Ruijs, A.H.C. (1990). Effects of postmenopausal oestrogen–progestogen replacement on serum lipids and lipoproteins: a review. *Maturitas*, **12**, 259–85
15. Goldman, L. and Tosteson, A.N.A. (1991). Uncertainty about postmenopausal estrogen – time for action not debate. *N. Engl. J. Med.*, **325**, 800–2
16. Farish, E., Rolton, H.A., Barnes, J.F. and Hart, D.M. (1991). Lipoprotein (a) concentrations in postmenopausal women taking norethisterone. *Br. Med. J.*, **303**, 694

3

Hormone replacement therapy and its current use in British specialist clinical practice

M.C. Ellerington and M.I. Whitehead

The management of the majority of patients requesting hormone replacement therapy is straightforward and can be undertaken by the primary health care physician, the general practitioner. However, difficulties and uncertainties may arise with some women because of their medical or family history, or when the women herself has doubts about the relative benefits and disadvantages of therapy. The hospital-based menopause clinic provides general practitioners with specialist advice in such circumstances. It should be able to offer up-to-date counselling for the patient and advice for her general practitioner. Treatment can be tailored to the patient's individual needs, such that side-effects are minimized. 'State-of-the-art' investigations, which may be deemed advisable, are often much more readily available to the specialist because they are being used for research in the specialist unit.

INTRODUCTION

Most women attending our menopause clinics request hormone replacement therapy for the relief of symptoms associated with oestrogen deficiency (Table 1). However, as public awareness of the menopause and its sequelae continues to grow, we are seeing increasing numbers of women who are

Table 1 Symptoms of the menopause

Hot flushes	Formication
Night sweats	Forgetfulness
Insomnia	Loss of confidence
Tiredness	Urinary frequency/urgency
Irritability	Loss of libido
Depressed mood	Vaginal dryness
Anxiety	Change in clitoral sensitivity
Aching limbs	Dyspareunia
Dry skin/hair	

seeking specialist advice about the use of hormone replacement therapy as preventive medicine to reduce their future risk of osteoporosis and, perhaps, arterial disease. Our advice is also sought where hormone replacement therapy has been associated with side-effects, or when the general practitioner is reluctant to prescribe because of certain factors which he/she considers to be a contraindication to therapy.

ASSESSMENT OF THE PATIENT

A history of typical climacteric symptoms, such as hot flushes, night sweats and vaginal dryness, will usually establish the diagnosis of oestrogen deficiency in most patients. It is stressed that such symptoms (particularly the flushes and sweats) often occur in women who are still menstruating and their onset may predate the menopause by several years. They then tend to occur for 7–10 days before menstruation.

Some women, however, are referred because the general practitioner is uncertain as to whether or not their complaints are indicative of oestrogen deficiency. Here, it is important to obtain accurate details of the duration and intensity of symptoms and their temporal relationship to changes in the menstrual pattern. The woman's medical history and/or family history may contain factors which might influence the decision to prescribe or withhold hormone replacement therapy. Additionally, certain factors (e.g. previous venous thromboembolic disease) may influence the choice of route of administration of hormone replacement therapy and dictate the necessity for certain investigations prior to initiation of treatment.

A complete physical examination (breast, abdominal and pelvic examination plus cervical smear, as appropriate) is then performed; this may be the woman's first such examination for several years and it provides an opportunity to screen for non-gynaecological conditions such as hypertension. Investigation of any such abnormalities discovered can usually be undertaken more quickly in the specialist unit than in general practice, because the former is usually hospital-based and has easier access to the relevant facilities. Endometrial biopsy may also be performed at this time, if indicated (see below).

Serum hormone assays (follicle stimulating hormone, luteinizing hormone and oestradiol) are not routinely performed in our clinics but are sometimes indicated when, from the history alone, the precise cause of the patient's symptoms is in doubt. They are essential to confirm premature menopause. Failure to recognize and treat this condition is, we believe, potentially serious because it results in an increase in risk of arterial disease (particularly myocardial infarction) and osteoporosis.

ORAL OR NON-ORAL THERAPY?

Oral oestrogens

Traditionally, the oestrogens used in hormone replacement therapy have been administered by mouth. Oral oestrogens are generally safe, effective and well-tolerated. The dose can be adjusted easily and rapidly and treatment can be withdrawn abruptly, if necessary. However, strictly speaking, the administration of oestrogen by mouth is 'unphysiological'. To obtain an adequate plasma concentration over the 24-hour period (which is essential for relief of daytime flushing and nocturnal sweats), the oestrogen has to be administered as a 'bolus'. This results in high peak plasma levels soon after ingestion, followed by a gradual decline in levels until the next tablet is taken. The ovary does not secrete oestradiol into the circulation once daily but releases small amounts at frequent intervals. Furthermore, due to the conversion of oestradiol to oestrone within the gut wall, all orally administered natural oestrogens give rise, in plasma, principally to oestrone.

Oral oestrogens also appear to have exaggerated effects on hepatic metabolism which are believed to be due to the first-pass effect of the single daily bolus dose. For example, oral oestrogens increase the production of renin substrate. In theory, this might increase the risk of hypertension, mediated through the renin–angiotensin–aldosterone system. However, at present, it is not clear whether the forms of renin substrate induced by oral oestrogens are those associated with hypertension[1]. Oral oestrogen administration has also been shown to enhance the production of certain coagulation and fibrinolytic factors. Thus, in our clinics, we tend to avoid their use in hypertensives, in those women who developed hypertension with use of the combined oral contraceptive, and in those with a history of unprovoked venous thrombo-embolic disease.

Conversely, it has been argued that oral oestrogen administration may enhance oestrogen benefits, as compared to non-oral oestrogens, upon reduction in arterial disease risk. The protection afforded by oestrogens upon arterial disease risk is, in part, lipid-mediated and some investigators have reported a more profound potentially beneficial effect upon lipid and lipoprotein metabolism with oral administration than with non-oral oestrogens. However, it has not been shown that orally administered oestrogens reduce arterial disease risk any more than those administered non-orally; conversely, the latter have not been shown to cause less hypertension than oral oestrogens. The required studies have not yet been performed.

Approximately 3–4% of patients suffer dyspepsia and/or nausea with oral oestrogens. Others appear to fail to absorb oestrogens effectively through the gut; in our experience this appears to be more common in patients with small bowel disease (e.g. Crohn's) particularly following extensive small bowel resection. However, in many women who fail to respond to oral oestrogens, there is no obvious reason. Non-oral therapy can overcome this problem, as well as producing a more physiological plasma profile. We would therefore recommend a therapeutic trial of non-oral hormone replacement therapy in women in whom oral oestrogens have not relieved typical oestrogen deficiency symptoms effectively.

Non-oral oestrogens

Transdermal oestrogens

Transdermal patches (Estraderm®: Ciba-Geigy, Horsham, UK) overcome the problem of poor absorption which is sometimes seen with oral oestrogens.

The incidence of nausea appears to be slightly less – around 2% – using patches. Nausea is a common symptom of early pregnancy, at which time it is most probably due to the sudden rise in plasma oestrogen concentrations. Thus, all forms of oestrogen, irrespective of the route of administration, are likely to cause nausea to some degree, especially during the first few days of treatment. It is important to explain to the patient that this symptom will usually subside within 2–3 weeks of commencing therapy, otherwise it may deter continued use.

Some women (up to 30%) develop skin reactions to the patch[2]. The majority of these are of mild erythema but blistering can occur and this leads to discontinuation of treatment in approximately 5% of women. Our advice to these patients, especially to those with only mild skin reactions, is to persevere with treatment because the skin reaction may subside with time. For those in whom it persists, moving the patch more frequently, e.g. daily, may eliminate or minimize the problem. It is believed that the skin irritation is caused by the alcohol in the patch reservoir. This problem is likely to be overcome with the advent of second-generation patches based upon a matrix dispersion system, which does not contain alcohol. Matrix dispersion systems are well advanced in development.

Patches should be changed every 3½ days – the lifetime of the patch. We have observed, in some patients, that oestrogen deficiency symptoms recur if the patch is left on for longer. Furthermore, some patients notice a recurrence of symptoms during the first 6–12 h following application of a new patch. We believe this is because it takes several hours for the fresh skin under the new patch to become fully saturated with ethanol and oestradiol. Only then will adequate diffusion into the dermal capillaries take place. In such patients, therefore, we recommend a half-day overlap when applying a new patch and removing the old one.

Subcutaneous implants

A small number of women appear to need higher plasma levels of oestradiol than can easily be achieved with tablets or patches. For these patients, oestradiol implants (Organon®: Cambridge, UK) are often very effective. Implants have one major advantage over other methods, namely guaranteed compliance. They are also non-oral and therefore avoid the problems experienced with oral oestrogens by some patients. The major disadvantage is that they cannot be easily removed if this is found to be necessary.

Two problems which are specific to implants warrant special mention. Following the insertion of an oestradiol implant, plasma levels rise rapidly, remain constant for 3–4 months and then decline gradually. Menopausal symptoms return as the plasma oestradiol level begins to fall, *not* when basal (pre-treatment) levels have been reached. Some patients, therefore, return earlier than planned, claiming that their implant has 'run out'. Reimplantation at this point, in a small number of patients, may lead to accumulation of oestradiol. Eventually, supraphysiological levels are reached (> 1200 pmol/litre) and these cannot be maintained for long periods. The patient's symptom-free intervals become gradually shorter, with further implants producing benefit for shorter and shorter periods. We have called this phenomenon 'tachyphylaxis'[3] and it is illustrated diagrammatically in Figure 1.

Management of these patients has proved extremely difficult. We would recommend the monitoring of plasma oestradiol levels with serial assays, the aim being to allow the plasma oestradiol to return to levels within the physiological premenopausal range. Therapy may then be reinstituted with either patches or tablets. It may take a year or more for the plasma oestradiol level to return to normal, and during this time the patient will almost certainly experience typical symptoms of oestrogen deficiency – despite the high plasma values. We commonly recommend the intermittent use of either oral conjugated equine oestrogens (Premarin®: Wyeth-Ayerst, Maidenhead, UK) up to 1.25 mg/day, or transdermal oestradiol up to 200 μg/day, which gives temporary relief of symptoms when they are severe. A thorough explanation of this treatment to the patient is also very important, and much psychological support will be required.

We have also recognized that implants, in some patients, may result in plasma oestradiol values above the threshold for endometrial stimulation for up to 3–4 years after insertion of the last implant[4]. It is necessary to continue cyclical progestogens during this time in women with an intact uterus until no further withdrawal bleeding occurs for 3 months. If the patients symptoms return 4–6 months after the last implant, it cannot be assumed that oestradiol levels have fallen below the threshold for endometrial stimulation. Although the above problems only seem to occur in small

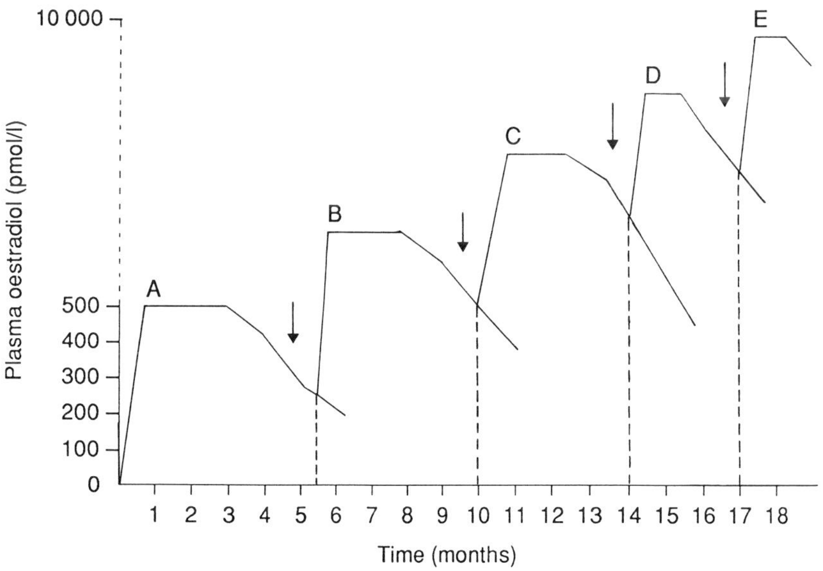

Figure 1 Diagrammatic representation of tachyphylaxis. A,B,C,D and E indicate the insertion of new implants. Arrows indicate the recurrence of menopausal symptoms. Note the ever-decreasing time intervals between implants

numbers of patients receiving implants, there is no way of predicting these individuals.

Vaginal oestrogens

These have been available for many years as either creams, gels or pessaries, and are prescribed mainly to relieve lower genital tract symptoms. However, because systemic absorption occurs readily through the vaginal epithelium[5,6] the long-term use of some of the older preparations at the manufacturers recommended dose (e.g. conjugated equine oestrogens; Premarin® cream: Wyeth, Maidenhead, UK) may lead to the development of endometrial neoplasia. There are many such cases reported in the literature. We would therefore recommend a regular course of progestogen if daily long-term use of this preparation at high dose is envisaged. Under these circumstances, after appropriate counselling, the patient may prefer to use either oral or transdermal hormonal replacement therapy as these are less messy than vaginal creams.

The vaginal epithelium responds well to extremely small doses of oestrogen. In women whose only symptoms are those associated with vaginal atrophy, we sometimes recommend intermittent use of very small doses of local oestrogen such as conjugated equine oestrogens, 0.1–0.2 mg, 2–3 times weekly. This very small dose will still produce premenopausal values for vaginal cytology. Recently, vaginal pessaries containing oestradiol, 25 μg (Vagifem®: Novo-Nordisk, Crawley, UK) have become available. This is a sustained release preparation which, according to the manufacturer, has not resulted in endometrial hyperplasia with over 2 years of use. However, it is not yet known whether such small doses in the very long term are sufficient to cause endometrial neoplasia.

There are some women in whom vaginal dryness persists, despite adequate doses of systemic hormone replacement therapy (oral conjugated equine oestrogens 0.625 mg/day or equivalent: transdermal oestradiol 50 μg/day) to control their other symptoms. We sometimes recommend that these women use a small dose of vaginal oestrogen cream in addition to their systemic hormone replacement therapy in an attempt to overcome this problem. It is to be remembered that oral conjugated equine oestrogens, 0.625 mg/day, and transdermal oestradiol, 50 μg/day, produce plasma oestradiol levels of around 200 pmol/l. The average plasma value during the menstrual cycle is approximately 500 pmol/l and some women seem to need more oestrogen to relieve vaginal dryness.

PROGESTOGENS

It is well recognized that the long-term use of unopposed oestrogens in women with an intact uterus results in an increase in risk of endometrial carcinoma. It is also well-documented that the addition of a 12–13-day course of progestogen each month[7,8] will reduce the incidence of endometrial hyperplasia to that seen in an untreated population[9] or possibly even lower[10].

Unfortunately, progestogens are associated with premenstrual syndrome-like side-effects, such as breast tenderness, abdominal bloating, greasy skin and mood disturbances in some women. A number of oestrogen/progestogen preparations are available in convenient calendar packs (which improve compliance) but these restrict the prescribing in terms of the dose and type of progestogen used. All currently available calendar packs in the UK contain only the C-19 nortestosterone progestogens, norgestrel or norethisterone. Prescribing the oestrogen and progestogen separately allows flexibility in the type and dose of progestogen prescribed. Women who are intolerant of a C-19 preparation may not experience side-effects with a C-21 derivative such as Duphaston® (Duphar Laboratories, Southampton, UK) or Provera® (Upjohn, Crawley, UK). By prescribing the oestrogen and progestogen separately, therapy can be tailored to the individual patient, thereby minimizing unwanted side-effects. Suitable daily doses of the currently available progestogens to oppose the effects of oral and transdermal oestrogens are shown in Table 2.

Due to the marked inter-patient variation in response to the progestogen, a non-invasive test is required to determine whether a given dose is adequate in an individual patient. It used to be commonplace for patients receiving hormone replacement therapy to undergo annual endometrial biopsy to ensure that their dose of progestogen was sufficient to provide adequate endometrial protection. However, Padwick and colleagues[11] demonstrated that with oral oestrogens the day of onset of withdrawal bleeding correlates well with the endometrial histology, and is dependent upon the daily progestogen dose. Thus, the latter can be titrated against the day of onset of bleeding. When the progestogen is added for 12 days each month, adequate endometrial protection is achieved, provided that the withdrawal bleed regularly starts on or after the 11th day of progestogen addition (Figure 2). With transdermal oestrogens, withdrawal bleeding starting on the 9th/10th day of progestogen addition is usually associated with an adequate endometrial response. The reason for this difference in timing between oral and transdermal oestrogens is presently unknown. There are no data correlating the day of onset of bleeding with the underlying endometrial status in patients receiving implants. Thus, where the day of onset of bleeding is known, the progestogen dose can be reduced to a minimum, thereby reducing or even completely overcoming any progestogen-related side-effects. Alternatively, changing the patient to a different type of progestogen may be beneficial.

At present, all progestogens except one have to be given orally. Cyclogest®

Table 2 Suitable doses of progestogens for use with oral/transdermal oestrogens

Progestogen	*Dose* (mg)
Norethisterone (Micronor®/Noriday®)	0.7–1.05
Norgestrel (Neogest®)	0.075–0.15
Dydrogesterone (Duphaston®)	10–20
Medroxyprogesterone acetate (Provera®)	5–10
Natural progesterone (Cyclogest®)	200–400

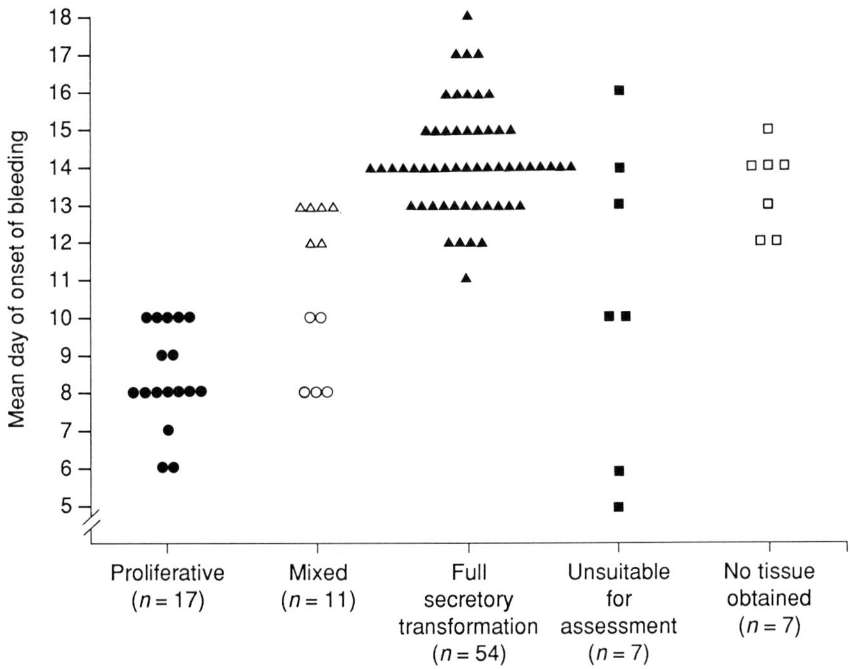

Figure 2 Correlation of endometrial histology day of onset of bleeding after addition of the progestogen. Number of samples shown in parentheses. (From ref. 11, reproduced with permission)

(natural progesterone; Hoechst, Hounslow, Middlesex, UK) is available for rectal or vaginal administration. Recently, we have studied the use of a transdermal patch which administers both oestradiol and the progestogen, norethisterone. We have shown that the dose of the latter, when given transdermally, can be safely reduced to a quarter of that given orally without compromising endometrial safety[12]. We have observed that the incidence of premenstrual syndrome-like side-effects with transdermal norethisterone is significantly less than with the minimum effective oral dose (M. C. Ellerington and M. I. Whitehead, unpublished data). It is anticipated that this combination patch (Estracomb®; Ciba-Geigy, Horsham, UK) will become available in the UK in mid-1992.

HORMONE REPLACEMENT THERAPY WITH AMENORRHOEA

One of the greatest drawbacks of hormone replacement therapy to many women is the re-establishment of vaginal bleeding. This occurs in approximately 85% of postmenopausal women on sequential oestrogen/progestogen therapy; the absence of bleeding in the remaining 15% does not, in our experience, signify endometrial pathology. Due to the anti-mitotic activity of progestogens in the endometrium, it has been suggested that continuous administration of both the oestrogen and the progestogen (every day in combination) will result in endometrial atrophy and therefore complete amenorrhoea. It should also be possible to use a lower dose of progestogen with continuous administration. However, in practice, this type of therapy has a number of drawbacks:

(1) It has not been demonstrated that continuous/combined hormone replacement therapy provides superior symptom relief to sequential/combined therapy;

(2) Despite using a lower dose of progestogen, progestogenic side-effects still occur in some women;

(3) Irregular bleeding is common; this is most frequent during the first 6 months of therapy, although it may persist, in some women, for up to 18 months;

(4) There is no correlation between endometrial histology and bleeding patterns. The presence of irregular bleeding does not signify endometrial pathology and, conversely, amenorrhoea does not guarantee the presence of normal endometrium;

(5) Data regarding endometrial safety are only available for up to 18 months of continuous use; no longer term data are available; and

(6) Data regarding the effects of continuous combined therapy on plasma lipids and lipoproteins are inadequate. Studies published to date are flawed by inadequate numbers of subjects, uncertain methodology and/or lack of control groups.

Despite the above, we have a small number of older postmenopausal women on this type of therapy. As our clinics are hospital based we have immediate access to endometrial biopsy. We regard continuous/combined regimens as experimental, and all our patients on such therapy undergo routine endometrial biopsy every 12–18 months.

Tibolone

Tibolone (Livial®: Organon, Os, Holland) is a unique derivative of a C-19 nortestosterone compound. It possesses oestrogenic, progestogenic and androgenic properties and was developed to avoid withdrawal bleeding in postmenopausal women.

Studies have shown that the recommended dose (2.5 mg/day) is as effective in controlling symptoms as oestradiol valerate (Progynova®: Schering, Burgess Hill, Sussex, UK) 2 mg/day or conjugated equine oestrogens (Premarin®: Wyeth-Ayerst, Maidenhead, UK) 0.625 mg/day[13].

In placebo-controlled studies, tibolone appears to conserve bone postmenopausally[14]. However, comparative data with conventional hormone replacement therapy are not yet available. Additionally, there are no data indicating whether or not tibolone reduces the risk of arterial disease.

ABNORMAL BLEEDING

Irregular perimenopausal bleeding and postmenopausal bleeding must be investigated prior to starting hormone replacement therapy. During therapy any bleeding which is inappropriately timed with respect to the 12-day course of progestogen or which is heavier and/or longer than the woman's normal menstrual bleed also demands investigation. If this continues after adjustment of the daily dose of progestogen then we perform an outpatient endometrial biopsy using a Vabra suction curette.

Oestrogen entering the liver, either via the portal vein or from the systemic circulation, is partially excreted in bile into the gut. Some is then reabsorbed from the gut and re-enters the liver via the portal vein, where some is then re-excreted in bile. This enterohepatic recycling may be an important secondary source of oestrogen. We have seen patients who have experienced breakthrough bleeding whilst taking antibiotics or during attacks of gastro-enteritis. Presumably, the resultant intestinal hurry interrupts the entero-hepatic recirculation, causing plasma oestrogen levels to fall below the threshold which maintains the endometrium. If breakthrough bleeding cannot be explained by the above or by non-compliance, a cervical smear and an endometrial biopsy should be performed. Sometimes an endometrial polyp will be missed by the outpatient suction curette and unscheduled bleeding continues. A formal dilatation and curettage under general anaesthesia is then indicated.

HORMONE REPLACEMENT THERAPY AS PREVENTIVE MEDICINE

Due to the rapid rate of bone loss in the early postmenopausal years, it is obviously better to start hormone replacement therapy at or soon after the menopause to achieve maximum prophylaxis against osteoporosis. However, an increasing number of women who are many years postmenopausal are now requesting preventive treatment for osteoporosis, probably because they have either recently read a magazine article about it or have a relative or friend who has just suffered a fracture. Although the benefits for these older women are likely to be less than those for the younger age-group, administration of hormone replacement therapy may still be of value. Fracture risk is correlated with bone density, and therefore stabilization of the skeleton by hormone replacement therapy in elderly women will still be beneficial. It will not replace the bone mass already lost but it will prevent further loss and thereby prevent a further increase in fracture risk[15].

Less than 50% of the reduction in the incidence of arterial disease observed in oestrogen users is explained by the beneficial effects of therapy on plasma lipids and lipoproteins. Doppler ultrasound with colour-flow mapping can be used to assess the flow velocity waveform of major arteries. Significant falls in the arterial pulsatility index (PI), which assesses the impedance to flow distal to the point of sampling, follow the administration of oestrogens to postmenopausal women. A 50% fall in PI has been reported in the uterine artery[16]. In untreated postmenopausal women, the PI of the internal carotid artery correlates with time since menopause; the longer the interval, the higher the value, i.e. the greater the impedance to flow (Figure 3). In this artery the response to oestrogens is dictated by the initial value – the higher the value, the greater its decline with oestrogen therapy[17]. These observations, together with the discovery of an oestradiol receptor-related protein in the muscularis of major arteries[18], suggest that oestrogens influence arterial tone. This may be an additional mechanism whereby oestrogens protect the arterial tree.

The minimum duration of hormone replacement therapy needed to reduce arterial disease risk is not known. Furthermore, the minimum effective dose has not been established. However, benefits have been reported in all age-groups: in the younger woman after premature menopause[19] and in women who are still taking hormone replacement therapy in their early 70s[20].

INITIATION, DURATION AND CESSATION OF THERAPY

Women who are still menstruating, albeit sometimes irregularly, are often referred to our clinics. As they have not yet reached menopause, the primary care physician may be uncertain as to whether the patient's complaints are due to oestrogen deficiency. As discussed above, symptoms of oestrogen deficiency may occur in premenopausal women, usually developing 7–10 days before menstruation. Relief of these symptoms may often be achieved by the administration of a small oestrogen *supplement* such as oestradiol

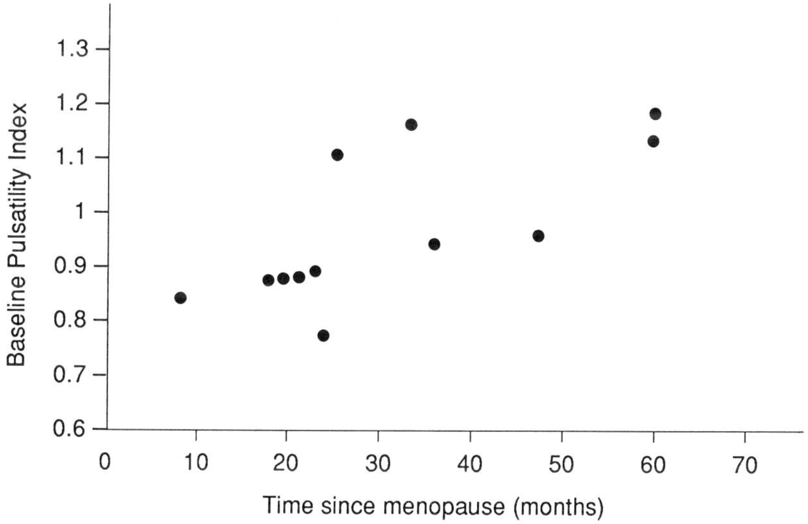

Figure 3 Correlation between baseline Pulsatility Index and time since menopause ($r = 0.74$, $p = 0.006$). (From ref. 17, reproduced with permission)

valerate, 1 mg/day (Progynova®: Schering, Burgess Hill, Sussex, UK) or transdermal oestradiol 25 μg/day (Estraderm®: Ciba-Geigy, Horsham, UK) during this time. However, it is important to ensure that the patient's progesterone level is measured in the premenstrual phase to ensure that levels are adequate for endometrial protection (20–30 nmol/l).

With progressive ovarian failure, the duration of the oestrogen deficiency symptoms gradually lengthens to occupy increasingly more time during the menstrual cycle. Continuous oestrogen/progestogen hormone replacement therapy is then required. However, in women who are still menstruating it is important that the exogenous hormone replacement therapy is synchronized with the patient's endogenous cycle. If this is not achieved, irregular bleeding may well occur. In a woman with a 21-day cycle, the progestogen should be added from day 9 (counting the first day of normal menstrual flow as day 1) to day 20. With a 28-day cycle, the progestogen is added from days 17–28, and so on. The oestrogen can be administered continuously without any break.

It is impossible to predict the duration of oestrogen deficiency symptoms. Approximately 70% of perimenopausal and early postmenopausal women will suffer vasomotor symptoms for up to 2 years; 25% of them experience such symptoms for up to 5 years and a small number remain symptomatic almost indefinitely. The converse applies with vaginal dryness and more women become symptomatic as the time-interval from the menopause lengthens. It is currently recommended that hormone replacement therapy be considered for a minimum of 5–6 years, as it has been calculated that this duration of therapy not only reduces fracture risk in later years by approximately 50%[21] (Figure 4), but does not appear, on the basis of current evidence, to increase the risk of breast cancer. Many general practitioners are reluctant to prescribe hormone replacement therapy for more than 1–2 years because of concerns about breast cancer.

Some of our patients have been on hormone replacement therapy for considerably longer than 10 years. The effects of such very long term therapy on breast cancer risk are a matter of controversy. Patients are reminded of this but we believe that their wishes must also be respected. We do not feel we have the right to withhold therapy from a symptomatic woman, or one with osteoporosis, who wishes to continue with it and is otherwise fit and well. Women who undergo a premature menopause are at increased risk of both osteoporosis and certain arterial diseases such as myocardial infarction. Unfortunately, many such women, and their doctors, are not aware of these consequences. This, once more, highlights the role of the specialist clinic in educating both patient and general practitioner. We feel that women undergoing a premature menopause should receive hormone replacement therapy *at least* until the average age of the menopause, which is 50 years.

When a patient wishes to stop hormone replacement therapy we advise her to reduce the dose of her oestrogen gradually over a period of 2–3 months. This is because, in our experience, abrupt withdrawal of therapy often results in a recurrence of oestrogen deficiency symptoms. We also advise that the monthly progestogen course should be maintained during this time. For patients who have been receiving implant therapy we

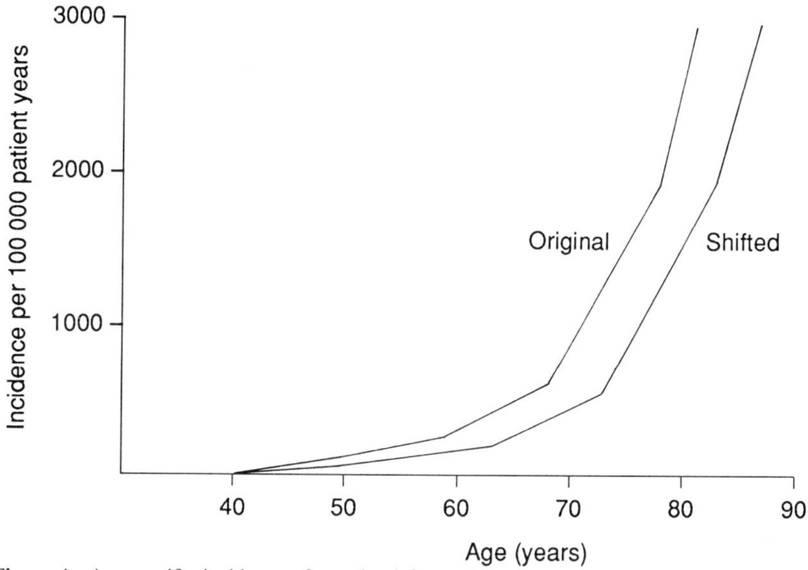

Figure 4 Age-specific incidence of proximal femoral fracture among women in Rochester, Minnesota as originally reported ('original') and as might appear ('shifted') if the onset of osteoporosis were delayed or progression slowed by 5 years. (Adapted from ref. 21)

recommend that the monthly course of progestogen be continued until all withdrawal bleeding has ceased for 3 consecutive months. As discussed above, this is the only way to ensure that plasma oestradiol levels have fallen below the threshold for endometrial stimulation.

RISKS AND CONTRAINDICATIONS

Many of the currently cited contraindications to hormone replacement therapy have been extrapolated from data derived from studies on the combined oral contraceptive pill. We believe this to be invalid because of the differences in potency between synthetic oestrogens, as used in the combined oral contraceptive pill, and natural oestrogens as used in hormone replacement therapy (Table 3).

Hypertension

The majority of women taking hormone replacement therapy experience no change, or even a slight fall, in blood pressure[23]. The 1–2% of patients who exhibit a rise in blood pressure with oral oestrogens are those with excessive weight gain. In such patients, and in women with pre-existing hypertension, we prefer the use of non-oral oestrogens. We do not believe that well-controlled hypertension should be a contraindication to non-oral oestrogens.

Table 3 Relative potency of various oestrogen preparations according to four specific parameters of oestrogenicity: follicle stimulating hormone (FSH); corticosteroid binding globulin-binding capacity (CBG-BC); sex-hormone binding globulin-binding capacity (SHBG-BC) and renin substrate (reproduced from ref. 22, with permission)

Oestrogen preparation	*Serum FSH*	*Serum CBG-BC*	*Serum SHBG-BC*	*Serum renin substrate*
Piperazine oestrone sulphate	1.1	1.0	1.0	1.0
Micronized oestradiol	1.3	1.9	1.0	0.7
Conjugated oestrogens	1.4	2.5	3.2	3.5
Diethylstilboestrol	3.8	70	28	13
Ethinyloestradiol	80–200*	1000*	614	232

* Estimated

Venous thromboembolic disease

Once again, this contraindication seems to have been carried over from the known effects of the more potent ethinyloestradiol contained in the combined pill. The biological activity of a number of pro-coagulant factors and coagulation inhibitors is adversely affected by this compound[24]. Oral administration of oestradiol valerate, a natural oestrogen, produces a small reduction in antithrombin III levels in postmenopausal women. However, menopause increases antithrombin III values and therefore the fall observed with hormone replacement therapy is to be expected.

Large-scale epidemiological studies have not demonstrated any significant increase in risk of venous thromboembolic disease among postmenopausal users of natural oestrogens[25]. Women with a past history of a deep venous thrombosis (DVT) and/or pulmonary embolism (PE) which occurred many years before the menopause and who were then exposed to endogenous (ovarian) oestradiol and yet have come to no further grief are, we believe, unlikely to be put at risk by non-oral hormone replacement therapy. The plasma oestradiol values achieved during the menstrual cycle are higher than those achieved by transdermal hormonal replacement therapy. Some women, following the DVT/PE, will have had at least one pregnancy during which oestradiol levels are many times higher than those in postmenopausal oestrogen users. Moreover, many venous thrombotic episodes have occurred after events such as surgery, trauma or immobilization which are much more likely to be responsible for the thrombotic episode.

However, we are concerned about those women who experienced unprovoked (i.e. spontaneous) venous thrombosis, especially during pregnancy or soon after starting the combined pill, when the rate of rise in plasma oestrogen concentrations may be more important than the absolute value. In these women we perform a fibrinolytic/coagulation profile to exclude an underlying abnormality. Even if the result of this is normal, we would prefer to avoid the use of oral oestrogens in these cases because the hepatic first-pass effect may cause a disturbance in the coagulation/fibrinolytic system. We believe, therefore, that non-oral oestrogens are preferable in these patients.

Fibroids

Fibroids may enlarge in some women taking hormone replacement therapy; we routinely perform annual pelvic examinations when this condition is suspected. If the fibroids enlarge with therapy and cause symptoms (e.g. menorrhagia, urinary frequency/urgency, tenesmus) the hormone replacement therapy would have to be withdrawn. Patients with symptoms due to large fibroids who wish to continue on hormone replacement therapy have to consider total abdominal hysterectomy.

Endometriosis

In women known to have had this condition we always try to establish the extent of the condition before offering hormone replacement therapy. It is helpful to establish whether or not residual disease was present following previous surgical treatment (e.g. hysterectomy). Endometriosis is oestrogen dependent and there is always a risk, albeit low, that it may be reactivated by hormone replacement therapy. In theory, this risk will be reduced if the oestrogen dose is kept to a minimum. We feel it helpful to question such patients, on every visit to the clinic, about symptoms or physical signs (e.g. dyspareunia) which may be indicative of reactivation of the disease. As with fibroids, annual pelvic examinations would seem advisable.

Benign breast disease and breast cancer

These topics are dealt with in greater detail in other chapters. The advice given to patients in our clinic conforms to the opinions of the other authors. To summarize, however, it would appear from current evidence that 5–6 years of hormone replacement therapy does not appear to increase the risk of breast cancer significantly, although very long term treatment (10 years or more) may be associated with a modest increase in risk.

Occasionally, we see patients who have had breast cancer themselves. Currently, there are no data to indicate that the risk of recurrence is increased if hormone replacement therapy is prescribed to these women. There are no data to the contrary because the required studies have not been performed. Progestogens alone, in moderate doses (e.g. norethisterone, 5–10 mg per day or equivalent) may be effective in controlling hot flushes and night sweats but do not benefit vaginal dryness or the psychological problems associated with oestrogen deficiency. In women with severe symptoms, progestogens alone are often inadequate for symptom relief. Therefore, provided that the woman is properly counselled and fully informed that she is 'sailing into uncharted waters', then we believe it unreasonable to withhold therapy with oestrogens. The same argument also applies to women with a history of endometrial cancer. Quality of life is often more important to these women than quantity.

CONCLUSION

As stated at the beginning of this chapter, the diagnosis, treatment and management of the majority of postmenopausal women requesting hormone replacement therapy is straightforward. Clearly, however, our specialist clinic, with its close association with research, will continue its important role in dealing with women who deviate from the 'norm'. We believe that there are very few women who *cannot* take hormone replacement therapy and hope that this present text has dispelled some of the myths that have arisen over the years.

ACKNOWLEDGEMENT

The financial assistance of ICRF to M.I. Whitehead is gratefully acknowledged.

REFERENCES

1. Laragh, J.H., Seeley, J.E., Leddinghum, J.G. and Newton, M.A. (1967). Oral contraceptives; renin aldosterone and high blood pressure. *J. Am. Med. Assoc.*, **201**, 918–22
2. Fraser, D.I., Parsons, A., Whitehead, M.I., Wordsworth, J., Stuart, T. and Pryse-Davies, J. (1990). The optimal dose of norethindrone acetate for addition to transdermal estradiol: a multicenter study. *Fertil. Steril.*, **3**, 460–8
3. Gangar, K.F., Cust, M.P. and Whitehead, M.I. (1989). Symptoms of oestrogen deficiency associated with supraphysiological plasma oestradiol concentrations in women with oestradiol implants. *Br. Med. J.*, **299**, 601–2
4. Gangar, K.F., Fraser, D.I., Whitehead, M.I. and Cust, M.P. (1990). Prolonged endometrial stimulation associated with oestradiol implants. *Br. Med. J.*, **300**, 436–8
5. Whitehead, M.I., Minardi, J., Kitchin, Y. and Sharples, M.J. (1978). Systemic absorption of oestrogen from Premarin vaginal cream. In Cook, I. (ed.) *The Role of Oestrogen/Progestogen in the Management of the Menopause*, pp. 63–71. (Lancaster: MTP Press)
6. Englund, D.E. and Johanssen, E.D.B. (1978). Plasma levels of oestrone, oestradiol and gonadotrophins in postmenopausal women after oral and vaginal administration of conjugated equine oestrogens (Premarin). *Br. J. Obstet. Gynaecol.*, **85**, 957–64
7. Persson, I., Adami, H.-O. and Bergkvist, L. (1989). Risk of endometrial cancer after treatment with oestrogens alone or in conjunction with progestogens: results of a prospective study. *Br. Med. J.*, **298**, 147–51
8. Whitehead, M.I., Townsend, P.T., Pryse-Davies, J., Ryder, T.A. and King, R.J.B. (1982). Effects of various types and dosages of progestogens on the postmenopausal endometrium. *J. Reprod. Med.*, **27**, 539–48
9. Studd, J.W.W., Thom, M.H., Paterson, M.E.L. and Wade-Evans, T. (1980). The prevention and treatment of endometrial pathology in postmenopausal women receiving exogenous oestrogen. In Pasetto, N., Paoletti, R. and Ambrus, J. (eds.) *The Menopause and Postmenopause*, pp. 127–39. (Lancaster: MTP Press)
10. Gambrell, D.R., Jr (1986). Prevention of endometrial cancer with progestogens. *Maturitas*, **8**, 159–68
11. Padwick, M.L., Pryse-Davies, J. and Whitehead, M.I. (1986). A simple method for determining the optimal dose of progestin in postmenopausal women receiving estrogens. *N. Engl. J. Med.*, **315**, 930–4
12. Whitehead, M.I., Fraser, D.I., Schenkel, L., Crook, D. and Stevenson, J.C. (1990). Transdermal administration of oestrogen/progestogen hormone replacement therapy. *Lancet*, **335**, 310–12

13. Crona, N., Samsioe, G., Lindberg, U.B. and Silverstolpe, G. (1988). Treatment of climacteric complaints with Org OD 14: a comparative study with oestradiolvalerate and placebo. *Maturitas*, **9**, 303–8
14. Lindsay, R., Hart, D.M. and Kraszewski, A. (1980). A prospective double-blind trial of a synthetic steroid (Org OD 14) for preventing postmenopausal osteoporosis. *Br. Med. J.*, **280**, 1207–9
15. Quigley, M.E.T., Martin, P.L., Burnier, A.M. and Brooks, P. (1987). Estrogen therapy arrests bone loss in elderly women. *Am. J. Obstet. Gynecol.*, **156**, 1516–23
16. Bourne, T., Hillard, T.C., Whitehead, M.I., Crook, D. and Campbell, S. (1990). Oestrogens, arterial status and postmenopausal women. *Lancet*, **335**, 1470–1
17. Gangar, K.F., Vyas, S., Whitehead, M.I. and Crook, D. (1991). Impedance to blood flow to the internal carotid artery is influenced by transdermal oestradiol and time since menopause. *Lancet*, **338**, 839–42
18. Padwick, M.L., Whitehead, M.I., Coffer, A. and King, R.J.B. (1988). Demonstration of an oestradiol receptor-related protein in female tissues. In Studd, J.W.W. and Whitehead, M.I. (eds.) *The Menopause*, pp. 227–33. (Oxford: Blackwell Scientific Publications)
19. Stampfer, M.J., Willett, W.C., Colditz, G.A., Rosner, B., Speizer, F.E. and Hennekens, C. (1985). A prospective study of postmenopausal estrogen therapy and coronary heart disease. *N. Engl. J. Med.*, **313**, 1044–9
20. Henderson, B.E., Ross, R.K. and Paganini-Hill, A. (1985). Estrogen use and cardiovascular disease. *J. Reprod. Med.*, **30** (suppl.), 814–20
21. Melton, L.J. (1988). Postmenopausal bone loss and osteoporosis: epidemiological aspects. In Zichella, L., Whitehead, M.I. and van Keep, P.A. (eds.) *The Climacteric and Beyond*, pp. 127–9. (Carnforth: Parthenon Publishing)
22. Maschchak, C.A., Lobo, R.A., Dozono-Takano, R., Eggena, P., Nakamura, R.M., Brenner, P.F. and Mishell, D.R., Jr. (1982). Comparison of pharmacodynamic properties of various estrogen formulations. *Am. J. Obstet. Gynecol.*, **144**, 511–18
23. Campbell, S. and Whitehead, M.I. (1977). Oestrogen therapy and the menopausal syndrome. In Greenblatt, R.B. and Studd, J.W.W. (eds.) *The Menopause: Clinics on Obstetrics and Gynecology*, Vol. 4, No. 1, pp. 31–47. (Philadelphia: Saunders)
24. Whitehead, E.M. and Whitehead, M.I. (1991). The pill, HRT and postoperative thrombo-embolism: cause for concern? *Anaesthesia*, **46**, 521–2
25. Boston Collaborative Drug Surveillance Programme. (1974). Surgically confirmed gall bladder disease, venous thromboembolism and breast tumours in relation to postmenopausal estrogen therapy. *N. Engl. J. Med.*, **290**, 15–19

4

Current use of hormone replacement therapy in general practice

M.A. Upsdell

This is a personal view of the prescribing of hormone replacement therapy in general practice and the overall management of the menopausal woman. Many doctors would question why we should treat the menopause at all, arguing that for women it is an inevitable life-event with no associated mortality.

However, the majority of women experience some symptoms during the climacteric which, although not life-threatening, have a considerable influence in reducing the quality of life and cause severe disruption in the home and at work. It is important to distinguish between symptoms that are truly hormonal in origin, and those which arise from mid-life events such as bereavement and partnership, family or employment difficulties. In practice, it may be virtually impossible to do so, in which case it is essential to discuss the situation with the woman to avoid unrealistic expectations from any chosen therapy.

In general practice, women consult more frequently than men, and the peak consulting rate occurs between 45 and 49 years of age, with many of these consultations relating to menopausal problems.

CLIMACTERIC SYMPTOMS

Vasomotor

The commonest climacteric symptoms are vasomotor, noticed in up to 75% of women as hot flushes, which are embarrassing and affect work and social life; night sweats causing insomnia and consequent diurnal irritability; and dizziness and palpitations which may provoke anxiety.

Urogenital atrophy

Vaginal dryness causes discomfort and dyspareunia which in turn aggravates sexual and marital problems. The vaginal epithelium is more susceptible to infections. Urinary symptoms are common, e.g. urgency, frequency and nocturia.

Psychological

These symptoms include emotional lability, poor concentration, loss of confidence and loss of libido. In this group it is often difficult to separate those symptoms that are truly due to perimenopausal hormonal changes and those that are psychological in origin. There is no evidence to indicate an association with true depression.

There are long-term effects of oestrogen deficiency, such as osteoporosis and cardiovascular disease.

Osteoporosis

Bone loss occurs at a rate of 1–3% per annum after the menopause, often resulting in fractures in later life. Of women over 65 years of age 35% will sustain a major fracture, usually of the hip, wrist or vertebral body; 25% of white women over 60 years have vertebral crush fractures on radiology.

Cardiovascular disease

The risk of arterial disease, particularly ischaemic heart disease, rises in the postmenopausal woman. Before the menopause the risk is one-fifth that of men of the same age. After the menopause the risks begin to approximate.

Climacteric symptoms, osteoporosis and cardiovascular disease are all reduced by hormone replacement therapy. Why then do only a minority of women take this therapy? There are two basic problems: firstly, that of uptake of hormone replacement therapy, and secondly that of continuation of therapy once started.

Wilkes and Meade, in a recent questionnaire to 1081 general practitioners in the Medical Research Council general practitioner research network, quote a 9% uptake of hormone replacement therapy among their patients aged 40–64[1]. This result is similar to Barlow's survey of Glasgow general practitioners of hormone replacement therapy use among women aged 40–60 with ever-use of 9% and current use of 7%[2]. In my own practice there is a similar uptake of 9%. Spector (1989) quoted an overall uptake of 10% in high-risk groups[3]. Continuation of therapy varies with time, with only 3% taking therapy for more than 3 years[4].

Barlow[2] has also shown differences with ever-use according to the clinical state of the woman (Table 1). Spector similarly quotes overall uptake of 30% in oophorectomized women[3].

There is no simple explanation but the attitudes of both doctors and patients are crucial. Many women remain suspicious and fearful of hormones, especially their side-effects, and worry about cancer and the continuation of

Table 1 Ever-use of hormone replacement therapy

Premenopause	8.5%
Postmenopause	15.4%
Hysterectomy	28.6%
Hysterectomy and bilateral salpingo-oophorectomy	45.5%

monthly bleeding. On the other hand, in recent years there has been much media attention on hormone replacement therapy, and many women have read widely and are sometimes almost as well-informed as the general practitioner they approach with their request to take therapy. They have a greater realization than before of the benefits of hormone replacement therapy in alleviating unpleasant symptoms, thus improving the quality of their lives and preventing the long-term sequelae discussed previously.

It is acknowledged that to make any impact on long-term sequelae, hormone replacement therapy must be provided on a large scale by general practitioners. There are insufficient specialist menopause clinics to cope with the possible 10 million postmenopausal women at risk. General practitioners offer easy access for consultation, 90% of all medical care being in the primary health sector.

Doctors' attitudes and knowledge are variable. A woman senses quickly if her general practitioner is sympathetic to her request for hormone replacement therapy. In a group practice it may be easy for her to consult with another doctor if the initial response is adverse to hormone replacement therapy. Indeed, many women will actively seek the female partner, if there is one, when she would usually see a male general practitioner, assuming that she will automatically understand and empathize. This is not necessarily so, as there are occasions where a female doctor who has never been bothered by menstrual or menopausal symptoms is less sympathetic than her male counterpart who has a partner who is being seriously afflicted.

The survey by Wilkes and Meade[1] shows that 9% of the female general practitioners and 15% of the male general practitioners prescribe hormone replacement therapy at the patient's request for relief of symptoms, with 84% of female and 76% of male general practitioners prescribing to prevent osteoporosis. However, female general practitioners treated more women than their male colleagues.

There are broadly three groups of doctors, which we may call non-prescribers, reluctant prescribers and enthuasiasts. Firstly, many general practitioners will not prescribe hormone replacement therapy on the grounds that:

(1) The menopause is a natural event which does not warrant intervention;

(2) Hormone replacement therapy simply postpones inevitable symptoms;

(3) The risks of taking therapy outweigh the alleged benefits;

(4) There is uncertainty about the different forms of hormone replacement therapy and which to choose;

(5) There is confusion over contraindications, particularly relative ones; and

(6) Very often there is inappropriate extrapolation of data on the combined oral contraceptive pill, and it is forgotten that hormone replacement therapy attempts to replace oestrogen and raise low to normal levels, whereas the combined oral contraceptive elevates oestrogen levels to suppress the ovarian–pituitary axis.

If I may quote from a letter from a woman who saw all three general practitioners in her practice:

> 'The first told me he did not like to mess about with nature. The second that God made women to cope with pain, discomfort and inconvenience all through their lives. The third that HRT would make me put on weight and make my blood pressure rise. He said I was already overweight. I am 51 years old, weigh 10 stone and am 5 ft 10 ins tall. I have headaches, hot flushes, can't sleep well, intercourse is painful as I am so dry. Once a month it all gets unbearable, I get so bad tempered.' She goes on to ask what should she do?

Secondly, there are general practitioners who will initiate therapy hesitantly, only to stop too readily for supposed contraindications, such as a slight rise in blood pressure, headaches, benign breast conditions, angina, rise in blood lipids, or forthcoming elective minor surgery. We are not helped by confusing recommendations from experts, such as a recent drug information letter advocating ethinyloestradiol as the oestrogen of choice and the use of hormone replacement therapy for as little as 1 month for symptom relief[5]. It is generally held that hormone replacement therapy should continue for 2 years for symptomatic relief and for 5–10 years for bone and arterial protection.

Thirdly, there are those general practitioners with a special interest in the menopause and hormone replacement therapy who see the benefits outweighing the risks and keep abreast of new developments and ideas. They will try to initiate uptake and encourage continuation with therapy wherever appropriate.

It is obvious that hormone replacement therapy offers the logical treatment for climacteric symptoms where it is not contraindicated. Alternative drugs, such as clonidine or β-blockers, are less effective in the relief of vasomotor symptoms. Terodiline, sometimes used for urinary symptoms, has recently been withdrawn by the manufacturers because of reported severe adverse cardiac reactions.

The evidence for the benefit in the prevention of osteoporosis is certain; the benefits in protection for the cardiovascular system are perceived as less clear-cut with the addition of progestogens, but the risks of cancer, especially of the breast, are worrying to many general practitioners.

How do we organize the delivery of advice to the menopausal woman? It can be opportunistic as she presents with or without symptoms and requests hormone replacement therapy, or target groups can be identified from age–sex and morbidity registers, e.g. women with a history of early menopause, hysterectomy, removal of ovaries or those on long-term steroid therapy. Women may be seen in general surgery consultations or at a designated menopause clinic. The choice of format of consultation will depend on the available time, resources of the practice and other professional personnel. The role of the practice nurse is invaluable in helping to provide a service acceptable to women, who will often find it easier to communicate with and confide in a nurse. This is not always entirely the doctor's fault, as many women feel that their symptoms are too trivial to consult a doctor. How many times do we hear a woman apologize for bothering her doctor, whose role she perceives as one of the treating of illness, not appreciating that illness prevention and the improvement of the quality of life are also valid roles for the modern general practitioner?

We are becoming involved increasingly in health education in the community by talking to women's groups. I have recently assisted a local Health Visitor to implement a Menopause Education Programme at a Health Centre Clinic[6]. She brought together groups of 20 women at six weekly evening sessions with a different topic and speaker at each. The sessions were organized as follows:

(1) What is the menopause? (with the health visitor as the resource);

(2) Diet (with a hospital dietician);

(3) Exercise (with a health educator);

(4) Coping with stress and anxiety (with a clinical psychologist);

(5) Hormone replacement therapy with a general practitioner (which task I undertook); and

(6) Evaluation of the course as a whole.

The health visitor feared a poor response but 70 women arrived at the first session following an article in a local newspaper. To date, I have helped her with three courses, with more to come. From questionnaires completed by the women, she found that 86% had consulted their general practitioner with menopausal symptoms and many were already on hormone replacement therapy. It was felt by 23% that they had received no help from the general practitioner, and a further 45% received limited help. The women wanted not only professional advice and information, but also to continue the group for the support they received from one another.

I sometimes found it frustrating to deal with the strange views of some of my colleagues, not being in a position to alter their management but being present in an educational role only.

I am now more convinced than ever that for general practitioners the team approach is necessary, working to an agreed common protocol in order to offer clear advice and to maximize help for women while being economical with medical time. It is the time that is required to evaluate counsel properly and then to appropriately prescribe, that deters many otherwise good general practitioners from providing a full service. With the accent on health promotion in the new general practitioner contract, this will hopefully become a less relevant reason for not providing better medical care to the perimenopausal woman.

The task in general practice, as I see it, and the basis for a protocol of management, can be based on the following model:

(1) Diagnosis that symptoms are truly due to the menopause: a role for the doctor.

(2) Providing information about the climacteric by the use of accurate and easily understood literature; health education about diet, exercise and smoking should be discussed, as well as hormone replacement therapy.

(3) Counselling, and the opportunity to discuss worries and fears, which may be undertaken by a practice nurse.

(4) To ask the woman if she wants to take hormone replacement therapy, a factor often mistakenly taken for granted. Surprisingly, many of those most at risk of osteoporosis or cardiovascular disease are resistant to embark on long-term therapy, despite careful counselling[7].

We should exclude absolute contraindications (Table 2), although even some of these would be disputed by some experts. Relative contraindications can usually be confirmed or discounted after careful investigation but may require a consultant's opinion. This may best be achieved by referral to a specialist menopause clinic. Heavy cigarette-smokers should be advised to stop or cut down because of the increased risk of cardiovascular disease in this group. Initial examination should include: height, weight and blood pressure management; urinalysis for protein and sugar; breast palpation and possibly mammography where indicated by age over 50 years or for clinical reasons; pelvic examination to assess the condition of the vagina, and the uterus for fibroids and pelvic masses; smear for cervical cytology (n.b. abnormal cytology is not a contraindication to hormone replacement therapy; indeed minor abnormal changes may resolve after a course of topical oestrogen); and blood tests if indicated. Routine follicle stimulating hormone measurement is unnecessary but may be helpful if the diagnosis is uncertain. Thyroid dysfunction is common at this age, so thyroid function tests are often useful and are best taken before hormone replacement therapy, which may alter them and make interpretation more difficult.

Table 2 Absolute and relative contraindications

Absolute	*Relative*
Breast cancer	Severe diabetes
Endometrial carcinoma	Past history of thromboembolism
Some ovarian carcinoma	Hyperlipidaemia
Severe liver or renal disease	Gynaecological conditions, e.g. fibroids or a pelvic mass
Severe thromboembolic disease	Breast lumps
Malignant melanoma	Gallbladder disease

PRESCRIBING HORMONE REPLACEMENT THERAPY

It is accepted practice in this country to give oestrogen alone where the woman has had a hysterectomy, but additional cyclical progestogen if the uterus is present, producing a monthly withdrawal bleed and avoiding the need for endometrial biopsies, unless irregular bleeding occurs. The route of administration of hormone replacement therapy will be chosen by doctor and patient together, depending on the circumstances and preferences.

Oral oestrogen is mostly taken daily, and cyclical progestogens added when indicated. Although relatively easy to use, all ingested compounds are absorbed via the portal system into the liver, and there is thus a first pass effect. This may adversely affect hepatic enzymes and coagulation factors, especially with the use of synthetic oestrogens, and for this reason the natural oestrogens, i.e. oestradiol and oestrone, are preferable. Proprietary blister packages aid compliance but fix the number of each tablet taken and are more expensive. It is occasionally necessary to tailor the number and type of progestogen for an individual woman by prescribing the oestrogen and progestogen separately. Tibolone is now available for the postmenopause where the return of regular bleeding is unacceptable, but full evaluation of its affects on long-term factors is awaited.

Vaginal oestrogen creams or pessaries may be used where the symptoms are predominantly urogenital, but some women find them messy to use. There may be erratic systemic absorption and, while short courses repeated up to 3–4 times per annum may be safe alone, longer treatment regimens will need additional cyclical progestogens in the presence of a uterus.

The transcutaneous route may be used with oestrogen creams or gels but these tend to be messy and the dosage inaccurate. Oestrogen patches are more acceptable and deliver a more reliable dosage. They are changed every 3–4 days and are used alone in the hysterectomized woman, but otherwise with additional cyclical progestogen tablets, usually for 12 days. We eagerly await a combined patch of both oestrogen and progestogen which women would find more convenient and acceptable. There are sometimes problems of skin irritation and detachment, particularly with the larger patches.

Subcutaneous implants have the advantage of not requiring daily attention, but the disadvantage of needing a minor surgical procedure, which may deter both patient and doctor. Because of the initial high oestrogen levels, symptoms may recur at diminishing intervals, leading to patient pressure for re-implantation sooner than is desirable: usually this should not be less than every 4–6 months.

Pregnancy must always be considered in the perimenopausal woman. Firstly, it is an absolute contraindication to hormone replacement therapy and must always be excluded if it is thought to be a possibility. Secondly, both doctor and woman must realize that hormone replacement therapy cannot be regarded as a method of preventing pregnancy. Careful contraceptive advice is therefore crucial.

Combined oral contraception should not be given in conjunction with hormone replacement therapy. However, it is often very useful to combine continuous natural oestrogen with a progestogen-only pill, thus providing both contraception and protection of the endometrium. The advent of lower-dosage combined oral contraception and the advice that there is no upper age-limit to its use (providing that there are no other risk factors of cardiovascular disease, e.g. smoking, hypertension, a strong family history or obesity) have led to the practice of women being kept on combined oral contraception until the menopause and then transferred directly to hormone replacement therapy. The difficulty lies in diagnosing accurately that the menopause has actually occurred. Many women may prefer to continue use of an intra-uterine device or a barrier method, either condom or cap. It is wise to discuss emergency contraception, previously misnamed 'morning after' or postcoital contraception; pills can be given or an intrauterine device inserted, up to, respectively, 72 h or 5 days after unprotected intercourse.

It is argued that while hormone replacement therapy undeniably improves climacteric symptoms, it is not cost-effective to treat all menopausal women as a prophylactic measure to prevent osteoporosis and cardiovascular disease. In general practice we are all now acutely aware of cost with Indicative Drug Budgets. However, with 35 000 hip fractures occurring in menopausal women and costing the National Health Service over £500 million in treatment in 1988 (not to mention the associated 20% mortality and decrease in the quality of life due to impaired mobility and loss of independence for the majority who do survive) we must surely put more effort as general practitioners into improving the uptake of less than 10% and the long-term continuation of hormone replacement therapy of less than 3% for chronic oestrogen deficiency. We would feel ourselves negligent, as indeed would our patients, if we failed to give maintenance thyroxine where there is proven hypothyroidism.

I do not advocate hormone replacement therapy for every woman; that is neither desirable nor feasible. Nor is it the elixir of youth. However, should we not be actively seeking out the women with high risk factors for osteoporosis and cardiovascular disease, the latter being the commonest cause of death in women in the UK, with breast cancer second? We now have the technology, with increased computerization in general practice, or at least manual age–sex registers, to identify this cohort of women and invite them to discuss menopausal problems and hormone replacement therapy with us. This has been carried out and well documented by Dr Jean Coope with considerable succes[8]. I confess to being daunted at the thought of this, especially when our practice computer listed 959 women aged 40–60 years, a figure which also did not include those others with a premature menopause nor those over 60 who might benefit from hormone replacement therapy. We have surprised the Department of Health, and ourselves I suspect, by the number of general practitioners reaching the top targets for cervical cytology and immunizations. We can do it again for our menopausal women, and we now have the framework of health promotion clinics in which to do so. Above all, we must try to improve long-term compliance of women taking hormone replacement therapy, where that is indicated, and this will involve the following:

(1) Patient and doctor education so that the balance in the benefit–risk ratio is on the benefit side;

(2) Careful screening for risk factors, both adverse and supportive of hormone replacement therapy;

(3) Regular monitoring and follow-up by the general practitioner or practice nurse, which will involve a 6-monthly (minimum) check of blood pressure and annual breast examination; and

(4) Regular auditing of women on hormone replacement therapy to check on its continued use for those most in need.

REFERENCES

1. Wilkes, H.C. and Meade, T.W. (1991). Hormone replacement therapy in general practice: a survey of doctors in the MRC's general practice research framework. *Br. Med. J.*, **302**, 1317–20
2. Barlow, D.H., Grosset, K.A., Hart, H. and Hart, D.M. (1989). A study of the experience of Glasgow women in the climacteric years. *Br. J. Obstet. Gynaecol.*, **96**, 1192–7
3. Spector, T.D. (1989). The use of oestrogen replacement therapy in high-risk groups in the UK. *Br. Med. J.*, **299**, 1434–5
4. Barlow, D.H. (1990). Should HRT be recommended in the community? In Drife, J.O. and Studd, J.W.W. (eds.) *HRT and Osteoporosis*, pp.373–83. (London: Springer-Verlag)
5. Mersey Regional Drug Information Service. Drug Information Letter. (1991). No. 84
6. Keymer, V. (1989–90). *The Menopause.* Certificate in Health Education dissertation
7. Coope, J. (1989). *Hormone replacement therapy*, p.34. (Royal College of General Practitioners)
8. Coope, J. and Roberts, D. (1990). A clinic for the prevention of osteoporosis in general practice. *Br. J. Gen. Pract.*, **40**, 295–9

General discussion I

(Chairman: Mr Ian Burn)

Mr I. Burn Can Professor Jacobs tell us anything about the effect of the combined oral contraceptive pill on osteoporosis?

Prof. H. S. Jacobs Trials comparing HRT and the oral contraceptive do not exist as yet. However, we have just completed a study at the Middlesex comparing a substantial number of young women on the combined oral contraceptive pill with age-matched controls. In this study, the birth control pill did not change vertebral bone mineral density.

Dr P.C. Somerville Regarding the increase in the high-density lipoprotein (HDL) levels and the reduction in the low-density lipoprotein levels with HRT, are there any data on the duration and strength of the progestogens used? Different authors advocate, for example, 5 or 10 mg of medroxyprogesterone acetate for 7, 12 or 14 days. What do we know of this dose–response relationship?

Prof. Jacobs The data that I have seen do seem to suggest a dose and duration relationship; if that is correct, it can be assumed that the smallest dose of a drug which has a harmful effect is probably the optimal one to use.

Dr E.C.G. Grant We should, I think, consider the broader subject of nutrients. I find that many of the women I see, most of whom have been on the pill, are very severely zinc- and magnesium-deficient. Magnesium is particularly important for cell membrane permeability. At least 30 nutritional substances which are needed for all normal cells to function are deficient in osteoporosis. Do we have comments on this broader aspect of the problem? *(Prof. Jacobs had no comment)*

Dr B.S. Hulka There is currently an ongoing double-blind clinical trial in the USA on the use of hormones in women – the Postmenopausal Oestrogen and Progestogen Intervention (PEPI) Trial. The end-points are various lipid fractions, hypertension, insulin, glucose and the lipoproteins which Prof. Jacobs discussed. The arms of the trial are placebo, oestrogen alone, and three different combinations of oestrogen/progestins; two of the latter include Provera®, one being continuous and the other cyclic, and the third is progesterone itself (a large dose in order to be absorbed through the gut). This trial includes some 800 women, all of whom have now been recruited and have been followed for at least one year. They will be followed for three years. Blood is being drawn at regular intervals, and they have physical examinations, endometrial biopsies if needed, for symptoms such as bleeding, and annual mammograms.

It is not a trial of a size that will be able to demonstrate clinical outcomes, whether they be adverse or beneficial, but it will certainly tell us what happens to various lipid fractions in relation to different doses and regimens of oestrogens and progestins.

Prof. S. Shapiro I do not think we can be quite as sanguine about the protective effect of HRT against coronary heart disease as Prof. Jacobs has suggested. I am aware that most of the epidemiological studies have suggested a protective effect, but several of them have serious methodological problems. There remains the possibility that there are so-called life-style factors, such as health consciousness among oestrogen users, which could account for the apparent protective effect. At the very least, it is possible that the amount of protection offered by oestrogens has been exaggerated. I can only endorse what Dr Hulka has said, that the only way to get around this problem is now by a randomized controlled trial.

As interesting and important as it would be to look at surrogates, such as plasma lipid fractions, I think the issue becomes so important that such a trial must be designed eventually to measure the end-points of myocardial infarction and death from ischaemic heart disease. That is the real challenge which faces us today.

Prof. Jacobs I agree, because the changing position of surrogates is a worrying factor, with new surrogates being developed all the time. For example, norethisterone does one thing to lipoprotein A and something else to HDL cholesterol.

Dr R.D. Gambrell I think the evidence is quite clear that oestrogen replacement therapy *does* protect from heart disease. All studies show this, with rare exceptions.

Professor Jacobs talked about lipids having a protective role. I also have recently had the privilege of hearing Trudy Bush's new 15-year data. She now estimates that the protective effect of hormone replacement on cardiovascular disease is mediated by lipids to about 25% of the total effects noted; she suggests that there are many other factors operating. There are data from King's College, London, showing oestrogen receptors in coronary vessel walls increasing blood flow. I would like to hear Professor Jacob's comments on this.

At the recent 13th World Congress in Singapore two studies were presented, one by Claus Christiansen, from Denmark, and the other by Bob Lindsay, formerly from the UK but now in the USA. These studies showed that the combination oestrogen/progestogen therapy is the only therapy that will actually promote new bone formation in women with established osteoporosis – so there is a benefit there. The other factors, other than lipids, mediated the protective effect.

Prof. Jacobs It seems, Dr Gambrell, that you are really supporting the argument that trials of hormone therapy must measure clinical events rather than surrogates. As I was trying to emphasize, the position on the importance of surrogates, and the surrogates that are used, changes all the time with advances in our knowledge. I agree with Prof. Shapiro that in the end we need clinical events as an indication of whether a hormone treatment is effective.

Prof. R.K. Ross It seems to me that the uterus is the only organ in postmenopausal women that really benefits very much from the use of progestogens. The bone seems not to improve very markedly, the heart certainly does not and, based on the data we have so far, it would appear that the breast does not either – and progestogens often make women feel bad. Could Professor Jacobs comment on the possibility of alternative delivery systems that might deliver progestogens only to the endometrium?

Prof. Jacobs I do not have any particular comments on giving progesterone directly to the uterus as a method of avoiding endometrial hyperplasia. It is obviously yet another technique that will be introduced. I cannot but think it will have its problems in that age group.

Some people do not feel worse on progesterone – they do, in fact, feel a great deal better. Progesterone stabilizes the temperature centre, and quite a few behavioural effects can also be shown. I think we should not just say it is a bad hormone; it is a hormone that the ovary makes regularly for most of its life, and I think it has a part to play in these therapies.

Dr Hulka Not only is the PEPI trial currently in progress in the USA, but there is also a plan for a trial of true cardiovascular end-points in 300 000 women. One of the arms of this trial will be some sort of hormone combination and the end-points will be cardiovascular disease events.

It is possible to ask whether there is a need for such a trial, given the data we currently have. If we have ever had convincing epidemiological data on any topic, use of ERT and reduction in risk of coronary events and death from these events have to be a fine example of such data. I think the epidemiological data are outstanding on that point. Despite everyone saying that we must have clinical trials, I would go so far as to say that we have excellent data already. However, the clinical trial that I have just mentioned will prove the point conclusively.

Prof. Jacobs Are there satisfactory data on oestrogen, or on oestrogen plus progestogen – which, in this country, is what women take?

Dr L. Rosenberg I think the evidence on oestrogen alone and coronary heart disease is not as convincing as it looks on the face of it. The people who have called for randomized trials often cite a randomized trial in the USA, the Coronary Drug Project, in which men were randomized to clofibrate or placebo. The very interesting result was that there was no significant difference in mortality between the drug- (clofibrate) takers and placebo. In fact, clofibrate did about 5% better than placebo. Some people said the results were analysed wrongly, and that we should really look at the people who stayed on their drug. When the clofibrate takers were compared with the clofibrate non-takers – that is, the people who did not comply with the drug to which they had been randomized – there was a very large difference in mortality. The clofibrate takers had a 40% lower mortality than the non-takers. This was very persuasive – until people looked at the placebo takers versus the non-takers, and also found a 40% difference. We are seeing reductions in coronary heart disease of the order of 40–50% in oestrogen users. I am not saying that it is all bias, but at least some of it, and possibly all of it, could be.

Prof. W.D. Dupont I would like to straddle the fence between Dr Hulka and Prof. Rosenberg. First, I am a strong proponent of doing clinical trials whenever possible. There is, however, a real problem with feasibility. If we take the analogue of the situation with cardiovascular disease, we should recall that when we started looking at men with a very high risk of heart disease we were impressed with the data from the Veterans' Administration trials which showed the intervention to be highly effective. When we started looking at much lower risk, such as in the Multiple Risk Factor Intervention Trial (MRFIT) there were enormous logistic difficulties in maintaining compliance and preventing the placebo group from migrating to the other group, and we ended up with highly equivocal results. Thus, I think it is premature to do a study of 300 000 women. It would be possible to do a randomized trial of women at very high risk of cardiovascular disease, because they had already had a myocardial infarction, for example. Such a randomized trial would be feasible, and would certainly strengthen the evidence in favour of oestrogens if it found beneficial effects. I fear that we will be spending an enormous amount of money on this very large trial of women who are not at an extremely high risk. Basically, it will provide epidemiological data and not much else.

Prof. Ross Mr Ellerington's study on risk of endometrial hyperplasia by number of days per month of progestogen therapy is obviously a slick one – the sort of study I wish I had done myself. Could Mr Ellerington tell us what he thinks the implications are, in terms of endometrial cancer risk, in relationship both to women using unopposed oestrogen and to women using no hormone replacement therapy at all? If progesterone is given for 12 days, hyperplasia can be eliminated. What does that mean in terms of endometrial cancer risk?

Mr M.C. Ellerington We do not feel confident enough to say that administering 12 days of progestin will reduce the risk of endometrial cancer to nil, because there are always those with silent disease before they start therapy. On the basis of studies which have been published in the past, it would seem that in the majority of those with silent disease, if there is any significant hyperplasia then the endometrial pathology seems to be reversed. But if there is already perhaps a small nidus of endometrial cancer, then that will almost certainly not be reversed by progestin therapy. We tell our patients, and advise their general practitioners, (GPs), that the administration of 12 days of progestin per month would appear to reduce the risk of endometrial cancer to that of untreated women, and possibly lower. I realize that a paper by Dr Gambrell some years ago suggested that it may reduce the risk of endometrial carcinoma significantly below that of untreated women.

Prof. Ross Secondly, I have heard Malcolm Whitehead suggest that there may be some sort of threshold effect of HRT on breast cancer risk, with risk increasing only after 5 or 10 years of treatment. I think we need to get rid of that notion, which is very unlikely to be correct. It is not very important to me whether or not we all agree that there is a duration-related increase in breast cancer risk associated with HRT, but if there is, it is very unlikely to be a threshold effect...

Mr Ellerington I agree. It has always baffled me why there should be a threshold effect... I feel it has to be duration-dependent, but it will be another 20 years, surely, before we find the answers we want accurately enough to satisfy us. The reason for this is that we do not have studies to answer the questions that challenge us with big enough numbers of patients to provide the necessary power.

Dr H.P. McEwan I was interested in Mr Ellerington's use of progestogens with vaginal creams because, as you know, these are not generally prescribed in the UK. In the older age-groups where the endometrium may be unresponsive, we do not get a high incidence of endometrial hyperplasia – but can we have further comments on this?

Mr Ellerington I do not think you can say specifically that the endometrium will be unresponsive. There does seem to be (going back to what we have said about threshold effects) such an effect, with respect to the endometrium, in terms of the serum concentration. If Premarin® is administered as a vaginal cream, 0.625 mg daily, even if only two or three times a week, serum levels sufficient to produce endometrial proliferation will be achieved. Therefore, if long-term use is envisaged, we advise that progestin is administered – perhaps not every month but certainly every 3 or 4 months.

Preparations for vaginal use are now available using significantly lower doses of oestrogens. The vaginal epithelium, after all, will respond and become premenopausal in terms of its cytology with as little as 0.1 mg Premarin®, so if we use the manufacturer's recommended dosage we are giving six times that. A new vaginal preparation, Vagifem®, a sustained-release preparation, has recently become available and provides 25 μg oestradiol. Although with the atrophic vagina there is initially a slight rise in serum levels (and slight suppression of follicle-stimulating hormone and luteinizing hormone), with longer-term use, and once there is a return to premenopausal vaginal cytology, there is no significant systemic absorption and endometrial proliferation apparently does not occur.

Dr McEwan Is there vaginal bleeding with women who are on progestogens in association with topical vaginal oestrogen? I would have thought it would be a very small percentage.

Mr Ellerington Yes, but it is in a very small percentage and the chances of vaginal bleeding decrease as women get older. In patients on sequential HRT in this country, my predecessors and Malcolm Whitehead found that only 85% of those with an intact uterus will bleed, and the older the woman becomes, the greater her postmenopausal age and the less chance she stands of bleeding. Indeed, some patients who start off bleeding on therapy will stop after several months or a few years. This is another cause for referral to our unit. The GP is worried in case this change signifies endometrial pathology, but we do not feel that it does.

Dr Upsdell, in her paper, seemed to suggest that every woman should go on to, or be offered, hormone replacement therapy once she had reached the menopause. It has to be accepted that every postmenopausal woman will be in a sub-oestrogenic state compared with premenopausal women. Is Dr Upsdell of the view that postmenopausal women should have HRT?

Dr M.A. Upsdell No – we do not consider all postmenopausal women to be in a state of chronic oestrogen deficiency that requires treatment. Some women do not seem to come to any great harm from their deficiency. [*Mr Burn* So you would wait for symptoms?] I would either wait for symptoms or start therapy for a woman who I thought was at risk of osteoporosis or possibly even cardiovascular disease, also targetting those who had undergone hysterectomy or oophorectomy.

Mr R. Badwe The present findings relate to cardiovascular protection and protection from osteoporosis, which may appear to be very convincing as far as the investigational studies are concerned, but their impact on the clinical end-points remain debatable. Whether those end-points should be used as the reason for giving HRT remains a matter of debate and conjecture. What is important from the patients' point of view is that they have symptoms of the menopause. Once patients are put on HRT, as Dr Upsdell rightly showed, the continuation rate beyond 3 years is less than 3%. What is the rate of recurrence of symptoms once these hormones have been stopped? If it is high, with the other benefits such as osteoporosis being still debatable, are you really justified in putting them on hormone replacement – and do you anticipate that a woman who does not have the ability to cope with the symptoms of the menopause at the age of 50 will have that ability, if there is a recurrence of symptoms, at the age of 60 when she stops hormone replacement?

Dr Upsdell If symptoms improve and we discontinue HRT, and then the symptoms return, I would put her back on HRT. I would simply re-prescribe the therapy. Clearly, we need to know the incidence of recurrence of symptoms if HRT is withdrawn – unless women are supposed to continue taking HRT until the end of their lives! I cannot give an accurate answer to your question.

Mr Ellerington It is an extremely difficult question to answer because many of those women who stay on long-term treatment – that is, for more than 5–10 years – have made up their minds to stay on it anyway. I can only speak personally, but I always remind them about the controversy over HRT and breast cancer and the possible link with long-term treatment. The women listen to what I have to say, and then reply that they are going to carry on with it anyway.

Some women get a recurrence of their symptoms when they stop HRT, which is why we feel it is very important to recommend that treatment is tailed off gradually. However, even doing that, a significant number (although I cannot quote a percentage) will get recurrence of symptoms. Those who do are that much older than when they first started treatment, and their symptoms can often be controlled with a much lower dose, certainly half or even a quarter of the dose originally given. We have patients from their late 60s right through to their late 70s who have been on HRT for nearly 20 years. They take a Premarin® tablet twice a week (or a quarter of a strip of Oestrogel® – a French preparation which some of our patients use, which goes back to a study they were on years ago) which is a minuscule dose, but sufficient to keep their symptoms at bay. I do not know whether these very tiny doses, which the elderly women tend to use more than the younger women, increase the risk of breast cancer. It seems unlikely that we have formal, organized data that address the question.

Prof. M. Elstein The King's College group has major experience of androgen (testosterone) implants in the climacteric woman. For women who have had a radical operation for endometriosis, I use an oestrogen and a testosterone implant, because the anti-oestrogenic action of testosterone is likely to serve as a good suppressant of any residual endometriosis that might remain. Would Mr Ellerington care to comment on that?

Mr Ellerington I have not seen data to support that – to show, that is, that the testosterone implant will provide endometrial protection. Progestogens will, and if we are being ultra-cautious with hysterectomized women who have a past history of endometriosis, we administer a daily progestogen as well (provided that the patient can tolerate it) in the form of either a small dose of norethindrone acetate or medroxyprogesterone acetate. I know of no data, though, that show that testosterone will reverse the proliferative effect of oestrogens and endometrium.

Professor Jacobs On the role of androgens in suppressing the endometrium, the evidence is not strong that they have an anti-proliferative effect.

Prof. Elstein With regard to the vaginal delivery system, there is a vaginal ring which delivers 5 μg of oestradiol and which has an adequate vaginal action without any endometrial effect. It is likely to be a matter of dose level and sensitivity of the end organ. The endometrium probably has a lower sensitivity than the vaginal epithelium in the postmenopausal woman. Perhaps both Mr Ellerington and Dr Upsdell might discuss this with regard to oestrogen therapy and let us know how they feel about it.

Another interesting development in vaginal delivery is a tablet that permits absorption from the vagina. This provides a first-pass effect without cutaneous irritation or the need for a skin patch, which some women find tiresome.

Mr Ellerington Silastic vaginal rings, and the new product Vagifem®, a sustained-release preparation recently released in the UK, cannot really be compared with the traditional practice of giving vaginal cream once daily or several times a week. With the latter, oestrogen will be absorbed as a bolus, whereas with the sustained-release preparation, whether it is the vaginal ring or Vagifem®, there is sustained release at a very low level. The vaginal epithelium will respond to extremely low levels of oestrogens, and therefore revert to its premenopausal cytological state. I think vaginal rings may prove useful. They certainly do not seem to be popular yet, but it remains to be seen whether they will become so when more research is done on them and when there has been more publicity.

Prof. R.E. Mansel I was very interested in both Mr Ellerington's and Dr Upsdell's work. I think they rather skated around the thorny issue of what is done about mammography in this context. It is a major problem. To give an example, we have surveyed our specialist breast clinic work-load, and 10% of it is due to HRT referrals. These women have nothing wrong with them. They are referred either for routine mammography, or for anxiety. Mr Ellerington said that the patients were surveyed carefully, but we have been given no information on what happens to the breast, either clinically or in imaging, when the woman is on HRT.

It is a very important topic because in the UK there are 24 000 new cases of breast cancer a year, which is 10% of the referrals. Thus, there are a quarter of a million referrals to breast clinics – and that is only a proportion of the women seen in general practice with breast problems. The work-load is enormous. I know that it has not been asserted today that the HRT specialist units demand that all HRT patients should undergo mammography, but there was an allusion by Dr Upsdell that if this facility was available it would be used. I think we need to be absolutely clear that if there is nothing wrong clinically with a woman, there is no indication for mammography, whatever the anxiety, because that is screening by another name and, as we all know, the government has said we should not screen under 50.

Mr Ellerington As you rightly say, Sir Donald Acheson recently advised that the results in the 50–64 year old age group in those areas that have commenced the screening programme, are encouraging. As far as I know, he has stated quite categorically that there is no evidence to support the use of screening in the under-50 year old age group.

However, I think this still does not address the question of the women with a strong family history; a sister or mother, say, who developed a premenopausal breast cancer. I would be interested to hear what some of the later speakers have to say about this. This may be a special risk group and it is not quite the same thing as population screening.

As far as HRT and mammography are concerned, as you will appreciate, the vast majority of our patients fall into the screening age group, so they will not be attending for mammograms any more frequently than if they were not taking HRT. It is still a very controversial issue, whether or not more frequent screening should be advocated in those patients who are at risk (perhaps by nature of either their family or personal history) of benign breast disease. Our unit at King's College Hospital has stopped offering mammography on a 2-yearly basis, which used to be done, and now offers it 3-yearly, but if a patient, even under 50, has a relevant risk factor, she may still be offered mammography, and more frequently than the Forrest Report recommends.

Dr Upsdell I would certainly not suggest routine mammography for every woman prior to putting her on HRT. We are told that under the age of 50 it is not as reliable and merely causes a great deal of unnecessary worry and morbidity. I believe it should be used where necessary in the woman over 50. The breasts should be examined by palpation on every woman before putting her on HRT as the basic initial examination.

Mr Burn Are there any figures on how many women under 50 – not premenopausal women, but those under 50 – are started on HRT? I specify the age of 50 because that is the cut-off point for breast screening.

Mr Ellerington That brings in the premature menopause group, and in a specialist practice we see quite a lot of them. It is perhaps 20–25%.

Prof. Mansel Studies on the effect of family history are now taking place in the UK on the initiative of the Royal Marsden Hospital in a prevention trial. This is now being extended with the support of the UK Cancer Research Campaign, and specialist breast family history clinics are being set up in many areas. We are about to start one in Manchester, so there will soon be plenty of studies on that.

Dr B.M. Campbell-Brown Regarding the more general aspects of HRT, does Prof. Jacobs know of any basis for the relative contraindication of otosclerosis which is found in so many HRT data sheets and research protocols? Depending upon the definition of otosclerosis, it would seem that up to 10% of the population may have inherited this problem.

Prof. Jacobs That is a difficult question. I think it has to be recognized that otosclerosis can get worse both in pregnancy and on the birth control pill. Data are lacking, but there are medico-legal implications. I think the argument comes from the experience of pregnancy and of the pill, and the anxiety that if hearing did get worse it would be difficult to distinguish from other factors and it might be attributed to oestrogen. I know of no formal studies of hearing in people with osteosclerosis on HRT.

Mr Ellerington I agree with Prof. Jacobs. All the evidence that we know of in our unit is purely anecdotal. The advice in our unit would be, if in doubt, to refer the patient to an ENT specialist – preferably one who is a colleague and works in menopause units.

When people ask me how they can get HRT because their GP will not prescribe it, I tell them to demand a second opinion; in my view a GP has no right to withhold it.

Mr M. Pugh In the woman with an oestradiol level of over 1000 pmol who has an implant with what has been described as tachyphylaxis, the idea of going 'cold turkey' seems a sort of iatrogenic torture. If such a woman is given nothing, she feels miserable. Might there be a place for using one of the new progestogenic preparations, such as Livial® (tibolone), perhaps on a 21-day basis, as an interim whilst the level falls?

Mr Ellerington That is a very interesting point. Livial® has only been made available in the last few months. In a year or so, when we have seen a few more tachyphylaxis patients, I might be able to give an answer. One thing we do for these patients is to allow them to use intermittent non-implant oestrogens, such as oral or transdermal, to tide them over their worst phases. If their oestradiol levels are measured, they plateau for a while and then become steady. They can be taken off the treatment for a while to allow the level to fall again. We are probably prolonging the duration of their 'cold turkey' phase (to use that expression) by doing this, but at least it makes life more bearable for them.

Prof. Jacobs The issue of tachyphylaxis is complicated. In this context I believe it is a misuse of a precise pharmacological term. A number of patients have told me that their 'implant' is running out. They feel depressed and have a number of symptoms that do *not* include flushing attacks, vaginal dryness or bladder symptomatology. I do not think therefore, that they are complaining of menopausal symptoms. They are often depressed people and doctors misdiagnose this symptomatology as being that of the menopause; they then give them increasing doses of oestrogens. Depression does not respond to oestrogen therapy. I think that this term 'tachyphylaxis' should be eliminated from this context because it is misleading and implies a precise scientific process, when what we actually have is clinical misdiagnosis and therefore clinical mistreatment.

Mr Ellerington We do see some patients with a recurrence of flushes after 3 months – genuine oestrogen deficiency symptoms – but I am sure this comment is helpful and that we should take care over this differential diagnosis.

5

Hormone replacement therapy and breast cancer risk: studies within the Breast Cancer Detection Demonstration Project

L.A. Brinton and C. Schairer

INTRODUCTION

A unique opportunity exists for evaluating the effects of menopausal hormone therapy within the context of the Breast Cancer Detection Demonstration Project, a multicentre screening project that recruited over 280 000 women for 5 years of breast screening. The cooperative nature of the study population as well as their inherently high rates of exposure to many factors have enabled evaluation of a number of potential breast cancer risk indicators, including exogenous hormones. This factor is especially amenable to evaluation, since a substantial proportion of the participants have reported usage, many for extended periods of time.

STUDY POPULATION

Women included in our studies were participants in the Breast Cancer Detection Demonstration Project, a breast cancer screening programme sponsored by the National Cancer Institute and the American Cancer Society. The screening project was begun in 1973 and by the close of recruitment in 1977 a total of 283 222 women at 29 centres throughout the United States had been enrolled for a 5-year programme of annual breast examinations. Initially, each annual screen included a clinical examination of the breast, two-view mammography, and thermography, although the use of thermography was later discontinued and the use of mammography was reduced beginning in 1977[1]. Subjects were recruited into the programme through a variety of methods of recruitment, including solicitation of friends and mass media campaigns. According to a 10% sample of participants, the majority heard about the programme through a friend (44%), a newspaper report (29%), or a television announcement (12%). Over 99% of the participants were between the ages of 35 and 74 years when they entered the screening programme, with a median age of 50 years. The majority of the participants were White (88.3%), with small percentages of Blacks (5.3%) and orientals (3.0%). Approximately 47% had household incomes of $15 000 or more as compared to a median household income in the US between 1973 and 1975 of $11 000. All but 5.6% had attended high school, and slightly over 40% had attended college. Approximately 5% of the women sampled reported an awareness of a breast lump at entry, and 17.6% reported previous breast surgery. Approximately 1% of the sample reported a previous breast cancer, and 17.6% reported a family history of breast cancer (grandmothers, mothers, sisters, half-sisters, aunts)[2].

CASE–CONTROL STUDIES

We have conducted two case–control investigations within the context of the Breast Cancer Detection Demonstration Project that enabled evaluation of the relationship of menopausal oestrogen use to risk of breast cancer[3,4]. The first study focused on women whose breast cancer was detected between July 1973 and May 1977, and included 881 menopausal breast cancer cases and 863 controls. The second study, which extended case ascertainment through January 1980, increased the sample size to 1960 cases and 2258 controls.

In the first study[3], use of oestrogen was associated with a relative risk of 1.24 (95% confidence interval (CI), 1.0–1.5), with higher risks observed among users of high-dose preparations. Hormone effects predominated among women who received them following bilateral oophorectomy (relative risk (RR), 1.54), obliterating the protective effect normally associated with the operation. In this group, risk increased with years of oestrogen use, reaching risks of 2–3 for users of 10 or more years. High risks were also observed among oophorectomized women who used hormones in the presence of other risk factors, including nulliparity, maternal family history of breast cancer and a history of benign breast disease.

In the second case–control study[4], no association was observed with ever-use of menopausal oestrogens (RR, 1.0), but a significant trend was seen with increasing use, such that users of 20 or more years were at a significant 50% excess risk. Dissimilar to the first study, elevations associated with long-term use were apparent across all menopause subgroups (natural, ovaries retained, ovaries removed). Although neither parity nor family history of breast cancer altered the effects of oestrogen use, there was some evidence of an interactive effect of hormone use and a history of benign breast disease. Hormone effects were particularly enhanced in women initiating use subsequent to a diagnosis of benign breast disease, particularly long-term users (RR, 3.0; 95% CI, 1.6–5.5), supporting a promotional role for oestrogens in the aetiology of breast cancer. This study also enabled an evaluation of interactive effects of usage of menopausal oestrogens and oral contraceptives[5], with no evidence of any synergism detected. Results from the study, however, indicated some predominance of oestrogen effects for the lower stage tumours, an observation similar to that observed for endometrial cancer[4].

COHORT STUDY

Since the end of the screening period in the late 1970s, we have been following the screenees in a prospective fashion to ascertain information on the development of various diseases as well as on changes in risk factors of interest. This study will provide the opportunity to prospectively assess information ascertained on a wide variety of potential risk factors in relation to risk of subsequent breast cancer. Of particular interest will be a comparison between results from this study and the previous case–control studies regarding effects of menopausal oestrogens. In addition, because of the timing of this cohort study, it will be possible to accrue important information on usage of combined oestrogen/progestin therapy, an exposure for which there is little conclusive data regarding breast cancer effects.

The follow-up effort, begun in 1979, was originally expected to last approximately 5 years, but was extended for another 5-year period, and plans are currently underway for another 5-year extension of follow-up (total follow-up after the end of screening of 15 years).

The study cohort enrolled in the follow-up study included women who remained active throughout the five annual screenings as well as those who did not return after their initial or any subsequent screening visit. Those included in the study were subdivided into four groups based on their status at the end of the screening programme.

Group 1 Cancers

This group included all participants who received a diagnosis of breast cancer while in the 5-year screening programme ($n = 4275$). Both project-detected cancers as well as cancers detected between screening visits were included.

Group 2 Benign biopsies/aspirations

This group included all participants who had biopsies, aspirations or other breast surgery performed during the screening period (whether recommended by the Project or not), with results indicating the presence of non-malignant breast disease ($n = 25\,115$).

Group 3 Recommended

This group included all participants who had recommendations by the Project for either biopsy or aspiration, but did not have the surgical procedure performed ($n = 9629$).

Group 4 Normals

This group was a sample of women who did not fall into the above three groups, i.e. had neither surgery nor recommendation for surgical consultation during the Breast Cancer Detection Demonstration Project programme ($n = 25\,166$). The women were individually matched to the surgical series (groups 1 and 2) on age at entry into the screening programme (5-year group), race, screening centre, time of entry into the screening programme (6-month periods), and length of participation in the screening programme. Because approximately 4000 of these women had been matched to both a cancer case and a benign case in the previously described case–control studies[4], the total number of subjects in this group is somewhat less than the total number of subjects in the benign and cancer cohorts.

Between the four cohorts, a total of 64 185 women were enrolled in the long-term follow-up study.

Data collection

A total of 61 437 of the eligible subjects (96%) for the long-term follow-up study completed a baseline interview, beginning in 1979. This telephone interview was administered as soon as possible after the beginning of the follow-up study for women who had already completed their fifth screening visit and at the fifth screening visit for the women who had not yet completed their screening visits. Subsequent to this baseline interview, yearly annual interviews were administered by telephone between 1980 and 1986.

A second phase of the study was begun in 1987. In this phase, all surviving members of the cohort ($n = 60\,079$) received a self-administered mailed questionnaire between 1987 and 1989, which was completed by 51 696 (86%) of the subjects.

Table 1 lists the information that was collected at the baseline interview.

Table 1 Information collected or updated during first phase of follow-up study

Ever-use of menopausal oestrogens; if yes, reasons for use, years taken, and age at first use
Ever-use of oral contraceptives; if yes, years taken and age at first use
History of biopsies for benign breast diseases before entering the screening programme; if yes, number and year of first biopsy
Family history of breast cancer in a blood relative, i.e. mother, sister, daughter, grandmother, aunt, including number affected
Age at menarche
Date and reason for periods stopping if no longer menstruating
Removal of uterus and/or ovaries; if yes, year of surgery
Number of livebirths and age at first livebirth
Physical examination of breast, mammographic examination of the breast, or thermographic examination of the breast since last screening visit or interview; if yes, reason for and number of examinations
Practice of breast self-examinations
Breast procedures (i.e. aspiration, biopsy, treatment surgery, primary radiation therapy, other primary therapy) since last examination by screening centre or last interview, date of procedure, breast side, and whether cancer was found

Table 2 Information collected or updated during second phase of follow-up study

Use of menopausal oestrogens since last interview; if yes, whether pills, shots, vaginal creams or suppositories; if pills, duration of use since last interview and regimen
Ever-use of oestrogen and progestin pills in the same month; if yes, age at first use, total duration of use, and number of days in the month progestin pills were taken
Changes in family history of breast cancer since last interview
Changes in menopausal status since last interview
Medical history, including osteoporosis, bone fracture, and cancer
Tobacco and alcohol use
Dietary habits and use of vitamins
Activity level and physical description, including usual and current height and weight and body shape
Marital status, race, education
Surgical procedures for breast conditions since last interview, including type of surgery (biopsy, lumpectomy, total removal of breast, aspiration), date of procedure, breast side, and whether cancer was found

Information subject to change was updated at each of the follow-up interviews. Table 2 lists the information collected in the second phase of the follow-up study. In addition to changes in exposure information from the last questionnaire (i.e. last annual interview), this new questionnaire obtained information on progestin usage (age at first use, total duration of use, number of days in the month that the pills were taken), medical history (including osteoporosis, bone fractures, cancers), tobacco and alcohol use, dietary habits and use of vitamins, activity level and physical description, including usual adult and current adult height and weight and body shape.

Hospital pathology reports and hospital discharge summaries were collected for all subjects who reported that they had a breast procedure during either phase of the follow-up study. During the first phase of the follow-up, 96% of self-reported breast cancers for which pathology reports were available were confirmed through medical record review. This figure rose to 99% for the breast cancers reported during the second phase of the follow-up study. In addition, death certificates were sought for all cohort members determined to be deceased.

Planned case–control within the cohort study

In order to evaluate the effects of oestrogen and progestin therapy on risk of breast cancer, a case–control study within the cohort is underway. This approach, rather than solely a prospective evaluation of the data, is being used for several reasons. First, all cases in the cohort provided information on progestin use after disease development. A case–control approach also allows inclusion of cases diagnosed during the screening programme and before the start of follow-up in 1979, thus increasing the size of the study.

Finally, because of deaths and losses to follow-up, information on progestin use was not obtained on all members of the cohort.

The case–control study will include cases of breast cancer from all four subgroup cohorts. Only first breast cancers will be included. Hospital pathology reports have been used to verify the self-reported breast cancers and to determine whether self-reported benign breast lesions were actually benign. Because 97% of self-reported breast cancers during the follow-up period (for which pathology reports were available) were confirmed by medical record review, self-reported breast cancers for which pathology reports could not be obtained (11% of cancers ascertained during the follow-up period) are being considered as cancers. Self-reported benign lesions for which hospital pathology reports indicated malignancy are being included as cases. Both *in situ* and invasive cases will be included.

Analyses focusing on menopausal oestrogen use without regard to concomitant progestin use will include over 5700 breast cancer cases who survived to answer the baseline interview: approximately 3900 cases identified during screening, 1000 cases reported during the first follow-up phase, and 800 cases reported during the second follow-up. Analyses assessing the effect of concomitant progestin use will include approximately 4400 cases who survived to answer the questionnaire that elicited information on progestin usage, including about 3000 detected during screening, 700 cases reported during the first follow-up phase, and 700 cases reported during the second follow-up phase. These 4400 cases are a subset of the 5700 cases available for the analyses of oestrogen use without regard to concomitant progestin exposure.

Four different controls will be sampled for each case from the non-cases. A risk set will include non-cases of the same race as the case, from the same cohort (i.e. normal, benign, recommended, or one from each of the other three cohorts for cases in the cancer cohort), from the same screening centre, and of the same age in the year the case was diagnosed. Incidence density sampling procedures will be used to select controls, such that controls for one case will not be excluded from subsequent selection as controls for another case. In addition, as recommended for this type of analysis[6,7], future cases will not be excluded from potential selection as controls for cases diagnosed earlier.

Analysis

For the purpose of analysis, study subjects will be divided into the following exposure groups: non-hormone users, users of oestrogens alone, and users of oestrogens combined with progestins. This latter group will be further divided into those who used the combined regimen only and those who used oestrogens alone in addition to the combined regimen.

Aspects of exposure that will be considered will include the following, each for both oestrogen use alone and use of combined oestrogen/progestin regimens:

(1) Ever-/never-use;

(2) Duration of usage;

(3) Age at first use; and

(4) Years since first use.

In addition, for progestin use, the number of days of each month during which exposure occurred will be considered. Duration of exposure, age at first and last use, years since first and last use, and number of days each month of progestin use will be considered as both continuous and categorical variables.

Confounding and effect modification variables that will be considered include a variety of standard breast cancer risk factors, notably menopausal status, age at menopause, number of previous breast biopsies, weight, height, Quetelet's index, history of breast cancer in a first-degree relative, number of livebirths and age at first livebirth, age at menarche, socioeconomic status, and oral contraceptive usage.

Other important variables that will be considered are the number of breast examinations since the last screening visit or interview and the reason for these examinations. These variables will be used to assess whether hormone users had more frequent breast examinations than non-users, a potential source of surveillance bias.

For the analyses, each control will be assigned a date identical to the date of diagnosis of the case to whom she was matched, and all events after that date will be ignored as they will be for the case. In addition, exposure data for both cases and controls will be lagged so that the exposure which most likely occurred after development of disease or the equivalent time-period for the matched control will not be included. For instance, exposure in the year immediately prior to the diagnosis of breast cancer will not be included. Odds ratios and 95% confidence intervals will be calculated using conditional logistic regression[8]. When examining specific subgroups (e.g. naturally menopausal women), it may be necessary to break the matching and to calculate odds ratios and 95% confidence intervals using unconditional logistic regression analyses which include the matching factors in the model. Confounding factors that individually change the estimated odds ratio associated with hormone use by more than 10% will be considered for inclusion in the final model. Effect modification will be considered under an additive model.

Initially, analyses will be performed separately in the normal, benign, recommended, and cancer cohorts. The benign and normal cohorts are of particular interest, given that they are groups at high and low risk of breast cancer, respectively. If exogenous hormones act to promote the growth of already transformed cells present in benign lesions, as some studies suggest[4,9–11], this will be most clearly revealed within the benign cohort. If, on the other hand, exogenous hormones act independently of benign breast disease, they will have the greatest relative influence in the normal cohort, a relatively low-risk group. Thus, examining risk in the four cohorts separately is one strategy to try to ascertain at which stage in the carcinogenic process the hormones are acting.

Patterns of risk associated with different aspects of exposure will also be examined to determine whether hormones act as early or late stage carcinogens. For instance, if hormones act at an early stage in the carcinogenic process, one would expect to observe a long interval between initial exposure and any increase in risk, with relative risks increasing even after exposure ceases[8]. On the other hand, if hormones act as late-stage carcinogens, the interval between first use and evidence of an effect would be shorter and relative risks should decrease rapidly after exposure stops.

Supplementary cohort analysis

To demonstrate that a case–control analysis using incidence density sampling yields results similar to a cohort analysis, a supplementary cohort analysis of risk associated with oestrogen use without regard to concomitant progestin use will be performed using the approximately 700 cases from the benign cohort, 400 cases from the normal cohort, and 200 cases from the recommended cohort incident during the follow-up period. Results from Poisson regression and Cox proportional hazards analyses will be compared to those from the case–control analyses on the same subset of study subjects.

Potential study limitations

A study limitation is that there is no validation of self-reported exposure to oestrogens and progestins or other risk factor information. However, several studies suggest that reliability of recall of menopausal oestrogen use is high. In two predominantly White, affluent retirement communities near Los Angeles, 89% of women were in agreement within 2 years on total duration of oestrogen use, based on a comparison between interview and medical chart data; for interview and pharmacy data, the agreement was 81%[12]. A study conducted in Sweden[13] found questionnaire information on oestrogen use to be highly concordant with prescription data with respect to brand (85%), dosage (88%), treatment schedule (88%), total duration of drug intake (months of treatment, correlation coefficient 0.98), and time of start of medication (correct month in 85%). In addition, in our previous case–control study[3], we found 94% agreement when validating the histories of recent hormone use against physician records. In addition, in checking self-reported ovarian status against hospital discharge summaries, operative reports, and pathology reports, the agreement rates were 95% for those reporting only a hysterectomy, 83% for a bilateral oophorectomy, and 77% for a hysterectomy with unilateral oophorectomy. In a recent case–control study in which menopausal oestrogen histories obtained through personal interviews were compared with information from the subject's physician or clinic records, the κ between users and physicians on ever-/never-use of oestrogens was 0.74, the intraclass correlation coefficient for duration of oestrogen use was

0.54, and the intraclass correlation for age at initial use of oestrogens was 0.57[14].

Related to the lack of validation is the possibility of recall bias due to the fact that some of the data were collected retrospectively and, for some cases, information was obtained many years after the diagnosis of breast cancer. It is reassuring that validation of the histories of recent hormone use against physician records in our previous case–control study showed identical agreement rates of 94% for cases and controls[3]. In addition, in a study of health-related information from multiple sources, there was no evidence that cases recalled more drug use or past disease than controls[12]. Finally, in a recent case–control study in which exposure information was validated, there was no differential misclassification by case–control status[14].

Preliminary exposure information and power of the study

Approximately 44% of the cohort reported ever-use of menopausal hormones at the baseline interview, with about 20% of the subjects reporting use of 10 or more years. Approximately 15% of those who answered the second phase questionnaire in 1987–1989 reported use of oestrogens in combination with progestins. Although the data on long-term combined treatment are undoubtedly limited, they probably reflect the patterns of use among US women and are sufficient to assess whether breast cancer risk is increased in users of the combined regimen for 6 or more years, as was found in a recent Swedish study[13].

SUMMARY AND CONCLUSIONS

The results of our case–control studies provide some concern regarding a potential adverse effect of long-term oestrogen use on the risk of breast cancer. The studies, however, highlight the difficulties in evaluating effects, since the overall association appears to be weak, leading to difficulties in evaluating risks within subgroups. For instance, the conclusion from our initial case–control study was that risk was particularly elevated in women receiving replacement therapy following a bilateral oophorectomy, an effect not confirmed with the accumulation of larger numbers of study subjects. In addition, results that oestrogen effects were higher in nulliparous women and those with a family history were not confirmed in the larger series, although there did appear to be consistency with respect to the possibility of enhanced risk among oestrogen users with a history of benign breast disease. The possibility of a promotional effect of oestrogens on benign breast disease warrants further attention, particularly with respect to specific histologic types of benign breast disease.

Concerns about the potential for recall bias with the findings of the case–control study raises the level of interest in the effects of menopausal hormones that will be available from the prospective study currently underway. The size and age of the women involved in the study will enable the accumulation of a large number of disease events following hormone exposure. Given the high rates of exposure to menopausal oestrogens within this population, there will be ample opportunity to evaluate usage patterns in detail. Of particular interest will be an evaluation of the effects of combined oestrogen/progestin usage on risk, since this exposure was not sufficiently common when the case–control studies were undertaken. We hope soon to report initial results from this prospective study. Based on results to date from the Breast Cancer Detection Demonstration Project, specific areas of interest will be the effects of hormone usage according to menopause subgroups, histories of benign breast disease, and characteristics of the tumours involved.

REFERENCES

1. Morrison, A.S., Brisson, J. and Khalid, N. (1988). Breast cancer incidence and mortality in the Breast Cancer Detection Demonstration Project. *J. Natl. Cancer Inst.*, **80**, 1540–7
2. Baker, L.H. (1982). Breast cancer detection demonstration project: five years summary report. *Cancer J. Clin.*, **32**, 194–225
3. Brinton, L.A., Hoover, R.N., Szklo, M. and Fraumeni, J.F. (1981). Menopausal estrogen use and risk of breast cancer. *Cancer*, **47**, 2517–22
4. Brinton, L.A., Hoover, R. and Fraumeni, J.F. Jr. (1986). Menopausal oestrogens and breast cancer risk: an expanded case–control study. *Br. J. Cancer*, **54**, 825–32
5. Stanford, J.L., Brinton, L.A. and Hoover, R.N. (1989). Oral contraceptives and breast cancer: results from an expanded case–control study. *Br. J. Cancer*, **60**, 375–81
6. Lubin, J.H. (1986). Extensions of analytic methods for nested and population-based incident case–control studies. *J. Chron. Dis.*, **39**, 379–88
7. Robins, J.M., Gail, M.H. and Lubin, J.H. (1986). More on 'biased selection of controls for case–control analyses of cohort studies'. *Biometrics*, **42**, 293–9
8. Breslow, N.E. and Day, N.E. (1987). *Statistical Methods in Cancer Research: The Design and Analysis of Cohort Studies.* (Lyon: IARC Publications)
9. Hoover, R., Glass, A., Finkle, W.D., Azevedo, D. and Milne, K. (1981). Conjugated estrogens and breast cancer risk in women. *J. Natl. Cancer Inst.*, **67**, 815–20
10. Ross, R.K., Paganini-Hill, A., Gerkins, V.R., Mack, T.M., Pfeffer, R., Arthur, M. and Henderson, B.E. (1980). A case–control study of menopausal estrogen therapy and breast cancer. *J. Am. Med. Assoc.*, **243**, 1635–9
11. Thomas, D.B., Persing, J.P. and Hutchinson, W.B. (1982). Exogenous estrogens and other risk factors for breast cancer in women with benign breast disease. *J. Natl. Cancer Inst.*, **69**, 1017–25
12. Paganini-Hill, A. and Ross, R.K. (1982). Reliability of recall of drug usage and other health-related information. *Am. J. Epidemiol.*, **116**, 114–22
13. Bergkvist, L., Adami, H.O., Persson, I., Hoover, R. and Schairer, C. (1989). The risk of breast cancer after estrogen and estrogen–progestin replacement. *N. Engl. J. Med.*, **321**, 293–7
14. Goodman, M.T., Nomura, A.M.Y., Wilkens, L.R. and Kolonel, L.N. (1990). Agreement between interview information and physician records on history of menopausal estrogen use. *Am. J. Epidemiol.*, **131**, 815–25

6

Postmenopausal hormone use and risk of breast cancer: 12-year follow-up of the Nurses' Health Study

G.A. Colditz, M.J. Stampfer, W.C. Willett, D.J. Hunter, J.E. Manson, C.H. Hennekens, B.A. Rosner and F.E. Speizer

INTRODUCTION

The increase in risk of breast cancer seen in association with early menarche and late menopause points to a potential role of ovarian hormones in the aetiology of this disease. Further, pregnancy is associated with increased risk of breast cancer, perhaps for up to 3 years after the delivery[1,2]. In case–control and cohort studies, urine or plasma oestrogen levels have been positively related to risk of breast cancer. Furthermore, obesity among postmenopausal women, which increases oestrogen levels, has been associated with higher risk of breast cancer incidence[3] and mortality[4]. Together, these data suggest that oestrogen levels may influence the risk of disease among postmenopausal women[5]. Oestrogens act as promoters of breast cancer in experimental animal models. Tamoxifen, a competitive inhibitor of oestrogen binding, has reduced the recurrence rate of breast cancer by about 25% in randomized trials[6].

Although exogenous oestrogens have long been suspected of increasing the risk of breast cancer, no relation has been observed in most studies. Previous case–control studies[7–21] and retrospective[22,23] and prospective cohort investigations[24–26], as well as studies using population rates for comparison[27–30] have focused primarily on ever-use, without distinction between current and past use of postmenopausal oestrogens. In a meta-analysis, the combined estimate of relative risk from 23 studies was 1.01 (95% confidence interval (CI), 0.95–1.08)[31], indicating virtually no relation between ever-use (which was predominantly past use) and risk of breast cancer. More recently, techniques of meta-analyses have been used to combine data addressing the question of duration of use and risk of breast cancer. Steinberg and colleagues found a 30% increase in risk (95% CI,

Material in this chapter draws on work reported in J. Am. Med. Assoc., (1990) **264**, 2648–53

1.2–1.6) after 15 years of use, based only on data from case–control studies[32]. In this meta-analysis, prospective data were not included because groups in some studies were not compatible to those in other studies. In another meta-analysis Dupont and Page assessed the overall relation between dose of oestrogen replacement therapy and risk of breast cancer, reporting no increase in risk with use of 0.625 mg per day (relative risk (RR), 61.06), and no increase in risk with higher doses. Further, they noted no significant increase in risk among women with prior benign breast disease (RR, 1.16; 95% CI, 0.89–1.5)[33].

The Nurses' Health Study was established in 1976 to study risk factors for cancer and other diseases, with particular emphasis on the potential effects of exogenous hormones and risk of breast cancer. We have previously reported an increased risk of breast cancer associated with current use, but no increase in risk among past users with even 15 or more years of use[34]. In this analysis we update our findings by adding an additional 2 years of follow-up, and specifically address the question of type of hormone used and risk of breast cancer.

METHODS

The Nurses' Health Study cohort was established in 1976, when 121 700 female registered nurses 30–55 years of age completed a mailed questionnaire that included items about known or suspected risk factors for cancer and cardiovascular diseases. Baseline information included details of breast cancer risk factors[35,36], postmenopausal use of hormones and history of use of oral contraceptive agents. Every 2 years, follow-up questionnaires have been mailed to the women to bring the information on risk factors up to date and to ascertain whether major medical events have occurred.

Data on postmenopausal hormone use

A history of postmenopause hormone use was elicited from respondents on the 1976 questionnaire. This information was updated by follow-up questionnaires sent in 1978, 1980, 1982, 1984, and 1986, that sought details of current use and duration of use since the preceding questionnaire. We used the response on each questionnaire to define current use status for the subsequent 2-year interval. However, as current use was not asked in 1976, for the 1976–1978 interval we defined a woman as a current user if her duration of menopause and her duration of use of postmenopausal hormones were within 12 months of each other. If the duration of menopause was more than 12 months greater than the duration of hormone use, she was classified as a past user for this 2-year interval of follow-up.

In biennial questionnaires sent in 1978 and subsequently, we asked each woman if she was currently using postmenopausal hormones and, if so, the type of hormones used. The daily dose of conjugated oestrogen (by far the most common form) was obtained from 1980 onwards and was classified as 0.3 mg, 0.625 mg, 1.25 mg, and more than 1.25 mg.

For past users, we calculated the time since last use; this information was updated every 2 years. The person-time of follow-up was reassigned according to the respondent's status at the beginning of each of the six 2-year intervals from 1976 to 1986. This procedure maintained the prospective nature of the study.

Identification of breast cancer cases

On each questionnaire, we inquired whether breast cancer had been diagnosed and, if so, the date of diagnosis. All women who reported breast cancer (or the next of kin for decedents) were contacted with permission to review the relevant hospital records and confirm the self-reported diagnosis. Pathology reports were obtained for 93% of the cases, and information on histologic tumour type, tumour size, and node involvement was extracted by physicians blinded to data on hormone supplement use reported by the participants. Although permission to review pathology reports and hospital records could not be obtained for 7% of cases, we based our analysis on all incident breast cancers because the rate of accuracy of self-reporting was extremely high (99.6%). We omitted the small number of carcinomas *in situ* from analysis.

Population for analysis

The end-point for the primary analysis was the occurrence of incident breast cancer. We therefore excluded from the analysis all women who reported breast or other cancer (excluding non-melanoma skin cancer) on the 1976 questionnaire. This left a total cohort of 118 300 women eligible for follow-up; the present analysis was limited to postmenopausal women. We classified a woman as postmenopausal from the time she returned a questionnaire on which she reported natural menopause or hysterectomy with bilateral oophorectomy. Self-report of menopause is highly reproducible in this cohort and is valid with regards to details of the extent of ovarian surgery[37]. In addition, we classified women reporting hysterectomy without bilateral oophorectomy as postmenopausal at the age when natural menopause had occurred in 90% of the cohort (54 years for current cigarette smokers and 56 years for non-smokers).

In 1976, 23 965 women met the criteria for classification as postmenopausal; these women entered the follow-up from 1976 to 1978. The report of menopause was updated every 2 years, and the population was expanded to include women who became postmenopausal and remained free from cancer. During the 12 years of follow-up from the return of the 1976 questionnaire to June 1, 1988, we accrued 480 112 person-years of follow-up among postmenopausal women; 1050 incident cases of breast cancer were identified among these postmenopausal women.

Follow-up of the cohort for the identification of non-fatal breast cancer, by questionnaire, telephone interview, and certified mail was 95% complete. For fatal breast cancer, follow-up was more than 98% complete.

Statistical analysis

The primary analysis used incidence rates with person-months of follow-up as the denominator. For each participant, person-months were allocated according to the 1976 exposure variables and were updated according to information on follow-up questionnaires. For women who developed breast cancer or died, person-months were assigned according to the covariate status reported on the most recent completed questionnaire, but follow-up terminated with the diagnosis of breast cancer or death. Women who reported a diagnosis of cancer other than non-melanoma skin cancer on the 1978, 1980, 1982, 1984, or 1986 questionnaire were excluded from subsequent follow-up. If no questionnaire was returned for a follow-up cycle, the most recently recorded covariate data were used for the subsequent follow-up interval. If the previous status was current postmenopausal hormone use, however, the updated status of use was classified as missing. For past use and never-use, the status of use was classified according to the most recent questionnaire.

We used relative risk as a measure of association, defined as the incidence of breast cancer among women who had used postmenopausal hormones divided by the corresponding rate among women who had never used these drugs. Additional stratified analyses were carried out to control for risk factors and to explore the possibility that the effect of current use of postmenopausal hormones might be modified by these factors. We used the Mantel test for linear trend to examine the relation between duration of current use of postmenopausal hormones and risk of breast cancer[38], and proportional hazards models to adjust for multiple risk factors simultaneously[39].

We also used proportional hazards models to analyse survival status among patients with breast cancer according to the history of use of postmenopausal hormones prior to diagnosis. Survival status for the 722 incident cases of breast cancer diagnosed between 1976 and June 1986 was ascertained as of June 1, 1990 for 702 women, the remaining 20 women were censored between June 1988 and June 1990. Overall, these women were censored for a total of 22.75 years of potential follow-up.

RESULTS

In 1976, 33% of postmenopausal women were current users of postmenopausal hormones, 18% were past users, 3.6% had missing information on use of postmenopausal hormones, and the remainder had never used these agents. During the 12 years of follow-up, postmenopausal women accrued 480 112 person-years of follow-up time. Current use of postmenopausal hormones accounted for 20.6% of this follow-up time, past use contributed 24.9%, missing information on hormone use contributed 4.0%, and never-use contributed 50.5% of the follow-up time.

Women who had never used postmenopausal hormones and current and past users had similar distributions for age at menarche and family history of breast cancer. Current users were slightly more likely to have reported a

Table 1 Age-standardized prevalence of risk factors for breast cancer in the Nurses' Health Study cohort according to use of postmenopausal hormones. Standardized to the age-distribution of person-time among never-users.

	Postmenopausal hormone use (%)		
Risk factor	*Never*	*Current*	*Past*
Age of $\leq$ 12 years at menarche	46.1	46.6	47.0
Nulliparity	5.9	9.6	7.9
Age (years) at first child's birth			
< 20	0.5	0.8	0.8
20–24	38.0	41.5	39.4
Parity			
1–2	29.6	34.9	32.6
$\geq$ 3	61.3	54.3	56.4
History of benign breast disease	5.2	9.3	6.4
Family history of breast cancer	8.6	8.2	8.4
Quetelet's index			
< 21 kg/m^2	12.8	18.0	13.0
> 29 kg/m^2	15.4	10.0	13.6
Alcohol intake			
never	34.5	30.8	33.1
$\geq$ 15 g/day	15.4	17.5	16.1

Table 2 Age-specific incidence rates of breast cancer by never-use and current use of replacement hormone therapy, Nurses' Health Study, 1976–1988

	Never-use			*Current use*			
Age	*Cases*	*Person-years*	*Rate**	*Cases*	*Person-years*	*Rate*	*Relative risk*
30–34	0	139	–	0	603	–	–
35–39	0	900	–	0	2 868	–	–
40–44	5	4 147	120	7	8 559	82	0.68
45–49	36	23 879	151	26	16 736	155	1.03
50–54	162	84 023	193	64	30 194	211	1.09
55–59	220	93 570	235	92	29 020	317	1.35
60–66	104	35 061	297	62	12 274	505	1.70
Overall	527	241 719		251	100 254		1.29
Multivariate							1.33

*χ^2 test for heterogeneity across the age strata = 6.16, $p > 0.10$

history of benign breast disease, to be lean, to consume alcohol, to be nulliparous, or to have given birth only once or twice (Table 1).

We examined the relation between current and past use of postmenopausal hormones and risk of breast cancer within 5-year age-groups (Table 2). The increased risk associated with current use of oestrogen replacement therapy was most evident among women 55 years of age or older. Overall, the age-adjusted relative risk of breast cancer among current users was 1.29

(1.11–1.50). The test for heterogeneity across age strata was not significant (χ^2 on 4 degrees of freedom = 6.16, $p > 0.10$). After adjusting for age of birth in single years, age at menopause, and type of menopause the relative risk increased slightly to 1.36 (1.15–1.61). Past use was not associated with increased risk of breast cancer. The relative risk, adjusted for age, age at menopause and type of menopause was 0.91 (0.78–1.07). In this model, the increase in risk of breast cancer associated with a 15-year delay in the age at natural menopause was between 30 and 40%.

We examined the association between current use of oestrogen replacement and risk of breast cancer among women reporting natural menopause, bilateral oophorectomy, and hysterectomy without removal of ovaries. After age-standardizing to the distribution of women with a natural menopause who never took replacement hormone therapy, the relative risk among the women with natural menopause was 1.33 (103 cases, 33 899 person-years), among women with a bilateral oophorectomy the relative risk was 1.35 (114 cases, 53 865 person-years), and among women with hysterectomy without oophorectomy the relative risk was 1.59 (35 cases, 7321 person-years).

To determine whether the association between current use and risk of breast cancer varied according to other risk factors we examined the age-adjusted relative risk within strata of parity, age at first birth, family history of breast cancer in mother or sister, personal history of benign breast disease, age at menarche, and body mass index. The relative risk varies little within strata of these risk factors providing little evidence for effect modification, and the relative risks adjusted for age and each risk factor one at a time were particularly stable (Table 3). The increase in risk among current users with late age at first birth, and the lack of association among women with a personal history of benign breast disease are noteworthy. After multivariate adjustment for all the established risk factors, age in single years, age at menopause in years, and type of menopause, the relative risk for current use was essentially unchanged at 1.33 (1.12–1.57) and the relative risk for past use was 0.92 (0.79–1.09).

We next examined duration of use and risk of breast cancer among current and former users (Tables 4 and 5). We observed no evidence of increasing risk with increasing duration of use among either current or past users. Among current users the test for trend in risk with increasing duration of use was 0.042, $p = 0.96$. The test for heterogeneity of trend across age strata was also null ($p = 0.5$). Among past users, women who had used replacement oestrogens for 10 or more years in the past had an age-adjusted relative risk of 0.79 (0.49–1.26) compared to women who had never used replacement hormones. Further adjustment for age and type of menopause did not materially alter these results.

Among past users of oestrogen replacement therapy, time since last use did not show any overall trend. Among women with natural menopause, those who had used replacement hormones less than a year in the past at the beginning of a follow-up interval had an age-adjusted relative risk of 1.54, however this increase was not seen among women with a bilateral oophorectomy (RR, 0.99). The age- and menopause-adjusted relative risk for these recent past users was 1.16 (0.72–1.87).

Table 3 Age-adjusted relative risk for current and past use of oestrogen replacement therapy within strata of established risk factors for breast cancer, Nurses' Health Study 1976–1988

	Current use	*Past use*
Family history		
yes	1.33	0.77
no	1.30	0.92
adjusted relative risk*	1.30	0.90
History of benign breast disease		
yes	0.97	0.81
no	1.42	0.91
adjusted relative risk	1.24	0.87
Menarche		
<13	1.37	0.85
13	1.36	0.96
>13	0.96	0.90
adjusted relative risk	1.28	0.89
Parity		
nulliparous	0.94	1.21
1–2	1.58	0.86
3+	1.17	0.86
adjusted relative risk	1.28	0.90
Age at first birth		
15–19	1.02	—
20–24	1.23	0.91
25–29	1.32	0.87
30–34	1.43	0.78
35–39	2.08	1.0
40+	2.79	1.47
adjusted relative risk	1.32	0.91
Body mass index (kg/m^2)		
<21	1.29	1.07
21–22.9	2.04	1.57
23–24.9	1.35	0.79
25–28.9	1.29	0.78
29+	0.57	0.68
adjusted relative risk	1.31	0.91

*Relative risk adjusted for age and breast cancer risk factor

In a previous study, Gambrell suggested that the addition of progestin was associated with a reduced risk of breast cancer of 0.3 (0.1–0.8)[40], therefore we examined this question using follow-up data from 1978 when type of oestrogen was first asked. During this 10-year follow-up period we observed 972 incident cases of breast cancer. Compared with never-users, women who were current users of conjugated oestrogen were at increased risk of breast cancer, as observed in the overall cohort analysis; the age-adjusted relative risk was 1.42 (95% CI, 1.19–1.70) (Table 6). During 6144 person-years of follow-up among women with current use of oestrogen and progestin, we observed 20 cases of breast cancer, giving an age-adjusted relative risk of 1.54 (0.99–2.39). Women who used oestrogen and testosterone were also at increased risk (RR, 2.45 (0.95–6.35)). We had insufficient information to

Table 4 Duration of current use of oestrogen replacement therapy and age-adjusted relative risk of breast cancer among postmenopausal women during 12 years of follow-up, Nurses' Health Study

Duration of current use (months)	*Number of cases*	*Person-years of follow-up*	*Age-adjusted relative risk*	*Multivariate relative risk*†
Never	527	241 718	1.0 (reference)	1.0 (reference)
Current*				
1–11	22	10 472	1.19 (0.79–1.82)	1.10 (0.72–1.72)
12–23	19	10 109	1.07 (0.69–1.69)	1.02 (0.62–1.66)
24–35	32	12 422	1.39 (0.97–1.99)	1.33 (0.93–1.90)
36–59	40	16 930	1.27 (0.92–1.75)	1.25 (0.90–1.75)
60–119	81	27 403	1.47 (1.16–1.85)	1.55 (1.21–1.99)
120–179	32	12 719	1.15 (0.80–1.64)	1.28 (0.88–1.86)
180+	24	6 899	1.53 (1.02–2.30)	1.48 (1.00–2.20)

*Test for linear trend in risk among current users = 0.042, $p = 0.96$; χ^2 test for heterogeneity in trend across age strata = 2.36, $p = 0.5$; †multivariate relative risk adjusted for age at menopause, current age, type of menopause, time period, age at first birth, parity, age at menarche, history of benign breast disease, family history of breast cancer, and body mass index

Table 5 Duration of past use of hormone replacement therapy and age-adjusted relative risk of breast cancer among postmenopausal women during 12 years of follow-up, Nurses' Health Study

Past duration of oestrogen replacement therapy (months)	*Cases*	*Person-years*	*Relative risk*
Never	527	241 718	1.0 (reference)
Past			
1–11	60	30 868	0.89 (0.69–1.15)
12–23	41	19 485	0.98 (0.73–1.32)
24–35	21	15 184	0.64 (0.43–0.96)
36–59	38	17 788	0.99 (0.73–1.33)
60–119	48	20 676	1.08 (0.82–1.42)
120–179	13	7 357	0.83 (0.50–1.37)
180+	5	2 636	0.81 (0.36–1.81)

Table 6 Type of hormone preparation used and age-adjusted relative risk of breast cancer among postmenopausal women 1978–1988, Nurses' Health Study

Type	*Cases*	*Person-years*	*Relative risk*
Never	493	222 270	1.0 (reference)
Conjugated oestrogen	158	56 182	1.42 (1.19–1.70)
Oestrogen and progestin	20	6 144	1.54 (0.99–2.39)
Other oestrogens	19	8 210	1.14 (0.72–1.81)
Progestins alone	2	400	2.52 (0.66–9.63)
Oestrogen and androgens	4	778	2.45 (0.95–6.35)
Other	43	27 706	—

provide informative risk estimates for other forms of replacement therapy. Adjustment for type of menopause in addition to age did not materially alter these relative risk estimates, nor did multivariate control for established breast cancer risk factors.

Dose of oestrogen therapy also has received considerable attention. We had little follow-up time among women using high doses of replacement oestrogen and hence cannot provide meaningful data on a dose of more than 1.25 mg per day. However, we observed a similar increase in risk among current users of 0.625 mg per day and 1.25 mg per day of conjugated equine oestrogen (Table 7).

Prior use of oral contraceptives before oestrogen replacement therapy has been raised as a possible modifier of breast cancer risk associated with oestrogen use. We examined this issue specifically, using data on past use of oral contraceptives reported by the participants on the baseline questionnaire and subsequent follow-up questionnaires. After age-standardizing to the age-distribution of women with a natural menopause and who never used replacement hormones, we observed that among never-users of oral contraceptives, current use of oestrogen replacement therapy was associated with a relative risk of 1.31 compared to never-users. Past users of oral contraceptives who had never used replacement hormones had an age-standardized relative risk of 1.16 compared to never-users of oral contraceptives, and women who had used both oral contraceptives in the past and were current oestrogen replacement users had a relative risk of 1.49.

To quantify the relation between prior use of oestrogen therapy and survival after diagnosis of breast cancer, we extended the mortality surveillance of the 722 incident cases diagnosed during the period from 1976 to June 1, 1986. With the added follow-up to June 1, 1990, we observed an additional 84 deaths, giving a total of 189 deaths. Exposure status was defined as of the questionnaire returned prior to the diagnosis of breast cancer. After adjusting for age in single years and body mass index, compared to women who had never used replacement hormones, the odds ratio for death among current users of oestrogen was 0.75 (0.52–1.10) and among past users the odds ratio was 0.84 (0.59–1.20). Addition of family history to the proportional hazards model did not alter these results. Because obesity is related to the

Table 7 Dose of conjugated oestrogen and age-adjusted relative risk of breast cancer 1980–1988, Nurses' Health Study

*Dose**	*Cases*	*Person-years*	*Relative risk*†
Never	452	195 512	1.0 (reference)
Vaginal	12	4 214	1.16 (0.66–2.07)
Current			
< 30	28	9 797	1.27 (0.86–1.85)
0.625	85	26 422	1.45 (1.16–1.83)
1.25	49	16 700	1.44 (1.07–1.93)
> 1.25	6	5 479	0.59 (0.26–1.31)

*Dose information missing for 38 cases arising during 19 039 person-years of follow-up; †age-adjusted relative risk and 95% confidence interval

likelihood of using oestrogen therapy and also related to survival after diagnosis, we retained body mass index in the model when we added tumour size and lymph node involvement at diagnosis. Consistent with our previous data showing that use of oestrogen therapy was not associated with tumour size or stage at diagnosis, when we added these variables to the model the odds ratio for death changed only slightly. For current use the odds ratio was 0.78 (0.54–1.15), and for past use the odds ratio was 0.84 (0.59–1.20).

DISCUSSION

In this 12-year prospective cohort study with 480 112 person-years of follow-up among postmenopausal women, we observed an elevated risk of breast cancer among current users of postmenopausal hormones. Further, we note that the addition of progesterone to oestrogen does not remove the elevation in risk that we observed, and the confidence interval did not overlap the previously reported protective association.

The prospective design of this study greatly reduces the possibility of bias due to the reporting of postmenopausal hormone use or other risk factors for breast cancer. Information on exposure to postmenopausal hormones depended solely on the self-report of the nurses prior to the onset of disease. Misclassification of postmenopausal hormone use should be minimal because subjects in this study were all registered nurses who had demonstrated a particular interest in medical research. The strong positive association between postmenopausal hormone use and endometrial cancer in this cohort[41] and the protective association of postmenopausal hormone use with coronary heart disease[42] – which agree with findings in other studies – also lend support to the accuracy of self-reported hormone use, because inaccurate self-reporting would tend to obscure associations with all end-points. Furthermore, a substudy of women who began menopause due to surgical procedures showed a high degree of concordance between the menopause information the participants provided in the questionnaire and their medical records[37]. Random misclassification of exposure would tend to attenuate any true effect; by reclassifying participants by exposure status every 2 years, we kept such misclassification at a low level. Furthermore, all medical records were reviewed by physicians blinded to the exposure status reported previously by the participants.

Differential completeness of follow-up was unlikely to have a major impact, since the rate of follow-up was high for both fatal and non-fatal breast cancer. Non-fatal follow-up was 95% of total potential follow-up time for both never-users and past users, and 98% for current users. The primary potential source of bias to be considered is increased breast cancer surveillance or detection among current users of postmenopausal hormones, who must be under the active care of a physician to receive their prescriptions. As we previously reported, during the 1986–1988 follow-up period current users had a slightly higher rate of mammography than did never-users. The overall rate of mammography in all three groups was far higher than the 24–29% among women reporting a mammogram in the preceding 2 years in two national surveys[43,44]. The difference between current users and never-users (15%), however, is not large enough to explain a relative risk of 1.33. Furthermore, when we conducted analyses delaying the diagnosis of breast cancer among current users by 2 years (allowing for early detection giving a lead time of 2 years) the relative risk remained unchanged. Although screening increases the early detection of breast cancer and decreases mortality[45–49], it does not appear to increase appreciably the diagnosis of 'pseudotumours' that would not otherwise come to medical diagnosis; in the Health Insurance Plan trial the total numbers of cases detected in screened (367 cases) and control women (364 cases) were virtually equal by the 6th year[50].

However, the reduction in mortality due to early diagnosis of breast cancer through screening may be as high as 30%. With a 15% difference in the rate of screening between never-users and current users of postmenopausal hormones, such a reduction would produce a relative risk for breast cancer mortality of only 0.95. In the present analysis, when we added tumour size and lymph node involvement at the time of diagnosis, the mortality ratio did not alter, consistent with the lack of association between these markers of screen-detected tumours and use of oestrogen therapy.

If the excess incidence of tumours observed among current users was only due to the diagnosis of 'pseudotumours' that would never be fatal, the expected relative risk for mortality would have been 1/1.33 or 0.75. This is very close to the observed mortality ratio observed for both current and past users of replacement oestrogen therapy. An alternative explanation is that oestrogen therapy stimulates the growth of otherwise slow-growing tumours that would be detected years later, perhaps growing less aggressively as is typical of tumours among older postmenopausal women. Our current data suggest that increased surveillance for breast cancer among women currently using oestrogen replacement therapy cannot explain their observed magnitude of excess risk of breast cancer or their relative survival. Further follow-up is needed to advance the understanding of these important relations.

Previous case–control and cohort studies have usually not differentiated current and past use of postmenopausal hormones, and all but three cohort studies have been based on fewer than 100 cases. Hunt and colleagues[29], following women attending menopause clinics in the UK for an average of 67 months, observed an increase in risk in predominantly current users compared to the incidence rates reported from the Birmingham Cancer Registry. Mills and co-workers[26] followed 20 341 Seventh-Day Adventist women for 6 years and detected 215 histologically-confirmed breast cancers. Current use of oestrogen replacement therapy among these women was associated with a significant increase in risk of breast cancer (RR, 1.69; 95% CI, 1.12–2.55) compared with never-users; however, there was no evidence of increasing risk with increasing duration of use among users.

The use of a combination of oestrogen and progesterone has been recommended to reduce the risk of uterine cancer among postmenopausal women taking replacement hormones. In addition, Gambrell and colleagues[28] reported that the combination of oestrogen and progestogens was associated with a relative risk of 0.3 (0.1–0.8) when they followed 5563 women and detected 53 cases of breast cancer during 37 236 person-years of follow-up. This finding was based on eight observed cases and comparison with an external tumour registry for expected incidence rates. In contrast, we found an age-adjusted relative risk of 1.54 based on 20 observed cases. Several other reports also fail to confirm the protective association due to combination oestrogens and progestogens. Ewertz[21] reported a relative risk of 1.36 (0.98–1.87) based on cases identified through the Danish Cancer Registry and a random sample of controls, although formulations available in Denmark differ from those in the United States. Bergkvist and colleagues[25] also reported that the addition of progestogens was associated with an increase in risk of breast cancer over that observed for oestrogens alone. Compared to never-users, women who used combination therapy for more than 6 years had a relative risk of 4.4 (0.9–22.4) based on ten cases.

In the study reported by Ewertz[21], the use of oestrogens plus androgens was associated with over a twofold increase in risk of breast cancer. In the present study, the combination of oestrogen plus androgen was associated with a relative risk of 2.45, consistent with that result. However, Brinton and co-workers[11] have not observed such an association in two large case–control studies. Further study is needed to clarify the magnitude of this association.

Despite a positive association between current postmenpausal hormone use and risk of breast cancer in this study, we found no association between dose of conjugated equine oestrogen and risk. This lack of a dose-dependent effect with up to 1.25 mg of Premarin® per day is consistent with reports by Hoover and colleagues[8] and Brinton and co-workers[11,21], although an earlier study by Hoover and colleagues[27] showed an increased risk of 1.9 among women taking more than 0.625 mg/day. Hoover and co-workers reported a relative risk of 1.5 for 1.25 mg or more/day, and Brinton and co-workers reported an increased risk of 1.70 for women taking 2.5 mg/day. The relation between dose of conjugated oestrogen and serum oestradiol levels shows that with a daily dose of 1.25 mg there is no increase in free oestradiol above the level observed for women taking 0.625 mg/day[51]. This finding is consistent with the observation that the relative risk of breast cancer is the same for women taking these different doses of conjugated equine oestrogen.

We observed no effect of duration of use of oestrogens on risk of breast cancer. The lack of a duration effect suggests that oestrogens may act acutely to increase risk, and that this effect is reversible within perhaps 2 years of cessation. This contrasts with the results of the recent meta-analysis, however, in that analysis data from cohort studies were excluded.

The magnitude of increase in risk of breast cancer associated with current use appears quite modest. Given the beneficial effect of postmenopausal oestrogen therapy on the risk of cardiovascular disease and hip fractures, Henderson and co-workers concluded (from a risk–benefit analysis allowing for a relative risk of 1.5 for breast cancer with long-term (> 20-year) use of postmenopausal oestrogens) that the benefits of oestrogen supplement therapy markedly outweigh the risks[52]. However, our data suggest greater complexity; elevated risk of breast cancer may appear before 20 years of postmenopausal hormone use but rapidly decline with cessation of use. Although this increase in risk will, in general, be counterbalanced by the cardiovascular benefits, these data suggest the need for caution in the use of oestrogens.

ACKNOWLEDGEMENTS

This work was supported by research grant CA40356 from the National Cancer Institute, NIH, Department of Health and Human Services. G.A. Colditz is supported by an American Cancer Society Faculty Research Award FRA-398.

REFERENCES

1. Williams, E.M.I., Jones, L., Vessey, M.P. and McPherson, K. (1990). Short term increase in risk of breast cancer associated with full term pregnancy. *Br. Med. J.*, **300**, 578–9
2. Bruzzi, P., Negri, E., La Vecchia, C., Decarli, A., Palli, D., Parazzini, F. and Del Turco, M.R. (1988). Short term increase in risk of breast cancer after full term pregnancy. *Br. Med. J.*, **297**, 1096–8
3. Tretli, S. (1989). Height and weight in relation to breast cancer morbidity and mortality. A prospective study of 570,000 women in Norway. *Int. J. Cancer*, **44**, 23–30
4. Tretli, S., Haldorsen, T. and Ottestad, L. (1990). The effect of pre-morbid height and weight on the survival of breast cancer patients. *Br. J. Cancer*, **62**, 299–303
5. Key, T.I.A. and Pike, M.C. (1988). The role of oestrogens and progestogens in the epidemiology and prevention of breast cancer. *Eur. J. Cancer Clin. Oncol.*, **24**, 29–43
6. Early breast cancer trialists' collaborative group (1988). Effective of adjuvant tamoxifen and of cytotoxic therapy on mortality in early breast cancer. An overview of 61 randomized trials among 28,896 women. *N. Engl. J. Med.*, **319**, 1681–92
7. Ross, R.K., Paganini-Hill, A., Gerkins, V.R., Mack, T.M., Pfeffer, R., Arthur, M. and Henderson, B.E. (1980). A case-control study of menopausal estrogen therapy and breast cancer. *J. Am. Med. Assoc.*, **243**, 1635–9
8. Hoover, R., Glass, A., Finkle W.D., Azevedo, D. and Milne, K. (1981). Conjugated estrogen and breast cancer risk in women. *J. Natl. Cancer Inst.*, **67**, 815–20
9. Hulka, B.S., Chambless, L.E., Deubner, D.C. and Wilkinson, W.E. (1982). Breast cancer and estrogen replacement therapy. *Am. J. Obstet. Gynecol.*, **143**, 638–44
10. McDonald, J.A., Weiss, N.S., Daling, J.R., Francis, A.M. and Polissar, L. (1986). Menopausal estrogen use and the risk of breast cancer. *Breast Cancer Res. Treat.*, **7**, 193–9
11. Brinton, L.A., Hoover, R. and Fraumeni, J.F. (1986). Menopausal oestrogens and breast cancer risk: an expanded case–control study. *Br. J. Cancer*, **54**, 825–32
12. Wingo, P.A., Layde, P.M., Lee, N.C., Rubin, G. and Ory, H.W. (1987). The risk of breast cancer in postmenopausal women who have used estrogen replacement therapy. *J. Am. Med. Assoc.*, **257**, 209–15
13. Rohan, T.E. and McMichael, A.J. (1988). Non-contraceptive exogenous oestrogen therapy and breast cancer. *Med. J. Aust.*, **148**, 217–21
14. Nomura, A.M.Y., Kolonel, L.N., Hirohata, T. and Lee, J. (1986). The association of replacement estrogens with breast cancer. *Int. J. Cancer*, **37**, 49–53
15. Kelsey, J.L., Fischer, D.B., Holford, T.R., LiVoisi, V.A., Mostow, E.D., Goldenberg, I.S. and White, C. (1981). Exogenous estrogens and other factors in the epidemiology of breast cancer. *J. Natl. Cancer Inst.*, 67, 327–33
16. Jick, H., Walker, A.M., Watkins, R.N., D'Ewart, D.C., Hunter, J.R., Danford, A., Madsen, S., Dinan, B.J. and Rothman, K.J. (1980). Replacement estrogens and breast cancer. *Am. J. Epidemiol.*, **112**, 586–94

17. Sartwell, P.E., Arthes, F.G. and Tonascia, J.A. (1977). Exogenous hormones, reproductive history and breast cancer. *J. Natl. Cancer Inst.*, **59**, 1589–92
18. Casagrande, J., Gerkins, V., Henderson, B.E., Mack, T. and Pike, M.C. (1976). Exogenous estrogens and breast cancer in women with natural menopause. *J. Natl. Cancer Inst.*, **56**, 839–41
19. Brinton, L.A., Hoover, R.N., Szklo, M. and Fraumeni, J.F. (1981). Menopausal estrogen use and risk of breast cancer. *Cancer*, **47**, 2517–22
20. Kaufman, D.W., Miller, D.R., Rosenberg, L., Helmrich, S.P., Stolley, P., Schottenfeld, D. and Shapiro, S. (1984). Noncontraceptive estrogen use and risk of breast cancer. *J. Am. Med. Assoc.*, **252**, 192–8
21. Ewertz, M. (1988). Influence of non-contraceptive exogenous and endogenous sex hormones on breast cancer risk in Denmark. *Int. J. Cancer*, **42**, 832–8
22. Hiatt, R.A., Bawol, R., Friedman, G.D. and Hoover, R. (1984). Exogenous estrogen and breast cancer after bilateral oophorectomy. *Cancer*, **54**, 139–44
23. Thomas, D.B., Persing, J.P. and Hutchinson, W.B. (1982). Exogenous estrogens and other risk factors for breast cancer in women with benign breast diseases. *J. Natl. Cancer Inst.*, **69**, 1017–25
24. Buring, J.E., Hennekens, C.H., Lipnick, R.J., Willett, W., Stampfer, M.J., Rosner, B., Peto, R. and Speizer, F.E. (1987). A prospective cohort study of postmenopausal hormone use and risk of breast cancer in US women. *Am. J. Epidemiol.*, **125**, 939–47
25. Bergkvist, L., Adami, H., Persson, I., Hoover, R. and Schairer, C. (1989). The risk of breast cancer after estrogen and estrogen-progestin replacement. *N. Engl. J. Med.*, **321**, 293–7
26. Mills, P.K., Beeson, W.L., Phillips, R.L. and Fraser, G.E. (1989). Prospective study of exogenous hormone use and breast cancer in Seventh-Day Adventists. *Cancer*, **64**, 591–7
27. Hoover, R., Gray, L.A., Cole, P. and MacMahon, B. (1976). Menopausal estrogens and breast cancer. *N. Engl. J. Med.*, **295**, 401–5
28. Gambrell, R.D., Maier, R.C. and Sanders, B.I. (1983). Decreased incidence of breast cancer in postmenopausal estrogen–progesterone users. *Obstet. Gynecol.*, **62**, 435–43
29. Hunt, K., Vessey, M., McPherson, K. and Coleman, M. (1987). Long-term surveillance of mortality and cancer incidence in women receiving hormone replacement therapy. *Br. J. Obstet. Gynecol.*, **94**, 620–35
30. Vakil, D.V., Morgan, R.W. and Halliday, M. (1983). Exogenous estrogens and development of breast and endometrial cancer. *Cancer Detection Prev.*, **6**, 415–24
31. Armstrong, B.K. (1988). Estrogen therapy after the menopause – Boon or Bane? *Med. J. Aust.*, **148**, 213–14
32. Steinberg, K.K., Thacker, S.B., Smith, S.J., Stroup, D.F., Zack, M.M., Flanders, W.D. and Berkelman, R.L. (1991). A meta-analysis of the effect of estrogen replacement therapy on the risk of breast cancer. *J. Am. Med. Assoc.*, **265**, 1985–90
33. Dupont, W.D. and Page, D.L. (1991). Menopausal estrogen replacement therapy and breast cancer. *Arch. Int. Med.*, **151**, 67–72
34. Colditz, G.A., Stampfer, M.J., Willett, W.C., Hennekens, C.H., Rosner, B. and Speizer, F.E. (1990). Prospective study of estrogen replacement therapy and risk of breast cancer in postmenopausal women. *J. Am. Med. Assoc.*, **264**, 2648–53
35. Romieu, I., Willett, W.C., Colditz, G.A., Stampfer, M.J., Rosner, B., Hennekens, C.H. and Speizer, F.E. (1989). A prospective study of oral contraceptive use and the risk of breast cancer in women. *J. Natl. Cancer Inst.*, **81**, 1313–21
36. London, S.J., Colditz, G.A., Stampfer, M.J., Willett, W.C., Rosner, B. and Speizer, F.E. (1989). A prospective study of relative weight, height, and the risk of breast cancer. *J. Am. Med. Assoc.*, **262**, 2853–8
37. Colditz, G.A., Stampfer, M.J., Willett, W.C., Stason, W.B., Rosner, B., Hennekens, C.H. and Speizer, F.E. (1987). Reproducibility and validity of self-reported menopausal status in a prospective cohort of women. *Am. J. Epidemiol.*, **126**, 319–25
38. Mantel, N. (1983). Chi-square test with one degree of freedom: extension of the Mantel–Haenszel procedure. *J. Am. Stat. Assoc.*, **56**, 690–700
39. Cox, D.R. (1972). Regression models and life-tables. *J.R. Stat. Soc. (B)*, **34**, 187–220
40. Gambrell, R.D., Maier, R.C. and Sanders, B.I. (1983). Decreased incidence of breast cancer in postmenopausal estrogen–progestogen users. *Obstet. Gynecol.*, **62**, 435–43
41. Stampfer, M.J., Colditz, G.A., Willett, W.C., Rosner, B., Hennekens, C.H. and Speizer, F.E.

(1986). A prospective study of exogenous hormones and risk of endometrial cancer. *Am. J. Epidemiol.*, **124**, 520 (abstract)
42. Stampfer, M.J., Willett, W.C., Colditz, G.A., Rosner, B., Speizer, F.E. and Hennekens, C.H. (1985). A prospective study of postmenopausal hormones and coronary heart disease in US women. *N. Engl. J. Med.*, **313**, 1044–9
43. Hayward, R.A., Shapiro, M.F., Freeman, H.F. and Corey, C.R. (1988). Who gets screened for cervical and breast cancer? Results from a national survey. *Arch. Int. Med.*, **148**, 1177–81
44. Heath, C.W., Funk, D.J., Strickland, R. *et al.* (1989). Trends in screening mammography for women 50 years of age and older – Behavioral Risk Factor Surveillance System, 1987. *Morbidity and Mortality Weekly Report*, **38**, 137–40
45. Tabar, L., Fagerberg, C.J.G., Gad, A., Baldetorp, L., Holmberg, L.H., Grontoft, O., Ljungquist, U., Lundstrom, B., Manson, J.C., Eklund, G., Day, N.E. and Pettersson, F. (1985). Reduction in mortality from breast cancer after mass screening with mammography. *Lancet*, **1**, 829–32
46. Shapiro, S., Venet, W., Strax, P., Venet, L. and Roeser, R. (1982). Ten-to-fourteen-year effect of screening on breast cancer mortality. *J. Natl. Cancer Inst.*, **69**, 349–55
47. Verbeek, A.L.M., Hendriks, J.H.C.L., Holland, R., Mravunac, M., Sturmans, F. and Day, N. E. (1984). Reduction of breast cancer mortality through mass screening with modern mammography. First results of the Nijmegen Project, 1975–1981. *Lancet*, **1**, 1222–6
48. Tabar, L., Fagerberg, G., Duffy, S.W. and Day, N.E. (1989). The Swedish two-country trial of mammographic screening for breast cancer: recent results and calculation of benefit. *J. Epidemiol. Commun. Health*, **43**, 107–14
49. Andersson, T., Aspegren, K., Janzon, L., Landberg, T., Lindholm, K., Linell, F., Ljungberg, O., Ranstam, J. and Sigfusson, B. (1988). Mammographic screening and mortality for breast cancer: the Malmo mammographic screening trial. *Br. Med. J.*, **297**, 943–8
50. Shapiro, S., Venet, W., Strax, P. and Venet, L. (1988). Periodic screening for breast cancer. *The Health Insurance Plan Project and its Sequelae*, 1963–1986. pp. 49–58. (Baltimore: The Johns Hopkins University Press)
51. Whitehead, M.I. (1978). The effects of oestrogens and progestogens on the postmenopausal endometrium. *Maturitas*, **1**, 87–98
52. Henderson, B.E., Ross, R.K., Paganini-Hill, A. and Mack, T.M. (1986). Estrogen use and cardiovascular disease. *Am. J. Obstet. Gynecol.*, **154**, 1181–6

7

An overview of the effect of oestrogen replacement therapy on breast cancer risk

W.D. Dupont and D.L. Page

INTRODUCTION

The effects of oestrogen replacement therapy are varied and complex. It provides relief for the symptoms of oestrogen deprivation associated with the menopause[1], is protective against osteoporosis[1], and reduces the risk of coronary heart disease[2,3]. On the other hand, unopposed oestrogens greatly increase the risk of endometrial cancer[1]. This risk can be reduced substantially by adding a progestin to oestrogen replacement therapy[4,5]. Unfortunately, progestins can adversely affect the favourable lipid balance induced by oestrogens[5], and it is currently not known if the protective effects of progestins on the endometrium are bought at the cost of decreased protection against cardiovascular disease.

It is within this context of the important known benefits and risks of oestrogen replacement therapy that the question of therapy and breast cancer risk must be considered. There are good biological reasons to hypothesize that oestrogen replacement therapy might adversely affect breast cancer risk. Oestrogens are known to promote breast cancer growth, and breast cancer is a disease with a long memory; events such as age at first childbirth can affect a woman's risk of breast cancer several decades after they occur. It is thus plausible that oestrogen replacement therapy given in a woman's 40s and 50s could enhance her risk of breast cancer decades later. The therapy's benefits for heart and bone suggest long-term therapy rather than a use restricted to the menopausal years. This fact makes the question of oestrogen replacement therapy and breast cancer risk one of great clinical importance.

The most definitive way of answering any scientific question is through tightly controlled experimentation. In medicine, this approach works best when the benefits or risks of therapy are large or can be quickly determined. To detect a small risk that will not become apparent for decades through a clinical trial can require vast numbers of subjects to comply with a randomly-assigned treatment for many years. Such trials are not usually feasible for economic, political and ethical reasons. Nevertheless, decisions concerning the use of therapies such as oestrogen replacement therapy must be made now by millions of patients. We are thus forced to rely on observational studies to make these decisions. In the absence of controlled experiments, it is not surprising that observational studies of oestrogen replacement therapy and breast cancer have reached variable conclusions. This diversity makes the task of interpreting this literature difficult. Quantitative overviews of the literature have an advantage over many conventional reviews in that they can avoid making an arbitrary and perhaps limited selection of studies for review. The challenge of conducting such overviews is to describe fairly the entire body of relevant literature while ensuring that one's conclusions are properly influenced by the quality, as well as the quantity, of the papers under study.

MATERIALS AND METHODS

This chapter is, in part, an update of a review which we published in 1991[6]. Our methods have been described in detail[6], and are briefly summarized here. We performed a search of the MEDLINE database[7] for studies of oestrogen replacement therapy and breast cancer. This search identified 556 papers, 35 of which were found to provide estimates of breast cancer risk associated with oestrogen replacement therapy. A conventional literature search identified an additional 17 papers giving a total of 52 papers for detailed review[8–59]. Of these 52 papers, we eliminated six small studies that had fewer than five breast cancer patients who had taken oestrogen[8–13]. This was done because overview methods tend to overestimate the precision of risk estimates from small studies. However, several of these papers had other methodological weaknesses that would have justified their exclusion on other grounds. Frequently, authors have published multiple papers on the same group of study subjects; for these studies we only retained the paper that had the longest follow-up on the largest number of women. This led to the exclusion of an additional 14 publications[14–27]. The remaining 32 publications[28–59] were subjected to a detailed methodological evaluation using the following criteria:

(1) Were explicit criteria used for patient selection?

(2) Was oestrogen replacement therapy confirmed by review of medical records?

(3) Were cases of breast cancer confirmed by review of histologic slides or medical records?

(4) Was the relative risk of breast cancer adjusted explicitly or implicitly for age and other confounding variables?

For case–control studies:

(5) Were all premenopausal women excluded from the case or control groups?

(6) Were patients with prior breast cancer excluded explicitly from the case group?

(7) Were patients with recurrent breast cancer excluded explicitly from the case group?

(8) Were control patients selected from a population-based reference group?

For cohort studies:

(9) Were all women recruited at or after their menopause?

(10) Were women with prior breast cancer excluded explicitly from the cohort?

(11) Were affirmative steps taken to minimize the number of patients lost to follow-up?

(12) Were criteria for determining the end of follow-up given explicitly?

The studies under review varied considerably with respect to these methodological strengths and weaknesses (Table 1). However, there were only two studies which we felt merited exclusion from our overview[28,29]. These papers apparently included substantial numbers of premenopausal subjects but did not evaluate breast cancer risk separately by menopausal status. They were excluded since the indications for non-contraceptive oestrogen therapy in premenopausal women are quite different from those of menopausal women, and these women may be subject to different cancer risks than those of postmenopausal patients. In our previous overview[6] we also excluded the study of La Vecchia and colleagues[51] since they failed to derive breast cancer risks separately for premenopausal and postmenopausal subjects. They did, however, provide risk estimates subdivided by type of menopause and duration of therapy. We have used these data in this review to estimate their relative risk of breast cancer in postmenopausal subjects associated with oestrogen replacement therapy. In the remaining 30 studies there was no apparent relationship between the estimates of breast cancer risk and the methodological strengths and weaknesses of these papers.

The statistical methods used in this paper are described in Dupont and Page[6] and Greenland[60]. Our preference is to use a fixed effects approach to summarize the relative risks from multiple studies. This approach provides a weighted geometric mean of the individual risks from the different studies together with the corresponding confidence interval. This mean can only be interpreted as the combined relative risk estimate from all studies when it is reasonable to infer that the different studies were all estimating the same relative risk. In this case, the mean's confidence interval estimates the plausible error of the combined relative risk estimate.

OVERVIEW OF THE LITERATURE

Figure 1 shows the relative risks of breast cancer associated with oestrogen replacement therapy that have been reported in the literature. The mean relative risk for these studies is 1.11. However, the variation between the relative risks reported in this figure is very large, and is far greater than

Table 1 Evaluation of methods used by the papers listed in Figure 1. Papers were evaluated using questions 1–12 given in the text (Y = Yes, N = No)

		Methodological questions											
		All studies				*Case–control studies*				*Cohort studies*			
First author	*Year*	1	2	3	4	5	6	7	8	9	10	11	12
Bergkvist[58]	1989	Y	Y	Y	Y					N	N	Y	Y
Brinton[50]	1986	Y	N	Y	Y	Y	N	Y	Y				
Byrd[33]	1977	Y	Y	N	Y					Y	N	Y	N
Casagrande[32]	1976	Y	Y	N	Y	Y	N	N	Y				
Colditz[59]	1990	Y	N	Y	Y					Y	Y	Y	Y
Dupont[56]	1989	Y	N	Y	Y					Y	Y	Y	Y
Ewertz[55]	1988	Y	N	Y	Y	Y	Y	Y	Y				
Gambrell[43]	1983	Y	Y	Y	Y					Y	N	N	N
Hiatt[47]	1984	Y	Y	Y	Y	Y	N	Y	Y				
Hoover[31]	1976	Y	Y	N	Y					Y	N	Y	Y
Hoover[38]	1981	Y	Y	Y	Y	N	N	N	Y				
Horwitz[46]	1984	Y	Y	Y	Y	Y	Y	Y	N				
Hulka[41]	1982	Y	N	Y	Y	Y	Y	Y	Y				
Hunt[53]	1987	Y	Y	Y	Y					N	N	Y	Y
Jick[36]	1980	Y	Y	Y	Y	Y	Y	Y	N				
Kaufman[45]	1984	Y	N	Y	Y	Y	Y	Y	N				
Kelsey[39]	1981	Y	N	Y	Y	N	Y	Y	N				
La Vecchia[51]	1986	Y	N	Y	Y	Y	N	N	N				
Mack[30]	1975	Y	Y	Y	Y	Y	N	N	Y				
McDonald[49]	1986	Y	N	Y	Y	N	Y	Y	Y				
Mills[57]	1989	Y	N	Y	Y					Y	N	Y	N
Nomura[48]	1986	Y	Y	Y	Y	N	Y	Y	Y				
Ravnihar[35]	1979	Y	N	Y	Y	N	N	N	N				
Rohan[54]	1988	Y	N	Y	Y	Y	Y	Y	Y				
Ross[37]	1980	Y	Y	Y	Y	Y	Y	Y	Y				
Sherman[44]	1983	Y	N	Y	Y	N	Y	Y	N				
Thomas[40]	1982	Y	Y	Y	Y					N	N	Y	N
Vakil[42]	1983	Y	N	N	Y					Y	N	N	N
Wingo[52]	1987	Y	N	Y	Y	Y	N	Y	Y				
Wynder[34]	1978	Y	N	Y	Y	Y	N	N	N				

could be reasonably expected due to chance variation between the studies ($p < 0.00005$). This suggests that either the women in these different studies differed in ways that affect breast cancer risk, or that the oestrogen therapy differed between these studies. To elucidate these differences, we looked at the effect of dose, type and duration of therapy on breast cancer risk. Figure 2 shows those studies that have reported breast cancer risks in women who received ≤ 0.625 mg/day of conjugated oestrogens. Note that all of these studies provide low, mutually consistent estimates of breast cancer risk. These risks do not differ significantly from each other ($p = 0.87$), and there is considerable overlap between the confidence intervals of all nine studies. This suggests that it is reasonable to combine these results into an overall estimate of breast cancer risk associated with conjugated oestrogen therapy at a dosage of ≤ 0.625 mg/day. This combined relative risk is 1.08, with a 95% confidence interval of 0.96–1.2. It provides strong evidence that low-dose conjugated oestrogen therapy does not appreciably increase breast

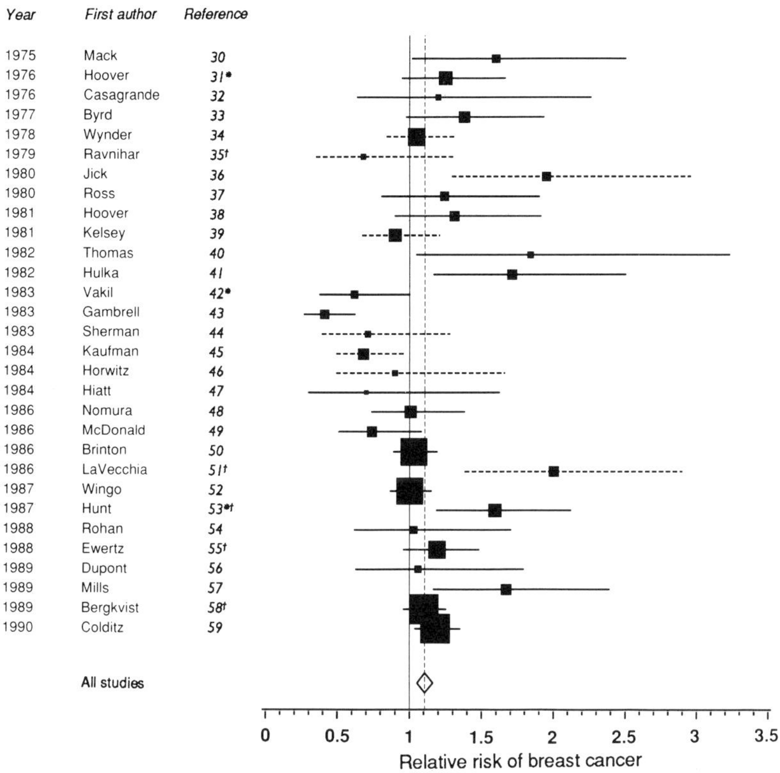

Figure 1 Relative risk of breast cancer associated with oestrogen replacement therapy that has been reported in the literature. Black squares denote relative risk estimates from each study and horizontal lines the 95% confidence intervals for these risks. Solid lines are used for studies with population-based control groups while dashed lines denote studies with hospital controls. The area of each relative-risk square is proportional to the information content of the study[6]. The diamond marks a weighted geometric mean of the individual relative risks from all studies, its width indicating the 95% confidence interval for this mean. The variation in risks reported in this figure is far greater than can be explained by chance and suggests that either different treatments were used in the different studies or that the study subjects varied among studies with respect to other factors that affected their risk of breast cancer. *Calculated using the general population as a reference group; all others calculated with respect to women who did not take oestrogens; †studies performed in Europe

cancer risk. It must be noted, however, that only a small proportion of the women in the studies from Figure 2 were followed for more than 10 years. Thus, the risk associated with longer-term therapy at this dose is less clear due to the limited number of studies that have reported such experience.

Studies of higher doses of conjugated oestrogens have reported variable levels of breast cancer risk[6]. The mean relative risk for this therapy was 1.10, with no study reporting a relative risk greater than 2.0. The variability in reported risks does not permit any strong inference from this literature. However, it is unlikely that the relative risk of breast cancer associated with $\geq$ 1.25 mg/day of conjugated oestrogens is greater than twofold.

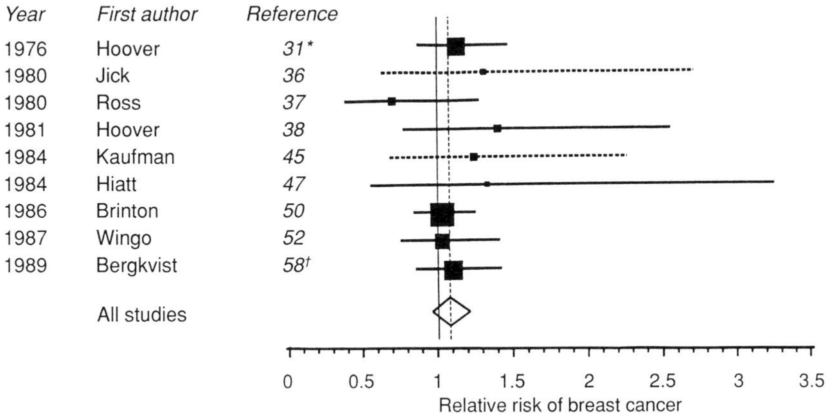

Figure 2 Breast cancer risk among women treated with ≤ 0.625 mg/day of conjugated oestrogens. These results are highly consistent among studies. The 95% confidence interval for the risk of breast cancer associated with this treatment is given by the diamond. These results provide strong evidence that this dose of conjugated oestrogens does not increase breast cancer risk. See Figure 1 for an explanation of the symbols in this figure (adapted from Dupont and Page[6])

A question of great clinical importance is whether the addition of a progestin to oestrogen replacement therapy affects breast cancer risk. It is certainly possible that progestins might enhance breast cancer risk since physiological proliferation of breast epithelium occurs during the luteal phase of the menstrual cycle when progesterone levels are high[61]. Unfortunately, there is very limited evidence concerning the effect of this combined therapy on breast cancer risk (Figure 3). Bergkvist and colleagues[58] found a fourfold (though insignificant) increase in breast cancer risk among women who took combined therapy for more than 6 years. Ewertz[55] found a 30% increase in breast cancer risk associated with this therapy which also lacked statistical significance. Gambrell and co-workers[43] reported a reduced risk of breast cancer associated with this therapy. It is possible, however, that their results may be affected to some extent by non-response bias. In view of the role of progestins in controlling the risk of endometrial cancer associated with unopposed oestrogens, it is important that we establish the effect of combined therapy on breast cancer risk.

Duration of therapy

Determining the effect of duration of oestrogen replacement therapy on breast cancer risk has acquired great importance given the known long-term benefits of this therapy. Figure 4 shows the effects of duration of therapy that have been reported in the literature to date; the relative risks from each study are denoted by a connected sequence of straight line segments and

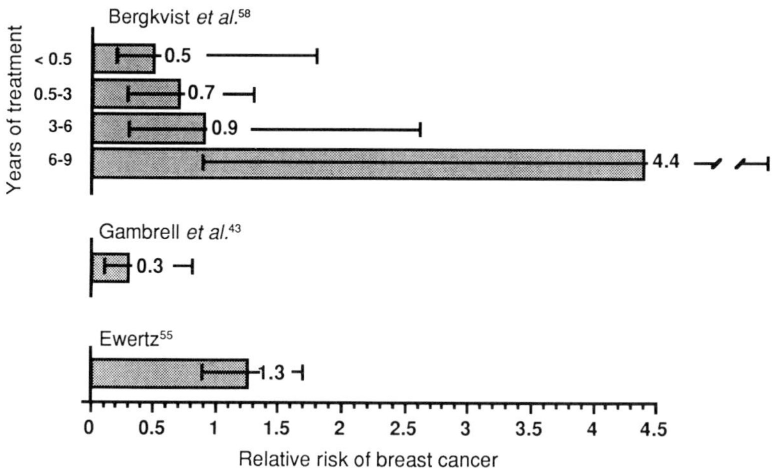

Figure 3 Risks of breast cancer associated with hormonal replacement therapy with oestrogen plus progestin that have been reported in the literature. The horizontal lines denote 95% confidence intervals

each pivot point on these lines denotes a relative risk of breast cancer associated with a specific interval of duration of therapy. The pivot points are centred over the corresponding duration intervals. For example, Brinton and colleagues[50] report relative risks of 1.28 and 1.24 associated with durations of oestrogen replacement therapy of 10–14 years and 15–19 years, respectively. In Figure 4, the risk line for this study has pivot points at 1.28 and 1.24 centred at 12.5 and 17.5 years, respectively. Final duration intervals that are reported as being greater than some number of years are drawn in this figure as having the same length as the corresponding penultimate duration interval. Nomura and co-workers[48] published risks for Caucasian and Oriental women in the same paper and these are denoted 48AP and 48BP, respectively, in Figure 4.

There are several points that are illustrated by Figure 4. First, there is a great deal of variability between the findings of the studies that have been published to date. Although studies such as those by Bergkvist and colleagues[58], Ewertz and colleagues[55] and Brinton and colleagues[50] have found consistent and significant trends of increasing breast cancer risk with increasing duration of treatment, there are other excellent studies that have not. It has been argued[62] that the failure to find a duration–risk relationship may be due to the bias induced by using hospital-based controls. However, eight of the 12 studies that did not find a significant trend used population-based control groups, including the large and excellent studies of Colditz

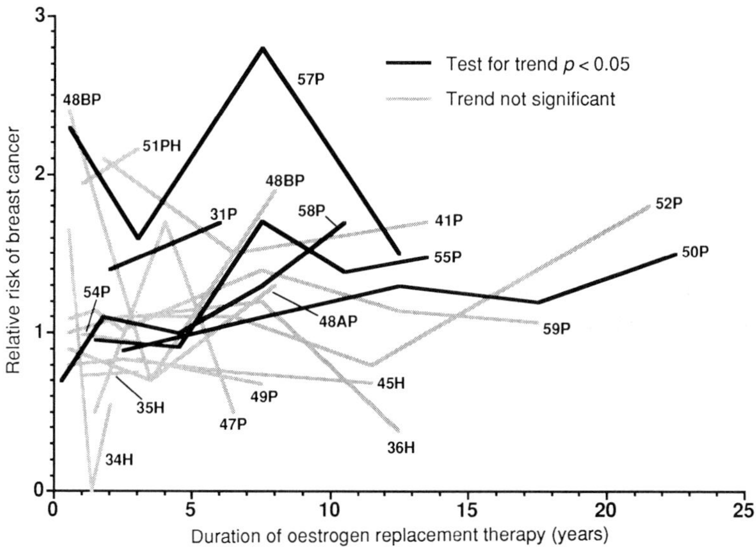

Figure 4 The effects of duration of oestrogen replacement therapy on breast cancer risk that have been reported in the literature. The number beside each duration–risk curve cites the reference from which it is obtained and the letters 'P' or 'H' indicate whether population- or hospital-based control groups were used, respectively. Studies that found a significant trend of increasing risk with increasing duration of oestrogen replacement therapy ($p < 0.05$) are indicated by black lines. Grey lines are used for all other studies. The results that have been published to date have been highly variable, with most studies having few patients who were followed for more than 15 years. Of the three studies with long-term follow-up[50,52,59] only Brinton *et al.*[50] have found a consistent and statistically significant trend of increasing risk with increasing duration of therapy. See text for additional explanation of this figure

and co-workers[59] and Wingo and co-workers[52]. It is thus difficult to draw any confident conclusions from the literature on the relationship between duration of oestrogen replacement therapy and breast cancer risk. It is interesting to note, however, that two of the studies which found a significant trend were done in Europe[55,58]. Oestradiol compounds are far more commonly used in Europe than in North America, and Bergkvist and colleagues[58] found a pronounced duration–risk relationship among women treated with these compounds that was not observed among women taking conjugated oestrogens. It is thus possible that the effect of duration of oestrogen replacement therapy on breast cancer risk may depend on the type of therapy used, with drugs that are similar or identical to human oestrogens being associated with a greater risk than those of equine origin. This would also be consistent with the evidence that breast cancer risk is elevated in women with longer than average exposure to endogenous oestrogens[63].

Another important point illustrated by Figure 4 is that the majority of studies that have looked at the effect of duration of oestrogen replacement therapy have only followed women for less than 10 years. There are only three studies that have observed substantial numbers of patients who have been treated for more than 15 years[50,52,59]. Of these, only Brinton and colleagues[50] have found a consistent and statistically significant trend of risk increasing with duration of therapy. Steinberg and co-workers[64] have recently published an overview on this topic that found a 30% increase in breast cancer risk at 15 years. They did this by fitting simple exponential models to the results from each study, and then taking a weighted average of the slope parameter estimates from these models to produce a single slope parameter estimate based on all studies. This had the effect of extrapolating duration–risk information from studies with limited duration times to estimate the effects of lengthy oestrogen replacement therapy. Their approach makes these estimates highly dependent on the validity of their simple exponential model. Looking at Figure 4, it is far from clear that such a model applies consistently across all studies.

Detection bias in observational studies of breast disease

The question of whether oestrogen replacement therapy increases breast cancer risk can only be addressed through observational studies. Such studies are most convincing in demonstrating major risk factors such as smoking for lung cancer. Determining the safety of oestrogen replacement therapy, on the other hand, requires that we are able to demonstrate risks of small magnitude – a task that is difficult to achieve with any observational approach. A description of the pitfalls of these studies can be found in any epidemiology text. We would like, however, to discuss briefly just one of these problems, that of detection bias. A particularly graphic illustration of this bias is given in Figure 5. Late in 1974, the wives of both the President and Vice President of the USA developed breast cancer. These two cases were given great publicity in this country and caused a great deal of concern among American women. As a result, either through increased physician, mammographic or self-examination, the incidence of breast cancer shot up 17% that year and then subsided to near previous levels (Figure 5). This suggests that many women have breast cancers that may be detected due to enhanced concern about this disease. It is not unreasonable to postulate that the decision to take oestrogen replacement therapy may provide such concern. For example, Colditz and colleagues[59] found a 36% increase in breast cancer risk among current oestrogen replacement therapy users but no increase in risk among former users. They found no evidence of a duration–risk relationship among current users. They hypothesize that this is because oestrogen replacement therapy acts to promote existing occult cancers but does not enhance the development of new ones. They also argue that their results are unlikely to be due to detection bias. It must be noted, however, that members of their nursing cohort who took oestrogen replacement therapy had a 31% increase in mammographic screening, and that it is not unreasonable to suppose that nurses may have a heightened concern about the risks of breast cancer associated with oestrogen replacement therapy. Colditz and colleagues[66] found a 36% increase in age-adjusted breast cancer incidence in patients who took oestrogen replacement therapy –

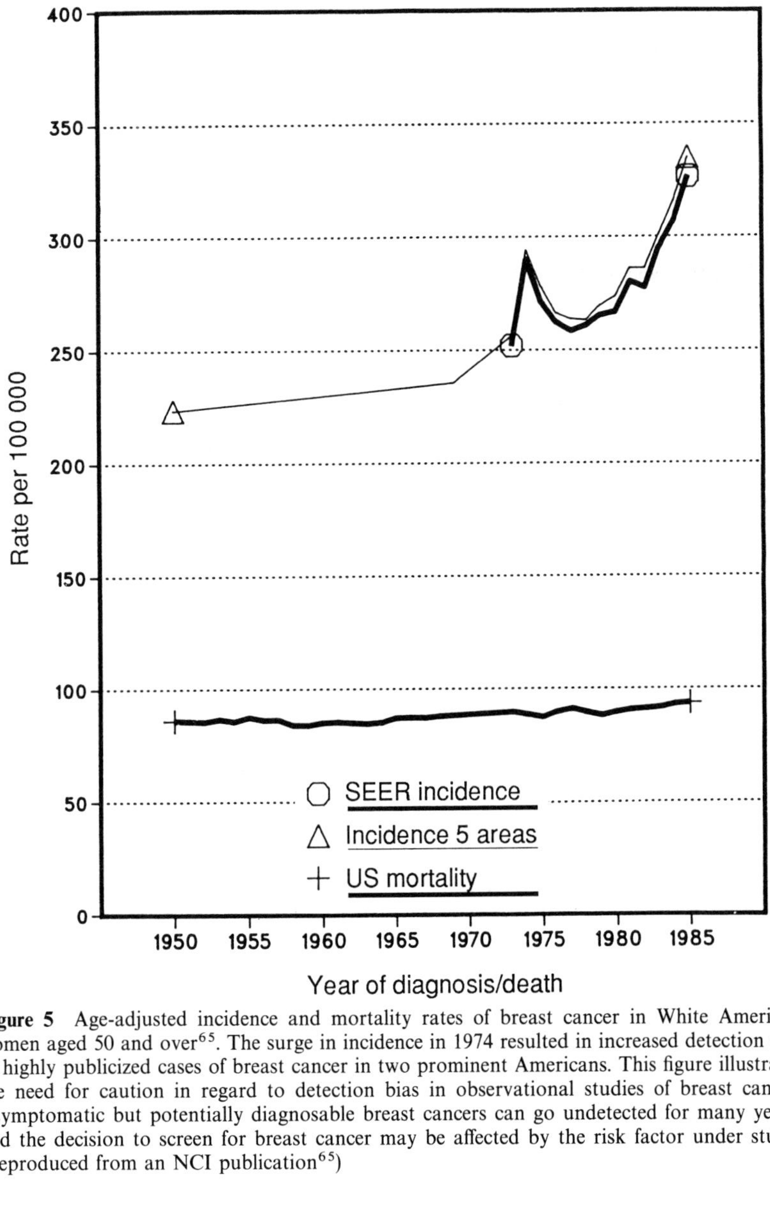

Figure 5 Age-adjusted incidence and mortality rates of breast cancer in White American women aged 50 and over[65]. The surge in incidence in 1974 resulted in increased detection due to highly publicized cases of breast cancer in two prominent Americans. This figure illustrates the need for caution in regard to detection bias in observational studies of breast cancer. Asymptomatic but potentially diagnosable breast cancers can go undetected for many years, and the decision to screen for breast cancer may be affected by the risk factor under study. (Reproduced from an NCI publication[65])

about twice the increase associated with the publicity over the breast cancers of Mrs Ford and Rockefeller. It is surely possible, therefore, that at least some of the increase in breast cancer risk reported by Colditz and colleagues[59] may be due to detection bias.

CONCLUSIONS

(1) Oestrogen replacement therapy consisting of 0.625 mg/day of conjugated oestrogens may be given for a decade to healthy menopausal women without increasing breast cancer risk.

(2) There is conflicting or limited evidence regarding the risk of breast cancer associated with:

   (a) high-dose conjugated oestrogen therapy;

   (b) oestrogen replacement therapy with synthetic oestrogens; and

   (c) oestrogen replacement therapy for more than a decade.

(3) There is no definitive proof at this time that any form of oestrogen replacement therapy causes breast cancer.

In view of the high proportion of postmenopausal women in our society, and the likelihood that ever larger numbers of these women will seek the benefits of oestrogen replacement therapy, it is imperative that more data on this topic be gathered. Of particular importance is the determination of the risks of long-term combination therapy with oestrogens and progestins. While it is to be hoped that the benefits of such therapy may be achieved at little or no risk of breast cancer, determining these risks with reasonable precision must be one of the higher priorities of epidemiology in the years to come.

ACKNOWLEDGEMENTS

We thank Walton D. Plummer, Jr for generating the computer graphics in this paper, Peggy A. Schuyler for editorial assistance, and Janelle Steele for assistance in preparing the manuscript. This work was supported in part by National Cancer Institute grants #RO1 CA50468 and #RO1 CA46492.

REFERENCES

1. Council on Scientific Affairs (1983). Estrogen replacement in the menopause. *J. Am. Med. Assoc.*, **249**, 359–61
2. Stampfer, M.J. and Colditz, G.A. (1991). Estrogen replacement therapy and coronary heart disease: a quantitative assessment of the epidemiologic evidence. *Prev. Med.*, **20**, 47–63
3. Stampfer, M.J., Colditz, G.A., Willett, W.C., Manson, J.E., Rosner, B., Speizer, F.E. and Hennekens, C.H. (1991). Postmenopausal estrogen therapy and cardiovascular disease: Ten-year follow-up from the Nurses' Health Study. *N. Engl. J. Med.*, **325**, 756–62
4. Persson, I., Adami, H.O., Bergkvist, L., Lindgren, A., Pettersson, B., Hoover, R. and Schairer, C. (1989). Risk of endometrial cancer after treatment with oestrogens alone or in conjunction with progestogens: results of a prospective study. *Br. Med. J.*, **298**, 147–51
5. Whitehead, M.I., Hillard, T.C. and Crook, D. (1990). The role and use of progestogens. *Obstet. Gynecol.*, **75**, 59S–76S
6. Dupont, W.D. and Page, D.L. (1991). Menopausal estrogen replacement therapy and breast cancer. *Arch. Intern. Med.*, **151**, 67–72

7. Feinglos, S.J.. (1985). *MEDLINE: A Basic Guide to Searching.* (Chicago: Medical Library Association)
8. Boston Collaborative Drug Surveillance Program (1974). Surgically confirmed gallbladder disease, venous thromboembolism, and breast tumors in relation to postmenopausal estrogen therapy. *N. Engl. J. Med.*, **290**, 15–19
9. Hammond, C.B., Jelovsek, F.R., Lee, K.L., Creasman, W.T. and Parker, R.T. (1979). Effects of long-term estrogen replacement therapy, II: neoplasia. *Am. J. Obstet. Gynecol.*, **133**, 537–47
10. Nachtigall, L.E., Nachtigall, R.H., Nachtigall, R.D. and Beckman, E.M. (1979). Estrogen replacement therapy, II: a prospective study in the relationship to carcinoma and cardiovascular and metabolic problems. *Obstet. Gynecol.*, **54**, 74–9
11. Wallach, S. and Henneman, P.H. (1959). Prolonged estrogen therapy in postmenopausal women. *J. Am. Med. Assoc.*, **171**, 1637–42
12. Wilson, R.A. (1962). The roles of estrogen and progesterone in breast and genital cancer. *J. Am. Med. Assoc.*, **182**, 327–31
13. Mustacchi, P. and Gordon, G.S. (1958). Frequency of cancer in estrogen-treated osteoporotic women. In Segaloff, A. (ed.) *Breast Cancer: The Second Biennial Louisiana Cancer Conference, New Orleans, Jan.* 22–23, 1958, pp. 163–9. (St Louis: C.V. Mosby Co.)
14. Burch, J.C. and Byrd, B.F., Jr (1971). Effects of long-term administration of estrogen on the occurrence of mammary cancer in women. *Ann. Surg.*, **174**, 414–18
15. Arthes, F.L., Sartwell, P.E. and Lewison, E.F. (1971). The pill, estrogens, and the breast. *Cancer*, **28**, 1391–4
16. Byrd, B.F., Jr, Burch, J.C. and Vaughn, W.K. (1973). Significance of postoperative estrogen therapy on the occurrence and clinical course of cancer. *Ann. Surg.*, **177**, 626–31
17. Henderson, B.E., Powell, D., Rosario, I., Keys, C., Hanisch, R., Young, M., Casagrande, J., Gerkins, V. and Pike, M.C. (1974). An epidemiological study of breast cancer. *J. Natl. Cancer Inst.*, **53**, 609–14
18. Burch, J.C., Byrd, B.F., Jr and Vaughn, W.K. (1974). The effects of long-term estrogen on hysterectomized women. *Am. J. Obstet. Gynecol.*, **118**, 778–82
19. Brinton, L.A., Williams, R.R., Hoover, R.N., Stegens, N.L., Feinelib, M. and Fraumeni, J.F., Jr (1979). Breast cancer risk factors among screening program participants. *J. Natl. Cancer Inst.*, **62**, 37–44
20. Bland, K.I., Buchanan, J.B., Weisberg, B.F., Hagan, T.A. and Gray, L.A., Sr (1980). The effects of exogenous estrogen replacement therapy of the breast: breast cancer risk and mammographic parenchymal patterns. *Cancer*, **45**, 3027–33
21. Gambrell, R.D., Massey, F.M., Castaneda, T.A. and Boddie, A.W. (1980). Estrogen therapy and breast cancer in postmenopausal women. *J. Am. Geriatr. Soc.*, **28**, 251–7
22. Brinton, L.A., Hoover, R.N., Szklo, M. and Fraumeni, J.F., Jr (1981). Menopausal estrogen use and risk of breast cancer. *Cancer*, **47**, 2517–22
23. Lawson, D.H., Jick, H., Hunter, J.R. and Madsen, S. (1981). Exogenous estrogens and breast cancer. *Am. J. Epidemiol.*, **114**, 710–13
24. Gambrell, R.D. (1982). Role of hormones in the etiology and prevention of endometrial and breast cancer. *Acta Obstet. Gynecol. Scand.*, **106**, (Suppl.), 37–46
25. Gambrell, R.D., Jr. (1984). Hormones in the etiology and prevention of breast and endometrial cancer. *South. Med. J.*, **77**, 1509–15
26. Nomura, A.M., Hirohata, T., Kolonel, L.N., Hankin, J.H., Lee, J. and Stemmermann, G. (1985). Breast cancer in Caucasian and Japanese women in Hawaii. *Natl. Cancer Inst. Monogr.*, **69**, 191–6
27. Buring, J.E., Hennekens, C.H., Lipnick, R.J., Willett, W., Stampfer, M.J., Rosner, B., Peto, R. and Speizer, F.E. (1987). A prospective cohort study of postmenopausal hormone use and risk of breast cancer in US women. *Am. J. Epidemiol.*, **125**, 939–47
28. Craig, T.J., Comstock, G.W. and Geiser, P.B. (1974). Epidemiologic comparison of breast cancer patients with early and late onset of malignancy and general population controls. *J. Natl. Cancer Inst.*, **53**, 1577–81
29. Sartwell, P.E., Arthes, F.G. and Tonascia, J.A. (1977). Exogenous hormones, reproductive history, and breast cancer. *J. Natl. Cancer Inst.*, **59**, 1589–92
30. Mack, T.M., Henderson, B.E., Gerkins, V.R., Arthur, M., Baptista, J. and Pike, M.C. (1975). Reserpine and breast cancer in a retirement community. *N. Engl. J. Med.*, **292**, 1366–71
31. Hoover, R., Gray, L.A., Sr, Cole, P. and MacMahon, B. (1976). Menopausal estrogens and

breast cancer. *N. Engl. J. Med.*, **295**, 401–5

32. Casagrande, J., Gerkins, V., Henderson, B.E., Mack, T. and Pike, M.C. (1976). Brief communication: exogenous estrogens and breast cancer in women with natural menopause. *J. Natl. Cancer Inst.*, **56**, 839–41
33. Byrd, B.F., Jr, Burch, J.C. and Vaughn, W.K. (1977). The impact of long-term estrogen support after hysterectomy. *Ann. Surg.*, **185**, 574–9
34. Wynder, E.L., MacCornack, F.A. and Stellman, S.D. (1978). The epidemiology of breast cancer in 785 United States Caucasian women. *Cancer*, **41**, 2341–54
35. Ravnihar, B., Seigel, D.G. and Lindtner, J. (1979). An epidemiologic study of breast cancer and benign breast neoplasias in relation to the oral contraceptive and estrogen use. *Eur. J. Cancer Clin. Oncol.*, **15**, 395–405
36. Jick, H., Walker, A.M., Watkins, R.N., D'Ewart, D.C., Hunter, J.R., Danford, A., Masden, S., Dinan, B.J. and Rothman, K.J. (1980). Replacement estrogens and breast cancer. *Am. J. Epidemiol.*, **112**, 586–94
37. Ross, R.K., Paganini-Hill, A., Gerkins, V.R., Mack, T.M., Pfeffer, R., Arthur, M. and Henderson, B.E. (1980). A case–control study of menopausal estrogen therapy and breast cancer. *J. Am. Med. Assoc.*, **243**, 1635–9
38. Hoover, R., Glass, A., Finkle, W.D., Azevedo, D. and Milne, K. (1981). Conjugated estrogens and breast cancer risk in women. *J. Natl. Cancer Inst.*, **67**, 815–20
39. Kelsey, J.L., Fischer, D.B., Holford, T.R., LiVolsi, V.A., Mostow, E.D., Goldenberg, I.S. and White, C. (1981). Exogenous estrogens and other factors in the epidemiology of breast cancer. *J. Natl. Cancer Inst.*, **67**, 327–33
40. Thomas, D.B., Persing, J.P. and Hutchinson, W.B. (1982). Exogenous estrogens and other risk factors for breast cancer in women with benign breast disease. *J. Natl. Cancer Inst.*, **69**, 1017–25
41. Hulka, B.S., Chambless, L.E., Deubner, D.C. and Wilkinson, W.E. (1982). Breast cancer and estrogen replacement therapy. *Am. J. Obstet. Gynecol.*, **143**, 638–44
42. Vakil, D.V., Morgan, R.W. and Halliday, M. (1983). Exogenous estrogens and development of breast and endometrial cancer. *Cancer Detect. Prev.*, **6**, 415–24
43. Gambrell, R.D., Jr, Maier, R.C. and Sanders, B.I. (1983). Decreased incidence of breast cancer in postmenopausal estrogen–progestogen users. *Obstet. Gynecol.*, **62**, 435–43
44. Sherman, B., Wallace, R. and Bean, J. (1983). Estrogen use and breast cancer: interaction with body mass. *Cancer*, **51**, 1527–31
45. Kaufman, D.W., Miller, D.R., Rosenberg, L., Helmrich, S.P., Stolley, P., Schottenfeld, D. and Shapiro, S. (1984). Noncontraceptive estrogen use and the risk of breast cancer. *J. Am. Med. Assoc.*, **252**, 63–7
46. Horwitz, R.I. and Stewart, K.R. (1984). Effect of clinical features on the association of estrogens and breast cancer. *Am. J. Med.*, **76**, 192–8
47. Hiatt, R.A., Bawol, R., Friedman, G.D. and Hoover, R. (1984). Exogenous estrogen and breast cancer after bilateral oophorectomy. *Cancer*, **54**, 139–44
48. Nomura, A.M.Y., Kolonel, L.N., Hirohata, T. and Lee, J. (1986). The association of replacement estrogens with breast cancer. *Int. J. Cancer*, **37**, 49–53
49. McDonald, J.A., Weiss, N.S., Daling, J.R., Francis, A.M. and Polissar, L. (1986). Menopausal estrogen use and the risk of breast cancer. *Breast Cancer Res. Treat.*, **7**, 193–9
50. Brinton, L.A., Hoover, R. and Fraumeni, J.F., Jr (1986). Menopausal oestrogens and breast cancer risk: an expanded case–control study. *Br. J. Cancer*, **54**, 825–32
51. La Vecchia, C., DeCarli, A., Parazzini, F., Gentile, A., Liberati, C. and Franceschi, S. (1986). Non-contraceptive oestrogens and the risk of breast cancer in women. *Br. J. Cancer*, **38**, 853–8
52. Wingo, P.A., Layde, P.M., Lee, N.C., Rubin, G. and Ory, H.W. (1987). The risk of breast cancer in postmenopausal women who have used estrogen replacement therapy. *J. Am. Med. Assoc.*, **257**, 209–15
53. Hunt, K., Vessey, M., McPherson, K. and Coleman, M. (1987). Long-term surveillance of mortality and cancer incidence in women receiving hormone replacement therapy. *Br. J. Obstet. Gynecol.*, **94**, 620–35
54. Rohan, T.E. and McMichael, A.J. (1988). Non-contraceptive exogenous oestrogen therapy and breast cancer. *Med. J. Aust.*, **148**, 217–21
55. Ewertz, M. (1988). Influence of non-contraceptive exogenous and endogenous sex hormones

on breast cancer risk in Denmark. *Int. J. Cancer*, **42**, 832–8
56. Dupont, W.D., Page, D.L., Rogers, L.W. and Parl, F.F. (1989). Influence of exogenous estrogens, proliferative breast disease, and other variables on breast cancer risk. *Cancer*, **63**, 948–57
57. Mills, P.K., Beeson, W.L., Phillips, R.L. and Fraser, G.E. (1989). Prospective study of exogenous hormone use and breast cancer in Seventh-Day Adventists. *Cancer*, **64**, 591–7
58. Bergkvist, L., Adami, H.O., Persson, I., Hoover, R. and Schairer, C. (1989). The risk of breast cancer after estrogen and estrogen–progestin replacement. *N. Engl. J. Med.*, **321**, 293–7
59. Colditz, G.A., Stampfer, M.J., Willett, W.C., Hennekens, C.H., Rosner, B. and Speizer, F.E. (1990). Prospective study of estrogen replacement therapy and risk of breast cancer in postmenopausal women. *J. Am. Med. Assoc.*, **264**, 2648–53
60. Greenland, S. (1987). Quantitative methods in the review of epidemiologic literature. *Epidemiol. Rev.*, **9**, 1–30
61. Anderson, T.J., Ferguson, D.J.P. and Raab, G.M. (1982). Cell turnover in the 'resting' human breast: influence of parity, contraceptive pill, age and laterality. *Br. J. Cancer*, **46**, 376–82
62. Key, T.J.A. and Pike, M.C. (1988). The role of oestrogens and progestagens in the epidemiology and prevention of breast cancer. *Eur. J. Cancer Clin. Oncol.*, **24**, 29–43
63. Kelsey, J.L. and Gammon, M.D. (1990). Epidemiology of breast cancer. *Epidemiol. Rev.*, **12**, 228–40
64. Steinberg, K.K., Thacker, S.B., Smith, J., Stroup, D.F., Zack, M.M., Flanders, W.D. and Berkelman, R.L. (1991). A meta-analysis of the effect of estrogen replacement therapy on the risk of breast cancer. *J. Am. Med. Assoc.*, **265**, 1985–90
65. National Cancer Institute Division of Cancer Prevention and Control (1988). 1987 *Annual Cancer Statistics Review*: *Including Cancer Trends*: 1950–1985, pp. II.69–82. (Bethesda: National Cancer Institute, NIH Publication No. 88-2789)
66. Colditz, G.A., Stampfer, M.J., Willett, W.C., Speizer, F.E., Hennekens, C.H. and Rosner, B. (1991). Letter to Editor. *J. Am. Med. Assoc.*, **265**, 1825

8

Breast cancer incidence and mortality after oestrogen and oestrogen–progestin replacement

H.-O. Adami, I. Persson, J. Yuen, L. Bergkvist and R. Hoover

INTRODUCTION

A follow-up study of women using hormone replacement has been going on in Uppsala, Sweden, since 1977. The cohort was recruited by means of prescription recordings of non-contraceptive oestrogens in a defined population from 1977 to 1980. This paper summarizes results already published based mainly on breast cancer diagnosed to the end of 1983[1,2]. Because hormone replacement may influence both the incidence of breast cancer and the prognostic outlook in women with oestrogen-associated breast cancer, we argue that mortality rates from the disease might be an important complementary outcome measure. Finally we describe briefly, without providing any results, a number of updated analyses of this cohort that are now underway.

METHODS

The methods of this study have been described extensively in previous publications[1–3]. All women for whom replacement oestrogens had been prescribed were identified from all the pharmacies in the Uppsala Health Care Region, Sweden, with about 1.3 million inhabitants. Recruitment began in April, 1977 and ended in March, 1980. The final cohort, identified from examination of 77 147 prescription forms, comprised 23 244 women 35 years of age or older, who had received at least one prescription. Complete follow-up with regard to cancer incidence and deaths was achieved through record-linkage procedures (based on the individually unique national registration number), to the national death register and cancer register in Sweden.

From the total cohort, a subgroup was selected in order to characterize the women more fully with respect to exposure to oestrogens and progestins and risk factors for breast cancer. This was done with a random sample of 735 women who were sent a questionnaire in 1980, which was answered satisfactorily by 89%. The questionnaire requested detailed information on exposure to oestrogens before, during and after the period in which the prescriptions were studied; compliance with drug treatment; the concomitant cyclic use of progestins; and information on the presence of other risk factors for breast cancer. Based on information mainly from the questionnaire study of the subcohort, the entire cohort could be further characterized as shown in Table 1. In 1982 and 1984, additional questionnaires were sent to the women who had answered the initial one to ascertain their exposure to estrogens after 1980.

To the end of 1983, all 253 women in whom invasive breast cancer developed after their inclusion in the cohort received a questionnaire that was identical to the one sent to the women in the subcohort. Complete answers were received for 196 (77%) of the women with breast cancer. All 253 patients were followed up till the end of 1986 through record-linkage procedures with a nationwide tax register. Similarly, vital status could be ascertained for 6617 cases of breast cancer diagnosed during the same period of time in the same geographical area of Sweden and notified to the Cancer Registry[2].

Hormonal exposure was considered in several different ways as shown in Table 2. Additional analyses were carried out to study latency and recency of use as possible determinants of breast cancer incidence, but because of the collinearity between these characteristics and duration of use, the former measures could not be assessed adequately.

The design of most of the incidence analyses of relative risk followed the case–cohort approach[1]. From the questionnaires, detailed data on hormone exposure were known for the women with breast cancer in the cohort and for all women in the subcohort. The number of person-years according to age and exposure strata in the subcohort were extrapolated to the total

Table 1 Features of the Uppsala prospective study of hormone replacement therapy

Characteristic	
Period of accrual	April, 1977–March, 1980
Number of oestrogen replacement prescription forms	77 147
Number of women in total cohort	23 244
Mean age at entry (years)	53.7
Average individual follow-up, to end of 1983 (years)	5.7
Menopausal status*	
premenopausal	6%
natural menopause	75%
surgical menopause	19%
Average height (cm)*	163.7
Average weight (kg)*	66.5
Compliance*	91%
Ongoing treatment at entry*	50%
Compounds prescribed*	
oestradiol	56%
conjugated oestrogens	22%
oestriol and other	22%
Combined oestrogen–progestin (7–10 days/cycle)*	31%

*Estimated from a questionnaire study to a 1/30 random sample, answered by 89% (653/735)

Table 2 The Uppsala prospective study of hormone replacement: classification of hormone replacement therapy

Class	*Characteristics*
1	Without regard to oestrogen compound or cyclically added progestin
2	With regard to progestins never always $\leq$ 5 years of oestrogen alone followed by combined > 5 years of oestrogen alone followed by combined any other pattern
3	With regard to types of oestrogens* oestradiol conjugated oestrogens other, mainly oestriol

*With and without regard to use of other types or of concomitant progestins

cohort. The relative risk was calculated as the ratio of the number of observed to expected cases.

In addition, a matched case–control analysis within the cohort was also performed. Although it did not permit a comparison with women who had not used hormones, this method allowed an evaluation of dose–response relations after control for a variety of potentially confounding variables[1].

Different statistical methods were used for survival analyses. Firstly, we computed relative survival rates to adjust for mortality attributable to the competing risks of deaths, without use of information on causes of death of individual patients. Secondly, we used the Cox's proportional hazard model to adjust for age and a number of other potentially confounding variables as described previously in detail[2].

RESULTS

Breast cancer incidence

Detailed tabulations of results based on follow-up to the end of 1983 have been published previously[1]. Overall, the relative risk of breast cancer among women in the oestrogen cohort compared with other women in the same region was 1.1 (95% confidence interval 1.0–1.3). In case–cohort analyses, the relative risk was close to unity in women who had used oestrogen replacement for 6 years or less, whereas it was significantly increased by about 70% (relative risk = 1.7; 1.1–2.7) in those who had used oestrogens for more than 9 years. Women who had used combination therapy during only 6 years or less showed no evidence of excess risk, whereas the relative risk following more than 6 years of use was 4.4 (0.9–22.4) on the basis of data from 10 patients.

In the matched case–control study within the cohort, we adjusted for education, biopsy for benign breast disease and type of menopause. When non-compliant women and those who reported oestrogen use for 6 months or less were used as a reference category, a significant trend ($p = 0.02$) was found with increasing duration of oestrogen treatment; a relative risk of 2.3 (1.1–4.8) was found in those who had used oestrogen for more than 9 years.

Prognosis following breast cancer in oestrogen users

The relative survival rate was significantly higher ($p = 0.02$) by about 10 percentage points at 8 years in patients who had received oestrogen treatment. The more favourable course could be confirmed only in patients aged 50 years or more at diagnosis, although we had a low statistical capability for detecting any effect in younger women due to small numbers. The most favourable outlook was seen in patients who were current users of oestrogen with or without progestin at the time of diagnosis; there was some evidence of benefit among those who had stopped taking hormones within 1 year preceding diagnosis, whereas patients who had finished their replacement more than a year before diagnosis had a relative survival rate virtually identical to that in cases from the background population. These associations were further confirmed and quantified in Cox's proportional hazards analyses in which the relative hazard among current users (compared with never-users) was 0.54 (0.34–0.86), and among those with a recency of 1–12 months, was 0.61 (0.30–1.20). We found no convincing evidence that latency or duration of oestrogen use were associated with prognosis[2].

COMMENTS

The strength of our study is its population-based design, its size, the ascertainment of exposure through prescription recordings during a 3-year period and the completeness of follow-up. However, there are also limitations in these data, namely the lack of a non-exposed cohort; incomplete information on exposure, confounders and modifiers; and the possibility for recall bias in case–cohort and nested case–control analyses. Based on data from our own and other recently published studies[4] and from updated pooled analyses[5,6], it seems reasonable to conclude presently that any association between hormone replacement and breast cancer within 10–15 years after menopause is likely to be small or moderate and confined to long-term and/or to current[4] users of hormone replacement. There is no firm evidence that any increased risk of breast cancer can be prevented by cyclically added progestins[1,7] (also, Persson and colleagues, unpublished results), but available data from the literature are sparse. Likewise, little is known about possible associations between hormone replacement and breast cancer at higher ages (after long-term treatment or after cessation of treatment). It has been generally assumed that oestradiol and conjugated oestrogens should have similar biological effects at the cellular level, but there are hints in the literature that these effects may in fact differ[1,5].

Besides the need to study in more detail the different dimensions of oestrogen exposure (duration, compound, dose, latency, recency) – and the

Table 3 Ongoing analyses of the Uppsala prospective study of hormone replacement therapy

Mortality analyses with external and internal comparisons
Mortality analyses using external comparisons with 'adjusted' expected rates
Cohort analyses based on prescription data (1977–1980) alone for exposure classification and follow-up to the end of 1988
Case–cohort analyses (update of ref. 1)
Cohort analyses based on (extensive) questionnaire data in a subcohort of about 12 000 oestrogen users born 1918 or later, and prescribed oestradiol and/or conjugated oestrogens
Analyses of survival among breast cancer cases compared with survival among cases arising in the background population (update of ref. 2)

impact of added progestins – as determinants of breast cancer risk, there is also a need to confirm the observation that hormone replacement might improve the prognostic outlook among patients exposed to exogenous hormones[2,4]. If this is the case, mortality rate might be an important outcome measure besides incidence. However, methodological difficulties arise because hormone replacement is considered contraindicated in women who have had a breast cancer. Thus, in practice, women prescribed such treatment may represent a 'screened' group with an almost zero prevalence of breast cancer and with a mortality from this disease which arises mostly (or even exclusively) due to breast cancers diagnosed after start of treatment. In contrast, mortality rates in the background population are derived from cases diagnosed over a lengthy period of time, sometimes with deaths occurring decades after initial diagnosis. Therefore, population mortality rates cannot be readily applied to cohorts of women on hormone replacement, since this would lead to an overestimation of expected rates and thus an underestimation of the standardized mortality ratio. Two approaches are pursued presently in the Uppsala cohort study to circumvent this problem. Firstly, we have calculated mortality rates based on internal comparisons, and these show a higher mortality rate in women given potent oestrogens than in those prescribed oestriol alone (Persson and colleagues, unpublished results). A second alternative is to recalculate expected mortality rates by removing (from the numerator) breast cancer cases diagnosed before a certain period of time, in order to provide standardized mortality rates for breast cancer in oestrogen users which are unbiased, in comparison with population rates.

Besides the calculation of mortality rates, the Uppsala cohort study is presently undergoing a whole series of updated analyses that are listed in Table 3. The results of these analyses are to be submitted for publication before the end of 1992.

REFERENCES

1. Bergkvist, L., Adami, H.O., Persson, I., Hoover, R. and Schairer, C. (1989). The risk of breast cancer after estrogen and estrogen–progestin replacement. *N. Engl. J. Med.*, **321**, 293–7
2. Bergkvist, L., Adami, H.O., Persson, I., Bergström, R. and Krusemo, U.B. (1989). Prognosis after breast cancer diagnosis in women exposed to estrogen and estrogen–progestogen replacement therapy. *Am. J. Epidemiol.*, **130**, 221–8

3. Persson, I., Adami, H.O., Johansson, E., Lindberg, B., Manell, P. and Westerholm, B. (1983). A cohort study on estrogen treatment and risk of endometrial cancer: methods, performance and applicability. *Eur. J. Clin. Pharmacol.*, **25**, 625–32
4. Colditz, G.A., Stampfer, M.J., Willett, W.C., Hennekens, C.H., Rosner, B. and Speizer, F.E. (1990). Prospective study of estrogen replacement therapy and risk of breast cancer in postmenopausal women. *J. Am. Med. Assoc.*, **264**, 2648–53
5. Steinberg, K.K., Thacker, S.B., Smith, J., Stroup, D.F., Zack, M.M., Flanders, W.D. and Berkelman, R.L. (1991). A meta-analysis of the effect of estrogen replacement therapy on the risk of breast cancer. *J. Am. Med. Assoc.*, **265**, 1985–90
6. Dupont, W.D. and Page, D.L. (1991). Menopausal estrogen replacement therapy and breast cancer. *Arch. Intern. Med.*, **151**, 67–72
7. Ewertz, M. (1988). Influence of non-contraceptive exogenous and endogenous sex hormones on breast cancer risk in Denmark. *Int. J. Cancer*, **42**, 832–8

General discussion II

(Chairman: Dr Barbara S. Hulka)

Prof. R.E. Mansel I wonder about the applicability of the population in Dr Brinton's study to the general population. Among the 64 000 women there were approximately 25 000 who had a biopsy or aspiration, 4000 with cancer, and 9000 with 'surgery recommended'. In the data from the Canadian study, the Nurses' Study and so on, the so-called 'normal' group had a much lower biopsy rate. Is this difference due just to changing trends, or will there be a problem in extrapolating Dr Brinton's data to the general population; that is, to the ordinary woman who is not solicited to go to the doctor by publicity?

Dr L.A. Brinton It has been a concern that this is a very specialized population, and I would be the last person to try to encourage the extrapolation of these results to a non-screened population. In our analyses we have attempted to focus on internal comparisons – that is, comparing users to non-users within the study population using controls derived from the same population. We would never attempt to compare this special population to an outside standard, because that could easily give erroneous results. We, however, have found associations for all the standard breast cancer risk factors that are almost identical to those of other studies. This lends some credence to the results, even though the study is in a very special cohort.

In terms of the biopsy rates, we need to be cautious about how we interpret our so-called 'normal' cohort. We will focus not only on the normal cohort but also on the women who have had recommendations for biopsy, and we will obviously need to consider carefully the detection issues when the effects of hormone usage are evaluated.

Prof. Mansel Secondly, and about the finding of increased *in situ* cancer early on, the Oxford group is doing some mathematical modelling of possible effects of the oral contraceptive on breast cancer rates. Would those findings not fit that very well? In other words, would we not expect to see, early on, a change in the *in situ* cancer rate which will later translate into increased invasive cancer?

Dr Brinton Unfortunately, I think we have to wait for time to pass before knowing the answer. It is certainly feasible, but it is too early to sort out what might be driving that association.

Dr D.W. Kaufman There remains concern about the Breast Cancer Detection

Demonstration Project (BCDDP) because although it was a screening programme, participation was voluntary. The possibility remains that women who were oestrogen users and had symptoms might preferentially be inclined to participate. The fact that the highest risk was found for low-stage cancer among oestrogen users is perhaps evidence of this kind of selection bias.

Dr Brinton The only way in which that issue can be sorted out is to have other investigators examine their data to see whether they find a similar association. I am not aware of other data currently available which would allow us to do that.

Prof. S. Shapiro I think that *in situ* cancer will present a problem which may well be intractable and beyond epidemiological skills. If it is the case that a woman with an itchy nipple or bleeding from the nipple is now going to present for biopsy, and if she tends selectively to present when taking oestrogens, perhaps because she is consulting her doctor for that reason, I cannot see any way in which a non-experimental study can be designed which will resolve whether this is a selection bias or cause and effect.

Dr R.D. Gambrell In the publication by Dr Colditz in 1990 reporting the 10-year study, there was a difference in alcohol consumption which was not mentioned today. Has that been looked at?

Dr G. Colditz It has not been looked at in this analysis because with only another 300 cases it was felt that we did not yet have the data to test the interaction that had been seen before. We are waiting for the next cycle of data in order to test that hypothesis in the independent data set from 1986–90.

Prof. N.S. Weiss Particular attention was paid in your analysis to current usage of oestrogens. One of the problems I suspect that we will have in reviewing this subject is that each of us tends to focus on the issue that interests us most. Dr Brinton emphasized long-term use; Dr Colditz has talked about current use. Perhaps Dr Colditz could also address two issues that relate to the total data: first, the effect of duration of use in the entire group of oestrogen users, whether current or not; second, the influence of progestogens, again whether or not they are being used currently. Have those analyses been done?

Dr Colditz We have not broken out past use of progestins. In respect of duration, I have the results for current and past use separately. For past use, 10 or more years of use, the relative risk is running at about 0.85, so clearly there is no increase in risk with long-term past use.

If the two are added together, the relative risk comes close to 1.1, but in fact because we are interested in the physiological effect of replacement on circulating levels of the hormones at the time, we have tried to separate out the past and current use, rather than mixing the two together at this stage. [*Prof. Weiss* Why is that important?]

I suppose I look at this from the point of view that replacement oestrogens raise the oestradiol levels almost back to premenopausal levels, so in some sense the maximum effect I would expect would be to shift women back into the premenopausal rates. I look at it as an acute effect rather than as a carcinogen, looking at oestrogen much more as a promoter.

Prof. Shapiro I think the data from your study are more compatible with detection bias than any other explanation. First, you said that according to the size of the tumour the risk remained the same. If I remember rightly, the size of the tumour selected was 1 cm diameter. Tumours far larger than that can escape detection unless women are selectively examining their breasts between examinations. You mentioned that mammography could not explain the finding, but there was information from mammography for only 2 years of the study. Also, no distinction was made between mammograms for screening and mammograms used to confirm the diagnosis when a lump was already present in the breast and the gynaecologist had made the diagnosis.

In addition, for use that had discontinued for as little as 1 year prior to diagnosis there was no longer an elevated risk... [*Dr Colditz* I did not say that] It is in your paper. [*Dr Colditz* No] When the evolution of breast lumps is taken into account – the period of time over which they evolve and when they are likely to be felt – even under a promotional hypothesis it is not plausible that use discontinued as little as one year previously could be associated with a non-significant elevation in the risk.

The question is whether epidemiological methods are capable of distinguishing between bias and confounding and causation for relative risks of the order of 1.33. (Incidentally, that is down from your previous estimate of 1.34.) With the inexact methods that we are obliged to use, I do not see how it is ever possible to make the distinction.

One further point in favour of the likelihood that your data are biased is that exactly the same association was found for current oral contraceptive use, and not for past use.

Until there is secure evidence that selection does not account for your findings, I suggest that it is risky to propose a promotional hypothesis.

Dr Colditz Women who had stopped taking oestrogens within 12 months prior to the follow-up interval had a relative risk of 1.16, but it is coming down.

I do not understand the comment about oral contraceptives, because we see a relative risk of 1.53 for current oral contraceptive use, where the tumours are more aggressive and more advanced at diagnosis – neither of which would be expected if there was merely detection bias for current use of oral contraceptives. I agree that detection is a major concern here. We routinely spend an enormous amount of time trying to make use of what data we have.

One problem you mention is mammography. I have spent a lot of time trying to work out how to tease out the screening versus the confirmatory mammograms. We now include on the questionnaire: 'mammogram for screening?' and 'mammogram for symptoms?', and also ask the women how their breast cancer was diagnosed. Neither of these solves the problem because a woman might detect a lump and go for a mammogram, so it is her self-examination which in large part has detected the tumour, but she takes the mammogram as the diagnostic test and says the cancer was diagnosed by mammogram.

We have a major problem, which is why at this stage I would lean more heavily on an analysis that looks at mortality – that takes into account the other causes of mortality in which we are interested in relation to oestrogens. However, the down side of this is that no importance is placed on the psychological effects of carrying a diagnosis of breast cancer. There is a problem in framing the risk–benefit analysis solely on mortality if it is not possible to take into account the quality of life issues that may go with having a heart attack versus being diagnosed with breast cancer. There are trade-offs. These are our incident data, and I think within 2 years we will be able to address more completely the total mortality.

Dr C. La Vecchia The possibility of detection bias is certainly a major problem. I think that Professor Adami published a very large series a few years ago showing that breast cancer survival was substantially higher around the age of the menopause and declined thereafter. The logical explanation is that female hormones have some promotional effect during the menopause. I would not, therefore, dismiss a promotional hypothesis in respect of Dr Colditz's data.

Mr I. Burn The observation about mortality was very interesting. We heard earlier that breast cancers are a relatively low cause of death, certainly in the USA, as compared with cardiac causes. I would expect, to date at any rate, that deaths from breast cancer are probably fairly low in your series, but are there any absolute figures on relative death rates from breast cancers in the groups that did and did not take hormone replacement therapy, as compared with other causes of death? It is understandable that there is some protective effect from the cardiac point of view.

Dr Colditz From a trade-off point of view, at the moment at least, there are about equal numbers of deaths from heart disease and breast cancer in the postmenopausal population. At this stage, all the analyses have not been done to be able to lay out the causes of death in the population of postmenopausal women.

Dr P.G. Wardle What number of cases was lost to follow-up – not from the survival group but from the total population?

Dr Colditz When women do not respond to a follow-up questionnaire the computer tape is sent to the National Center for Health Statistics with name, date of birth, etc. Three days later, we get back (by express mail) a tape with a cascade of levels of matching that we then work through to try to identify potential participants who were in the study and are deceased. More than two-thirds of the deaths are notified to us by the Post Office and the next of kin, but we need to search for the remaining non-responders. A test of the sensitivity of that computer base estimated that it was over 96% sensitive. The non-fatal complete follow-up time for this 12-year analysis is running around 95%. All the non-fatal cases lost to follow-up in this 12-year period have been searched, most of them multiple times, if they have not answered a couple of cycles. There could be a few cancers that have been missed, but it will be only about five. It is probably also worth mentioning that our incidence is within two or three cases of the expected number of breast cancers, based on tumour registry rates for White women.

Dr Wardle How many of the original 121 700 have been lost to follow-up?

Dr Colditz It depends upon what level of loss you mean. There are about 5000 women who now refuse to participate in the study, which does not stop us searching for their cause of death, for example. While they are not updating their exposure information, we can still look at their past exposure and keep them under surveillance for mortality. In 1988 we had an 88% response, so about 12 000 women did not answer the 1988 follow-up questionnaire. They are not all postmenopausal but are distributed across all ages.

Prof. Mansel I was interested in listening to Dr Dupont in the idea that benign breast disease could be so easily labelled. I know it is being taken from an overview, but as the co-author of a bench-mark series of papers, I think it perhaps needs to be dissected slightly more. I presume you mean by ‘benign breast disease’ a woman who tells you she has had a benign biopsy. This makes no conclusion about the relationship of hyperplasia with atypia or with family history.

Prof. W.D. Dupont That is correct. My justification is based on our own study in which a very careful histological analysis was made of the original slides showing benign lesions. We found that breast cancer risk is associated with the type of benign breast disease and, in particular, that women with atypical hyperplasia have about a fourfold increase in breast cancer risk. However, when we looked at the effect of oestrogen replacement therapy (ERT) adjusted for the type of benign breast disease, we failed to find an elevation in breast cancer risk – that is, women with atypical hyperplasia had about the same risk of breast cancer whether or not they took ERT. In this particular case, I feel it is not unreasonable to talk about benign breast disease as an entity with respect to ERT, although it is correct to say that it is in no sense a single disease.

Mr Burn I have always understood that by undertaking meta-analyses we allow ourselves the luxury of coming to a decision. Prof. Dupont has certainly come to a decision, but I question whether it is the right one. If the relative risk is 1.1 as distinct from 1 and we have a million women with breast cancer, why does your conclusion show that there is no increased risk?

Prof. Dupont The problem is, of course, the difference between statistical significance and clinical significance or clinical relevance. From the point of view of the individual patient, it is far from clear that a risk of that magnitude, an increase in relative risk of, say, 10%, is large enough to be of sufficient concern to modify either her behaviour or the way she is treated by her physician. If there are enough observations on enough patients it can certainly be shown that there is a statistically significant difference between groups of patients defined by virtually any risk factor. It is important to bear in mind what is considered to be the minimal clinically meaningful elevation in cancer risk – a question which only the clinicians can address.

In a very real sense, this null hypothesis of relative risk of 1, against which we calculate p values, is a straw man. The only reason for having this null hypothesis is because statisticians are not clever enough to come up with simple computational methods of dealing with more relevant measures of meaningful variation in risk.

Dr La Vecchia With regard to the exponential curve, I would suggest that there is no increased risk with short-term use, but there might be some modest increase with longer-term use. I wonder whether this might open some discussion on a possible interaction with age? Women who use oestrogens for 5 years or less tend to use them at the age of, say, 50, whereas women who use replacement treatment for 15 years or so are using them up to age 60. Could an interaction with age suggest an explanation for this unusual finding in epidemiology?

Prof. Dupont Interaction between age and dose or between age and actually taking any form of therapy? [*Dr La Vecchia* Between age at use and duration of use] That is certainly a possibility. Of course, these results are obviously age-adjusted, but even so...

Dr La Vecchia It is not a problem of age adjustment, but an innate problem because women who use oestrogens for a longer period tend to use them until an older age.

Prof. Dupont It is well known that the age of menopause is a risk factor for breast cancer, with women who have a late age of menopause being at increased risk. There may well be a confounding between the effects of duration of treatment and of age at which treatment starts. The problem of elucidating this is exceedingly complicated. We are probably pushing the data further than we should in trying to extrapolate what is going on with respect to the duration effect. To try to look at duration by age of onset will be a formidable problem.

Prof. R.K. Ross I liked the Steinberg paper[1]; they rated my study the second highest quality next to their own, so it must have been a really good analysis! They came to a slightly different conclusion, in fact. You are critical of those authors for taking a lot of studies that had little data in the 10–15-year interval to make inferences about the risk of long-term usage. Had they not done this, would their estimates of long-term risk have been much different from those they reported?

Prof. Dupont My guess is that the curves would probably not have been too dissimilar, but that the confidence intervals would have been considerably wider. It turns out, perhaps through good luck as much as good judgement, that their exponential curves are not wildly divergent from the studies of Colditz, Wingo or Brinton. However, the confidence intervals placed on those curves are certainly affected to a large degree by the many earlier studies – the studies with limited duration – which, in my opinion, is inappropriate.

Prof. Shapiro The question has been raised about a relative risk of 1.1. For a disease as common as breast cancer, it is correct to say that a 10% increase in risk would pose a public health problem. I think this gets to the heart of this meeting; we simply lack the skills or the competence to decide whether or not an elevation of 1.1 is causal. It may be an awkward situation in which to be, but it is one that has to be faced.

Prof. Dupont That is certainly the case. Admittedly, from the point of view of a government trying to allocate scarce dollars, a 10% increase in risk in an ideal world might well be highly significant. Of course, if we were talking about risk factors such as smoking and lung cancer or heart disease, which are vastly greater risks – or for that matter, protective effects of ERT on the heart, which are vastly smaller – there is perhaps a 50% reduction in risk of cardiovascular disease, then there would be no question of the importance of their risks; however, I cannot get very excited about two relative risks of such small magnitude.

Let us suppose that we are able, somehow, to prove that this relative risk of 1.1 is real; to go to the next step of asking whether this is causal is a profoundly difficult question. I do not expect to live to see the day when epidemiologists can solve this question. Hopefully, the basic scientists will eventually understand the real aetiology of breast cancer, at which time they may be able to say whether or not a relative risk of 10% is causal.

Dr R.D. Mann We should not forget that with HRT the benefit–risk ratio for long-term use relates to *prophylaxis*, not therapy. HRT is not being given to treat disease, in a situation in which the patients endure either the discomfort of the disease or of the drug; long term HRT is used as a form of preventive medicine, so we have to be rigorous in evaluating the significance of any possible increase of breast cancer risk. We need to be deeply concerned if any woman suffers cancer of the breast who would not otherwise have had this disease, or if it is promoted in women in whom it would not have become manifest.

Dr B.S. Hulka Dr Adami's *American Journal of Epidemiology* article[2] would suggest that survival has been better in oestrogen-using women than in non-users. When you correct this problem of prescribing and non-prescribing for women who already have cancer, do I understand that there is actually a somewhat higher overall mortality from breast cancer amongst oestrogen users?

Prof. H.-O. Adami Yes – and that difference may be higher than would be assumed since, in terms of mortality, we are seeing the sort of net effect of incidence and prognosis.

Dr Hulka I believe this is different information than we have had previously and have gathered from the published literature.

REFERENCES

1. Steinberg, K.K., Thacker, S.B., Smith, S.T., Stroup, D.F., Zack, M.M., Flanders, W.D. and Berkelman, R.L. (1991). A meta-analysis of the effect of estrogen replacement therapy on the risk of breast cancer. *J. Am. Med. Assoc.*, **265**, 1985–90
2. Bergkvist, L., Adami, H.-O., Persson, I., Bergström, R. and Krusemo, U.B. (1989). Prognosis after breast cancer diagnosis in women exposed to estrogen and estrogen–progestogen replacement therapy. *Am. J. Epidemiol.*, **130**, 221–8

9

Oestrogen replacement treatment and breast cancer: update of an Italian case–control study

C. La Vecchia

INTRODUCTION

The biological rationale for a possible association between postmenopausal hormonal therapy and breast carcinogenesis is based on a series of indirect pieces of evidence: the age curves in breast cancer incidence and mortality show a flattening of the slope after the menopause, following the decline of the levels of sexual steroids[1,2], and postmenopausal obese women (who have elevated levels and availability of endogenous oestrogens) have an elevated risk of breast cancer[3]. There are receptors for oestrogens and progestins in the breast tissue (and a proportion of breast tumours), and cellular mitoses and turnover are influenced by the levels of sexual hormones throughout various phases of the menstrual cycle[4]. Further, serum and urine oestrogen levels in various populations are a correlate of breast cancer risk[5].

There is, however, biological evidence that the link between oestrogens and breast cancer is complex, and it is not possible to postulate a simple association between excess oestrogen and elevated breast cancer risk. In particular, there is no convincing epidemiological support for the 'oestrogen window' hypothesis[6] for perimenarchal and perimenopausal periods. This attempted to explain the association between early menarche or late menopause and breast cancer in terms of excess oestrogen levels, unopposed by progestins. Early menarche, however, implies early and more regular menstrual cycles, and late menopause causes prolonged ovulation[7–9]. Further, there is no defined relationship between menstrual irregularities and breast cancer, and one study suggested that women with frequent irregular menstrual cycles are at a lower risk of breast cancer[10].

Over the last 15 years, more than two dozen epidemiological studies of menopausal replacement treatment and breast cancer have been published[11–35]. Although the overall incidence does not consistently indicate any association between ever-use of oestrogen replacement treatment and subsequent breast cancer risk, several uncertainties persist. In particular, all studies (except four conducted in the 1970s[13,14,20,22]) found elevated relative risks among long-term users.

Thus, available epidemiological evidence for oestrogen replacement treatment allows the exclusion of appreciable increases in risk in the short- to medium-term after stopping short-term use (up to 5 years), while the relative risk appears elevated by 30–70% for long-term use.

A first report of the case–control study conducted in Northern Italy[36], based on 1108 cases and 1281 controls collected between 1983 and 1985, showed an association apparently (though not significantly) higher than in most other studies, with a relative risk of 1.8 for ever-use and of 2.0 for long-term use. In this article, we have reconsidered the relationship between oestrogen replacement treatment and breast cancer from an update of the same study to the end of 1990, for a total of 3037 cases and 2569 controls.

SUBJECTS AND METHODS

The data were derived from a case–control study of breast cancer conducted since January 1983 in the Greater Milan area, Northern Italy, the general design of which has previously been described[36].

The cases included in the present analysis were 3037 women with histologically-confirmed breast cancer admitted to the National Cancer Institute, to several university clinics (chiefly surgical) and to the Ospedale Maggiore, which includes the four largest teaching and general hospitals in Milan. The age range was 23–74, and median age was 53 years.

The control group consisted of 2569 women admitted with a wide spectrum of acute conditions to several specialized university clinics and the Ospedale Maggiore of Milan. They had diseases which were not malignant, gynaecological or hormone-related, and which had been diagnosed within the year prior to the interview. Of these, 29% were admitted for traumatic conditions (mostly fractures and sprains), 26% had non-traumatic orthopaedic disorders (mostly low back pain and disc disorders), 16% were admitted for acute surgical conditions (mostly abdominal, such as acute appendicitis or strangulated hernia), and 30% had other miscellaneous illnesses, such as ear, nose and throat and dental disorders. The age range of the comparison group was 21–74 (median age 54 years). The age distribution of cases and controls is given in Table 1. Less than 3% of the eligible women (cases or controls)

Table 1 Distribution of 3037 cases of breast cancer and 2569 controls according to age; Milan, Italy, 1983–90

	Breast cancer		*Controls*	
Age-group (years)	*Number*	(%)	*Number*	(%)
< 40	325	(10.7)	393	(15.3)
40–49	845	(27.8)	586	(22.8)
50–59	887	(29.2)	718	(27.9)
60–69	727	(23.9)	642	(25.0)
70–74	253	(8.3)	230	(9.0)

refused to be interviewed. Most subjects, 85% of the cases and 94% of the controls, resided in the same region, Lombardy.

A structured questionnaire was used to obtain information on major known and potential breast cancer risk factors and, specifically, lifetime history of use of selected drugs, including oral contraceptives, non-contraceptive oestrogens for menopausal replacement treatment, and female hormones for other indications. The time and duration of each episode of use were recorded, as well as the brand name, whenever available.

Standard methods of analysis for case–control studies (stratification and the Mantel–Haenszel procedure and unconditional multiple logistic regression[37]) were used to obtain relative risks and the corresponding 95% confidence intervals (CI) for breast cancer in relation to various measures of non-contraceptive oestrogen use. Included in the regression equations were terms for age, geographical area, marital status, education, history of benign breast disease, family history of breast cancer, nulliparity and age at first birth, age at menarche and at menopause, type of menopause, body mass index and oral contraceptive use.

RESULTS

Table 2 gives the distribution of breast cancer cases and the comparison group according to various measures of oestrogen replacement treatment. Ever-use was reported by 148 (4.9%) of cases and 90 (3.5%) controls, corresponding to an age-adjusted relative risk of 1.4 (95% CI, 1.1–1.8), and a multivariate relative risk of 1.3 (95% CI, 1.0–1.8).

The most commonly used preparations were conjugated oestrogens (43%), followed by synthetic oestrogens (14%) and combinations of oestrogens and progestins or other steroid hormones (12%). The type of formulation used was undefined for 31% of cases. There was no significant heterogeneity across different types of hormones, but the data were insufficient for meaningful inference on each type of preparation.

There was some evidence of a duration–risk relationship, since the multivariate relative risk was 1.2 for use lasting less than 3 years and 1.5 for longer use; the trend in risk with duration was of borderline significance ($\chi^2 = 3.87, p < 0.05$), but there was no consistent pattern across more detailed strata of duration, since the relative risk was already above unity (1.3) among the 77 cases and 46 controls who had used oestrogen for less than 12 months. Moreover, there was no consistent pattern of risk with reference to time elapsed since first use (relative risk = 1.3 for less than 10 years and 1.4 for 10 years or more), or since last use (relative risk = 1.4 for less than 10 years and 1.5 for 10 years or more).

Table 3 gives the risk estimates for ever- and long-term (≥ 3 years) oestrogen replacement treatment in strata of age and other selected covariates, including the best recognized correlates of breast cancer risk. Because of the smaller absolute numbers in various strata, the risk estimates were somewhat variable. However, most of the relative risks were above unity, and the variations observed were largely within the limits of random variation,

Table 2 Distribution of 3037 breast cancer cases and 2569 controls according to various measures of oestrogen replacement treatment use; Milan, Italy, 1983–90

	Breast cancer		*Controls*		*Relative risk estimates (95% confidence interval)*	
	Number	(%)	*Number*	(%)	*M–H**	*MLR*†
Ever-use						
no	2889	(95.1)	2479	(96.5)	1‡	1‡
yes	148	(4.9)	90	(3.5)	1.4 (1.1–1.8)	1.3 (1.0–1.8)
Duration of use (years)						
< 3	105	(3.5)	65	(2.5)	1.3 (1.0–1.8)	1.2 (0.9–1.7)
≥ 3	38	(1.3)	22	(0.9)	1.5 (0.9–2.5)	1.5 (09–2.6)
unknown	5	(0.2)	3	(0.1)	—	—
χ^2_1 (trend)					5.27†	3.87†
Time since first use (years)						
< 10	59	(1.9)	33	(1.3)	1.5 (1.0–2.3)	1.3 (0.8–2.0)
≥ 10	87	(2.9)	55	(2.1)	1.4 (1.0–2.0)	1.4 (1.0–2.0)
unknown	2	(0.1)	2	(0.1)	—	—
Time since last use (years)						
< 10	68	(2.2)	43	(1.7)	1.3 (0.9–1.5)	1.2 (0.8–1.8)
≥ 10	75	(2.5)	43	(1.7)	1.5 (1.1–2.3)	1.5 (1.0–2.3)
unknown	5	(0.2)	4	(0.2)	—	—

*Mantel–Haenszel estimates adjusted for age in decades; †$p < 0.05$, estimates from multiple logistic regression equations including terms for age, geographical area, marital status, education, benign breast disease, family history of breast cancer, nulliparity and age at first birth, age at menarche and at menopause, type of menopause, body mass index and oral contraceptive use; ‡Reference category

indicating no significant heterogeneity across strata of any of the variables considered. Nevertheless, the association was appreciably stronger in the first 3 years of data collection (previously reported elsewhere[36]) than in subjects interviewed between 1986 and 1990.

Table 4 gives the age-adjusted relative risks of breast cancer according to separate strata of duration and time since last use. Although the risk estimate was appreciably higher for long duration (10 or more years since last use), no consistent pattern of risk was observed across strata of the two time-factors.

DISCUSSION

The updated analysis of this case–control study confirms a moderate association between oestrogen replacement treatment and subsequent breast cancer risk. The overall relative risk of 1.3 was significantly above unity, but there was little evidence of a duration–risk relationship.

The risk estimate, moreover, was lower than the 1.8 observed during the first 3 years of the study, on a total of 1108 cases, and the relative risk in the subsequent cases was only 1.2. In the discussion of the first report, we observed that the relative risk of 1.8 was apparently (though not significantly) higher than that reported for several other studies, mostly conducted in

Table 3 Relative risk of breast cancer according to oestrogen replacement treatment use in strata of selected covariates, Milan, Italy, 1983–90

	*Relative risk estimates (and 95% confidence intervals)**	
Covariate	*Ever-use*	*Use ≥ 3 years*
Age (years)		
< 60	1.3 (0.9–1.8)	1.1 (0.6–2.2)
≥ 60	1.6 (1.1–2.4)	2.2 (0.9–5.0)
Parity		
0	1.2 (0.7–2.2)	1.3 (0.5–3.5)
1–2	1.0 (0.7–1.5)	1.3 (0.6–2.3)
≥ 3	4.5 (2.1–9.6)	7.0 (0.9–57.7)
Age at first birth (years)		
< 25	1.9 (1.2–3.1)	1.9 (0.8–4.8)
≥ 25	1.2 (0.8–1.9)	1.4 (0.6–3.5)
History of benign breast disease		
no	1.3 (1.0–1.8)	1.6 (0.9–2.9)
yes	1.8 (0.8–4.0)	0.7 (0.1–3.1)
Family history of breast cancer		
no	1.4 (1.0–1.8)	1.5 (0.9–2.7)
yes	1.5 (0.5–4.1)	0.9 (0.2–4.6)
Education (years)		
< 7	1.5 (1.1–2.3)	1.9 (0.9–4.0)
≥ 7	1.2 (0.8–1.7)	1.0 (0.5–2.2)
Body mass index (kg/m^2)		
< 25	1.1 (0.8–1.5)	1.3 (0.7–2.5)
≥ 25	2.1 (1.3–3.4)	1.8 (0.7–4.4)
Type of menopause		
natural	1.6 (1.1–2.2)	2.4 (1.1–5.3)
surgical or radiant	1.5 (0.9–2.6)	1.0 (0.5–2.3)
Age at menopause (years)		
< 50	1.6 (1.1–2.3)	1.6 (0.8–3.1)
≥ 50	1.6 (1.0–2.6)	1.8 (0.7–4.4)
Period of data collection		
1983–85	1.9 (1.3–2.7)	2.0 (1.0–4.0)
1986–90	1.0 (0.4–2.2)	1.2 (0.7–2.2)

*Mantel–Haenszel estimates adjusted for age, reference category: never-users

North America, whose main results are summarized in Table 5. The most likely interpretation was in terms of random variation, and this is confirmed by the flattening of the association in subsequent periods of the study, with a 'regression towards the mean' of overall results from other studies.

The risk estimates, however, tended to be elevated systematically in other European countries also[30–32], possibly because of the different types of preparations used, with higher prevalence of synthetic oestrogens and oestrogen–progestin combinations[38,39].

Considering the short average duration of oestrogen replacement treatment in this Italian population, the risk estimate may well be somewhat overesti-

Table 4 Relative risk (and 95% confidence intervals) of breast cancer in separate strata of duration and time since last oestrogen replacement treatment use, Milan, Italy, 1983–90. Mantel–Haenszel estimates adjusted for age; reference category: never-users

	Duration of use (years)	
	< 3	*≥ 3*
Time since last use (years)		
< 10	1.4 (0.8–2.2)	1.2 (0.6–2.3)
≥ 10	1.4 (0.9–2.1)	2.0 (0.8–5.3)

Table 5 Relationship between menopausal replacement treatment and breast cancer risk in selected studies

		Relative risk	
Study, year	*Reference*	*Ever-use*	*Long-term use*
Hoover *et al.*, 1976	11	1.3	2.0
Casagrande *et al.*, 1976	12	0.8	—
Sartwell *et al.*, 1977	13	0.8	0.6
Wynder *et al.*, 1978	14	1.1	0.4
Ravnihar *et al.*, 1979	15	0.8	—
Ross *et al.*, 1980	16	1.1	1.9
Jick *et al.*, 1980	17	1.1	—
Brinton *et al.*, 1981	18	1.2	1.3
Hoover *et al.*, 1981	19	1.4	1.8
Kelsey *et al.*, 1981	20	0.9	0.7
Hulka *et al.*, 1982	21	1.8	1.7
Sherman *et al.*, 1983	22	0.7	—
Hiatt *et al.*, 1984	23	0.7	1.8
Kaufman *et al.*, 1984	24	1.0	1.3
Talamini *et al.*, 1985	25	0.9	—
Brinton *et al.*, 1986	26	1.0	1.5
Nomura *et al.*, 1986	27		
Caucasian		1.0	1.3
Japanese		0.9	1.9
Wingo *et al.*, 1987	28	1.0	1.5
Buring *et al.*, 1987	29	1.1	1.3
Ewertz, 1988	30	1.2	1.5
Hunt *et al.*, 1987	31	1.6	1.3
Bergkvist *et al.*, 1989	32	1.1	1.7
Dupont *et al.*, 1989	33	1.5	—
Mills *et al.*, 1989	34	1.7	1.5
Colditz *et al.*, 1990	35	1.2	1.1

mated. This may be partly due to the low frequency of menopausal hormonal therapy (3.5% of the comparison group), and the consequent possible greater selection of users, in terms of higher social class and other potential correlates of breast cancer, i.e. possible confounding factors[36,38]. Nevertheless, allowance for indicators of socioeconomic status and other major known or potential determinants of breast cancer only partially accounted for the association between oestrogen replacement treatment and breast cancer.

Another possible reason for overestimating the association in this study was the inclusion of orthopaedic and traumatic conditions which may, at least in part[40], be associated with low oestrogen levels and be inversely related to oestrogen use, and hence may have inflated the risk estimates. However, the frequency of use of menopausal replacement treatment across various categories of controls was not appreciably different, and a previous separate analysis of controls by diagnostic subcategories did not show any material difference in risk[36].

Other strengths and weaknesses of this study are common to most hospital-based case–control investigations[37]. More specifically, although this study was not population-based, cases were identified in the major teaching and general hospitals of the area under surveillance, thus reducing the scope for selection bias. Further, the hospital-based design may improve the comparability of recall of drug histories by cases and controls. Nevertheless, the absence of a strong duration–risk relationship suggests the possibility of recall bias, since short-term use may be potentially influenced by more accurate recall by the cases.

Among the strengths of this study are the satisfactory participation rate, the comparable catchment area of case and controls, and, *a posteriori*, the observation that the established risk factors for breast cancer[41] emerged consistently.

Besides the absence of a strong and clear duration–risk relationship, no consistent pattern of risk emerged for the other time-factors considered. A cohort study found that current use may be particularly relevant[35], in that oestrogens may have a late-stage effect on breast carcinogenesis, as on other female hormone-related neoplasms, such as endometrial cancer[42,43]. In another cohort study[27], however, the highest risk was observed in cases who had first used replacement treatments more than 10 years earlier. In this study, the risk estimates were comparable for shorter and longer time since first or last use.

In conclusion, the low prevalence of oestrogen replacement treatment use in this Italian population seriously hampered analysis, and particularly any inference on subgroups, time factors, dose or type of preparation. Nevertheless, the large size of the dataset, the originality of the population, in terms of baseline breast cancer incidence and patterns of hormone use[38,44], and the consistency of its results with the overall evidence from other studies[39] add useful information to a debate of major public health relevance.

While further epidemiological data will be available within the next few years on the long-term effects (i.e. after long latency) of postmenopausal hormonal treatment, it is important to recognize that the cost–benefit analysis of such treatment must be considered in a broader epidemiological and public health perspective, including cancer as well as cardiovascular disease and bone metabolism[45,46].

ACKNOWLEDGEMENTS

This work was conducted within the framework of the National Research Council (CNR), Applied Projects 'Oncology' (Contract No. 87.01544.44), and

'Prevention and Control of Disease Factors' (Contract No. 91.00285.PF41), with the contributions of the Italian Association for Cancer Research, the Italian League against Tumours, Milan and Mrs A. Marchegiano Borgomanerio, and with grants-in-aid from the Italian Ministry of Health and the Europe against Cancer Programme of the Commission of the European Communities. The authors wish to thank Mrs J. Baggott, Mrs M.P. Bonifacino, and the G.A. Pfeiffer Memorial Library for editorial assistance.

REFERENCES

1. Pike, M.C. (1987). Age-related factors in cancers of the breast, ovary, and endometrium. *J. Chron. Dis.*, **40**, Suppl. 2, 59–69S
2. Decarli, A., La Vecchia, C., Mezzanotte, G. and Cislaghi, C. (1987). Birth cohort, time, and age effects in Italian cancer mortality. *Cancer*, **59**, 1221–32
3. Parazzini, F., La Vecchia, C., Negri, E., Bruzzi, P., Palli, D. and Boyle, P. (1990). Anthropometric variables and risk of breast cancer. *Int. J. Cancer*, **45**, 397–402
4. Ferguson, D.J. and Anderson, T.J. (1981). Morphological evaluation of cell turnover in relation to the menstrual cycle in the 'resting' human breast. *Br. J. Cancer*, **44**, 177–81
5. Henderson, B.E. (1985). Hormones as a cause of human cancer. In Fortner, J.G. and Rhoads, J.E. (eds.) *Accomplishments in Cancer Research*, pp.152–68. (Philadelphia: Lippincott Co.)
6. Korenman, S.G. (1980). Oestrogen window hypothesis of the aetiology of breast cancer. *Lancet*, **1**, 700–1
7. Apter, D. and Vihko, R. (1983). Early menarche, a risk factor for breast cancer, indicates early onset of ovulatory cycles. *J. Clin. Endocrinol. Metab.*, **57**, 82–6
8. MacMahon, B., Trichopoulos, D., Brown, J.B., Andersen, A.P., Aoki, K., Cole, P., deWaard, F., Kauraniemi, T., Morgan, R.W., Purde, M. Ravnihar, B., Stormby, N., Westlund, K. and Woo, N.-C. (1982). Age at menarche, probability of ovulation and breast cancer risk. *Int. J. Cancer*, **29**, 13–16
9. Olsson, A., Landin-Olsson, M. and Gullberg, B. (1983). Retrospective assessment of menstrual cycle length in patients with breast cancer, in patients with benign breast disease, and in women without breast disease. *J. Natl. Cancer Inst.*, **70**, 17–20
10. La Vecchia, C., Decarli, A., Di Pietro, S., Franceschi, S., Negri, E. and Parazzini, F. (1985). Menstrual cycle patterns and the risk of breast disease. *Eur. J. Cancer Clin. Oncol.*, **21**, 417–22
11. Hoover, R., Gray, L.A., Sr, Cole, P. and MacMahon, B. (1976). Menopausal estrogens and breast cancer. *N. Engl. J. Med.*, **295**, 401–5
12. Casagrande, J., Gerkins, V., Henderson, B.E., Mack, T. and Pike, M.C. (1976). Exogenous estrogens and breast cancer in women with natural menopause. *J. Natl. Cancer Inst.*, **56**, 839–41
13. Sartwell, P.E., Arthes, F.G. and Tonascia, J.A. (1977). Exogenous hormones, reproductive history, and breast cancer. *J. Natl. Cancer Inst.*, **59**, 1589–92
14. Wynder, E.L., MacCornack, F.A. and Stellman, S.D. (1978). The epidemiology of breast cancer in 785 United States Caucasian women. *Cancer*, **41**, 2341–54
15. Ravnihar, B., Seigel, D.G. and Lindtner, J. (1979). An epidemiological study of breast cancer and benign breast neoplasias in relation to the oral contraceptive and estrogen use. *Eur. J. Cancer Clin. Oncol.*, **13**, 395–403
16. Ross, R.K., Paganini-Hill, A., Gerkins, V.R., Mack, T.M., Pfeffer, R., Arthur, M. and Henderson, B.E. (1980). A case–control study of menopausal estrogen therapy and breast cancer. *J. Am. Med. Assoc.*, **243**, 1635–9
17. Jick, A., Walker, A.M., Watkins, R.N., D'Ewart, D.C. Hunter, J.R., Danford, A., Dinan, B.J. and Rothman, K.J. (1980). Replacement estrogens and breast cancer. *Am. J. Epidemiol.*, **112**, 586–94
18. Brinton, L.A., Hoover, R.N., Szklo, M. and Fraumeni, J.F., Jr (1981). Menopausal estrogen use and risk of breast cancer. *Cancer*, **47**, 2517–22

19. Hoover, R., Glass, A., Finkle, W.D., Azevedo, D. and Milne, K. (1981). Conjugated estrogens and breast cancer risk in women. *J. Natl. Cancer Inst.*, **67**, 815–20
20. Kelsey, J.L., Fischer, D.B., Holford, T.R., LiVolsi, V.A., Mostow, E.D., Goldenberg, I.S. and White, C. (1981). Exogenous estrogens and other factors in the epidemiology of breast cancer. *J. Natl. Cancer Inst.*, **67**, 327–33
21. Hulka, B.S., Chambless, L.E., Deubner, D.C. and Wilkinson, W.E. (1982). Breast cancer and estrogen replacement therapy. *Am. J. Obstet. Gynecol.*, **143**, 638–44
22. Sherman, B., Wallace, R. and Pean, J. (1983). Estrogen use and breast cancer. Interaction with body mass. *Cancer*, **51**, 1527–31
23. Hiatt, R.A., Bawol, R., Friedman, G.D. and Hoover, R. (1984). Exogenous estrogen and breast cancer after bilateral oophorectomy. *Cancer*, **54**, 139–44
24. Kaufman, D.W., Miller, D.R., Rosenberg, L., Helmrich, S.P., Stolley, P., Schottenfeld, D. and Shapiro, S. (1984). Noncontraceptive estrogen use and the risk of breast cancer. *J. Am. Med. Assoc.*, **252**, 63–7
25. Talamini, R., La Vecchia, C., Franceschi, S., Colombo, F., Decarli, A., Grattoni, E., Grigoletto, E. and Tognoni, G. (1985). Reproductive and hormonal factors and breast cancer in a Northern Italian population. *Int. J. Epidemiol.*, **14**, 70–4
26. Brinton, L.A., Hoover, R. and Fraumeni, J.F., Jr (1986). Menopausal oestrogens and breast cancer risk: an expanded case–control study. *Br. J. Cancer*, **54**, 825–32
27. Nomura, A.M.Y., Kolonel, L.N., Hirohata, T. and Lee, J. (1986). The association of replacement estrogens with breast cancer. *Int. J. Cancer*, **37**, 49–53
28. Wingo, P.A., Layde, P.M., Lee, N.C., Rubin, G. and Ory, H.W. (1987). The risk of breast cancer in postmenopausal women who have used estrogen replacement therapy. *J. Am. Med. Assoc.*, **257**, 209–15
29. Buring, J.E., Hennekens, C.H., Lipnick, R.J., Willett, W.C., Stampfer, M.J., Rosner, B., Peto, R. and Speizer, F.E. (1987). A prospective cohort study of postmenopausal hormone use and risk of breast cancer in US women. *Am. J. Epidemiol.*, **125**, 939–47
30. Ewertz, M. (1988). Influence of non-contraceptive exogenous and endogenous sex hormones on breast cancer risk in Denmark. *Int. J. Cancer*, **42**, 832–8
31. Hunt, K., Vessey, M., McPherson, K. and Coleman, M. (1987). Long-term surveillance of mortality and cancer incidence in women receiving hormone replacement therapy. *Br. J. Obstet. Gynaecol.*, **94**, 620–35
32. Bergkvist, L., Adami, H.O., Persson, I., Hoover, R. and Schairer, C. (1989). The risk of breast cancer after estrogen and estrogen–progestin replacement. *N. Engl. J. Med.*, **321**, 293–7
33. Dupont, W.D., Page, D.L., Rogers, L.W. and Parl, F.F. (1989). Influence of exogenous estrogens, proliferative breast disease, and other variables on breast cancer risk. *Cancer*, **63**, 948–57
34. Mills, P.K., Beeson, W.L., Phillips, R.L. and Fraser, G.E. (1989). Prospective study of exogenous hormone use and breast cancer in Seventh-Day Adventists. *Cancer*, **64**, 591–7
35. Colditz, G.A., Stampfer, M.J., Willett, W.C., Hennekens, C.H., Rosner, B. and Speizer, F.E. (1990). Prospective study of estrogen replacement therapy and risk of breast cancer in postmenopausal women. *J. Am. Med. Assoc.*, **264**, 2648–53
36. La Vecchia, C., Decarli, A., Parazzini, F., Gentile, A., Liberati, C. and Franceschi, S. (1986). Non-contraceptive oestrogens and the risk of breast cancer in women. *Int. J. Cancer*, **38**, 853–8
37. Breslow, N.E. and Day, N.E. (1980). *Statistical Methods in Cancer Research*, Vol. 1. The analysis of case–control studies. *IARC Sci. Publ.*, **32**
38. Franceschi, S., La Vecchia, C., Tudisco, A. and Tognoni, G. (1982). Patterns of hormonal therapy during the menopause: a retrospective survey on 500 women in Lombardy. In Fioretti, P., Martini, L., Melis, G.B. and Yen, S.S.C. (eds.) *The Menopause: Clinical, Endocrinological and Pathophysiological Aspects*, pp. 579–84. (London: Academic Press)
39. Steinberg, K.K., Thacker, S.B., Smith, S.J., Stroup, D.F., Zack, M.M., Flanders, W.D. and Berkelman, R.L. (1991). A meta-analysis of the effect of estrogen replacement therapy on the risk of breast cancer. *J. Am. Med. Assoc.*, **265**, 1985–90
40. La Vecchia, C., Negri, E., Levi, F. and Baron, J.A. (1991). Cigarette smoking, body mass, and other risk factors for fractures of the hip in women. *Int. J. Epidemiol.*, **22**, 671–7
41. Boyle, P. (1988). Epidemiology of breast cancer. *Bailliere's Clinical Oncology*, **2**, 1–57

42. Day, N.E. and Brown, C.C. (1980). Multistage models and primary prevention of cancer. *J. Natl. Cancer Inst.*, **64**, 977–89
43. La Vecchia, C., Franceschi, S., Decarli, A., Gallus, G. and Tognoni, G. (1984). Risk factors for endometrial cancer at different ages. *J. Natl. Cancer Inst.*, **73**, 667–71
44. Levi, F., Maisonneuve, P., Filiberti, R., La Vecchia, C. and Boyle, P. (1989). Cancer incidence and mortality in Europe. *Soz. Präventivmed.*, **34**, suppl.2, S1–84
45. Henderson, B.E. (1989). The cancer question: an overview of recent epidemiologic and retrospective data. *Am. J. Obstet. Gynecol.*, **161**, 1859–64
46. Mack, T.M. and Ross, R.K. (1989). Risks and benefits of long-term treatment with estrogens. *Schweizerische Medizinische Wochenschrift*, **119**, 1811–20

10

Osteoporosis: prevalence, prediction and prevention

M.A. Smith and J.O. Drife

INTRODUCTION

The alliteration in the title of this paper covers a subject which includes a wide range of complex issues associated with what is, in itself, a complex disease. We must therefore limit ourselves to specific aspects of the title and so it is important to clarify the scope of this paper. The first issue to consider is our use of the word 'osteoporosis'. The basic definition was given in 1941 by Albright[1], who stated that osteoporosis was: 'too little bone, but what bone there is, is normal'. With the known loss of bone after the menopause, or indeed the decrease in bone mineral after the age of 35 years[2], it could be said that some of the bones of the majority of the female population are, to some extent, osteoporotic. For practical clinical purposes it is important to differentiate between the underlying process of the disease and the symptoms experienced by the patient. In this review of the prevalence of osteoporosis we will concentrate on the symptoms that are of most concern to both patients and healthcare services; these are bone fractures, particularly of the neck of the femur and the spine.

The current debate about the possible use of hormone replacement therapy for treating patients who may be at risk from osteoporosis stems from the upsurge in interest in the use of bone mineral measurement techniques to 'predict' women at risk early in life, usually around the time of the menopause, before significant bone loss has occurred. It will be seen that major technological developments have occurred over the last 2 years such that it is now possible to perform measurements on patients and measure the bone mineral in the spine and neck of the femur with a higher degree of precision. The availability of such equipment has lead a number of groups to propose and offer a screening service for osteoporosis for women at around the time of the menopause. It will be seen that in many cases the basis of screening programmes may be based more on wishful thinking than on sound scientific data.

As this conference is concerned with hormone replacement therapy, we will limit our discussion about the prevention of osteoporiosis to the role and effect of hormone replacement therapy as a preventative therapy to reduce the risk of osteoporotic fractures.

PREVALENCE

The prevalence of osteoporotic fractures of the neck of the femur varies widely between different racial groups, between men and women and with the age of the population. In addition, the incidence within a particular racial age-group will vary with time, even when the changing age-distribution of the population is taken into account. Table 1 lists the fracture incidence obtained from a number of published studies of different countries and racial groups. The data are for all fractures of the neck of the femur for men and women over the age of 35 years, and indicate a dramatic difference in fracture risk between different racial groups. The clearest racial difference occurs between White and non-White women, the former having a much higher prevalence of osteoporotic-induced fractures than either Black, Asian, or other non-White groups; the most substantial difference is demonstrated in a South African study[4], although it is likely that the life-styles of the two groups will be much more dissimilar than the groups of White and Blacks in the American study.

Caution must be applied when considering the figures in Table 1. Not only will the quality of the epidemiology data vary, but the incidence can change dramatically with time. This is best illustrated by considering the data from the United Kingdom study of Oxford which was initially carried out over the period 1954–1958[5] and then subsequently in 1983[6]. This study demonstrated a 75% increase in fractures of the proximal femur in less than 20 years, due, it is imagined, to a change in the age-spectrum of the population during that time. A similar dramatic increase in incidence over a 30-year interval in the Swedish study has been shown[7].

Table 1 Femoral neck fractures in men and women over 35 years of age; number per 100 000 population per annum[3]

Location of study	*Women*	*Men*
Washington, USA		
Whites	232	82
Blacks	119	110
Finland	213	136
Oslo, Norway	421	231
Malmo, Sweden	237	101
Oxford and Dundee, UK		
1954–1958	142	69
1983	260	125
New Zealand		
Whites	220	99
Maoris	104	84
Johannesburg, South Africa		
Whites	257	99
Bantu	14	14

The variation in the incidence of fractures of the neck of the femur with age is dramatic but the published results are not entirely consistent. One feature to be noted, which will have an impact if hormone replacement therapy is considered as a prophylactic measure, is the relationship between any increase in fracture incidence and the menopause. An often-quoted study[8] considers all limb fractures and demonstrates a clear increase in fracture incidence around the time of the menopause in women (44–54 years) and a similar increase approximately 10 years later in men. However, a study of the age-specific fracture incidence using national hospital discharge survey data[9] shows a gradual increase in fracture incidence until the age range 65–69 years, after which the increase is more noticeable (Table 2). There is no sharp increase at or around the time of the menopause; in fact the increase is approximately exponential. The fact that there is an acceleration in the increase of incidence at a time some years after the menopause does not, of course, invalidate the argument that the menopause is a key factor in osteoporotic fracture.

An indication of the magnitude of the prevalence of osteoporosis is given in a recent paper[10] which states that in England in 1985, nearly a quarter of all orthopaedic beds in the National Health Service were committed to people over 65 years with hip fractures; the total number of patients with hip fractures over the age of 65 years were 30 900 and 6740 for women and men, respectively. The larger number of fractures in women compared with men is influenced significantly by the longer life-expectancy of women. It is interesting to note that the cumulative probability of a person aged 45 years sustaining a hip fracture is, for women and men respectively, 3% and 2% at 75 years, 11% and 5% at 85 years and 22% and 11% at 90 years. This illustrates that osteoporosis is not only a problem for women, as there is only a twofold difference of probability that a woman will suffer a hip fracture compared to a man, if both were to live to the same age.

Table 2 Incidence of femoral neck fractures (per 100 000/annum) in the USA in the years 1974–1979 based on hospital discharge statistics[9]

	Women		*Men*	
Age-group	*Whites*	*Non-Whites*	*Whites*	*Non-Whites*
30–34	4	12	12	18
35–39	3	10	15	19
40–44	22	14	25	15
45–49	34	11	23	31
50–54	50	18	25	56
55–59	89	31	41	81
60–64	153	38	67	61
65–69	237	102	117	23
70–74	531	167	222	213
75–79	1018	409	434	335
80–84	1731	881	735	179

PREDICTION

There has been much discussion and debate concerning risk factors associated with osteoporosis and possible biochemical indicators of the disease. However, this chapter will be concerned with the current issue of prediction, which is the identification of women potentially at risk before symptoms of the disease occur. As osteoporosis affects the bone mineral matrix, it has long been recognized that a quantitative measurement of bone mineral mass, or bone mineral content, may be of value in the study of osteoporosis. Many techniques have been developed to measure bone mineral at various sites of the body[11] including the femur, radius, os calcis, lumbar spine, neck of femur and whole body. These techniques have been improved, particularly over the last 4 years. There are bone scanners now available which use two X-ray energies to obtain a quantitative measurement of bone in the spine, the hip or in the whole body[12]. Such systems are referred to as DEXA (Dual Energy X-ray Absorptiometry) scanners and they can either measure the bone mineral in grams, referred to as bone mineral content, or in g/cm^2, referred to as bone mineral density. Bone mineral content will be influenced by the size of the patient, whereas the bone mineral density is the area-normalized bone mineral content, and tends to be less influenced by size; the coefficient of variation of lumbar spine bone mineral density for a specific age in the normal population is around 12–14%. The dose received by the patient is low, and so the technique has potential as a mass screening tool. It must be remembered that the aim is to predict women who may eventually suffer the most severe symptoms of osteoporosis, i.e. a major bone fracture, rather than to predict osteoporosis itself.

In order to predict patients at risk from fractures, a number of hypotheses have been proposed, and extrapolations made from these, with the view to establish a practical screening regimen, often based on some pragmatic assumption.

FRACTURE THRESHOLD

A fracture threshold can be postulated from the fact that, over a period of time, a patient suffering from osteoporosis will experience a gradual reduction in bone mineral and an increased propensity to fracture. Given the fact that the bone mineral matrix supplies the strength for the bone, it was felt that there may be a relationship between the bone mineral value itself and the risk of fracture. The basis for the concept of a fracture threshold is illustrated in Figure 1. It can be seen that there is a decrease in bone mineral after the menopause in normal subjects and that patients suffering from an osteoporotic fracture tend, as a group, to have a lower bone mineral level. A level can be set, below which the likelihood of fracture increases. Such a level is arbitrary because there is no separation between the groups of women at a similar age with and without fracture.

If such a fracture threshold exists, it may be possible to perform a bone mineral measurement earlier than the usual age of fracture and predict whether a patient is likely to cross the threshold as they get older, from their

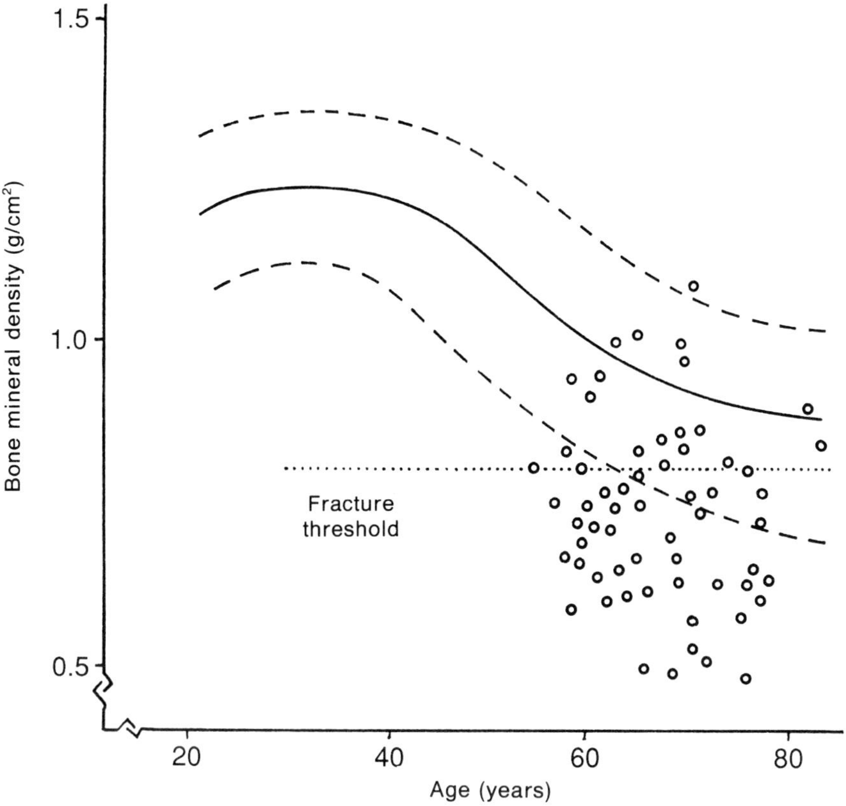

Figure 1 Typical results obtained when bone mineral density is measured in the spines of healthy women and women suffering from an osteoporotic fracture. Solid line = mean bone mineral density in the lumbar spine in normal healthy women; dashed lines = $\pm$ 1 SD of mean bone mineral density; circles = women who have suffered osteoporotic fractures; dotted line = possible fracture threshold. It can be seen that considerable overlap exists between the normal values and the fractures

peak bone mineral density value and their subsequent rate of loss (Figure 2). Women could be screened around the time of the menopause to assess whether they have a high or low bone mineral level and whether they are fast or slow losers. The latter is an over-simplification as there would be a spectrum of rates of loss. From the research of a number of centres, the consensus was that an appropriate level for the fracture threshold could be 60% of the mean premenopausal bone mineral density.

The concept of a fracture threshold is weakened by the fact that there is a large amount of overlap between bone mineral measurements obtained in women who have suffered a fracture of the neck of the femur and age-matched controls. A compilation of all the high-quality published studies[10] has shown that the mean difference in bone mineral measurement between patients with a fracture and normal controls is only half a standard deviation

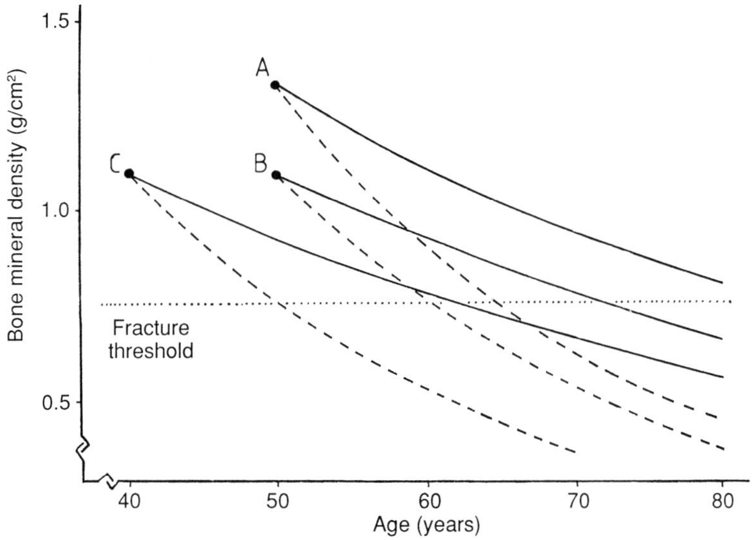

Figure 2 The likelihood of crossing a 'fracture threshold' will be related to the peak bone mass prior to the menopause, the rate of loss after the menopause and the age of the menopause. Subject A has a peak bone mineral density 1 SD above the mean and a menopause at 50; subject B has a peak bone mineral density 1 SD below the mean and a menopause at 50; and subject C has a peak bone mineral density 1 SD below the mean and a menopause at 40. The solid line indicates a bone loss of 1.5%/annum; the dashed line indicates a bone loss of 3%/annum; and the dotted line is a nominal fracture threshold set at 60% mean peak bone mineral density value

in each group. Consequently, the implications for screening are not good, because even if women were measured late in life the bone mineral density measurements of the femur would always have a high level of false-positive results. For example, a 30% detection rate would result in a 15% false-positive rate. If the percentage detection rate were to be increased, then the proportion of false-positives would increase to greater than half the detection rate. The separation obtained using lumbar spine or forearm bone mineral density is even worse.

The absence of a discrete fracture threshold could be related to a number of factors. The first is that bone strength is related to both bone mineral content and bone architecture. The latter may contribute perhaps 30–40% to the strength of the bone. Thus a simple measurement of bone mineral itself will not be completely related to bone strength. Secondly, low bone mineral is only one of the risk factors associated with a fractured neck of femur, and many of the women with a low bone mineral level may simply be waiting to experience a slight trauma to produce the fractures.

MATHEMATICAL MODEL OF RISK ASSESSMENT

A mathematical technique has been proposed relating fracture risk to a number of potential risk factors. This technique is referred to as stochastic modelling[13], so-called because it uses mathematical techniques which obey the laws of statistical probability. The postulated stochastic model has specifically been used to consider the relationship between peak bone mineral density or the rate of bone loss and the probability of fracture of the neck of the femur. The perimenopausal peak bone mass was found to be a better predictor of such a fracture than the rate of bone loss after the menopause. The mathematical model suggested that 66% of women who would suffer a fracture of the neck of the femur were in the lower quartile of the peak bone mass values at the time of the menopause, compared with 31% in the higher quartile of bone mass loss[14]. This suggests that rate of bone mineral loss has a far lower impact on fracture risk than peak bone mass.

The stochastic model has not been validated experimentally, although it has led to a number of screening programmes being set up which measure women around the age of 50 years and define those in the bottom quartile, i.e. the lower 25% of the population, as at risk from osteoporosis; such categorization requires validation in a long-term study to determine whether the sensitivity of 66% is correct.

PREVENTION

The prevention of a disease as widespread as osteoporosis can be tackled in one of two ways. The first is to use the predictive techniques discussed previously to identify the women at high risk and then prescribe appropriate preventive therapy. The second approach is to recommend preventive measures for the whole population, or for a clearly defined subset such as women over 45 years of age. The latter would be the appropriate course of action if a high-risk subset could be clearly defined, and if any medication that was to be prescribed was free of harmful side-effects. In most health-care systems the cost of such medication would also have to be taken into account, and this, along with the magnitude of any side-effects, would influence whether the former, more selective, approach should be adopted. However, as was seen in the previous section, the efficacy of the necessary predictive screening technique has not yet been fully evaluated.

The disease of osteoporosis is known to be associated with a number of independent risk factors. Conclusions about the risk factors are based on both relative risk of fracture and changes in bone mineral. The latter can be measured and studied over a relatively short period of time but it must be remembered that bone mineral measurements alone do not discriminate between fracture patients and normals. The direct effects of various interventions or changes in life-style on fracture incidence, as opposed to bone mineral content, have not been studied adequately yet; such studies require large numbers and a long time-scale which could be around 20–30 years or more.

Calcium in the diet has been shown to reduce fracture incidence. One study investigated two comparable populations in Yugoslavia which differed in their dietary intake of calcium[15]. Although this demonstrated the importance of calcium intake, it raised the additional question of whether there may be a need to influence risk factors much earlier in life, for example in childhood, than has traditionally been considered necessary with osteoporosis. There is no epidemiological evidence to show that an increase in dietary calcium later in life, at around the time of the menopause, has a direct effect on fracture reduction. A beneficial effect on bone mineral of additional dietary calcium late in life has, however, been demonstrated as has the effect of exercise.

This chapter is not the place to discuss the various drug treatments for osteoporosis, but there is clear consensus that oestrogen is by far the most effective treatment for preventing the condition. We have therefore concentrated on the role of hormone replacement therapy, which could be used either in conjunction with a screening programme or recommended to all women. The importance of oestrogen therapy for the management of osteoporosis was first recognized in the 1940s[16]. It is now believed that the primary action of oestrogen is to inhibit bone resorption, so a reduction in oestrogen level will tend to reduce bone mass. It is accepted that there is an age-related osteoporotic effect on bone in both men and women, producing a gradual reduction in bone mineral and therefore, eventually, an increased fracture risk. In women this is compounded by the reduction in oestrogen at the time of the menopause[17]. The age-related bone loss may commence before the menopause in some sites of the body, such as the neck of the femur, whereas in the spine, any age-related loss is not apparent before the menopause.

The effect of oestrogen therapy on bone mineral has been demonstrated in a large number of studies. Of these, the research by Lindsay and colleagues[18,19], Nachtigall and colleagues[20] and Christiansen and colleagues[21,22] are worthy of special mention. The Glasgow study by Lindsay and co-workers started in 1968 and studied 217 women following surgical menopause. Sophisticated techniques for measuring bone mineral were not available at that time, but using a simple radiographic technique to study the metacarpal bones in the hand they were able to demonstrate that mestranol could maintain bone mass compared to placebo. However, when the therapy was stopped, significant bone mineral loss occurred. Essentially the same conclusions were obtained in studies of women following a natural menopause using oral conjugated equine oestrogens[20] and using oral oestradiol with calcium supplement[21,22]. The bone mineral mass of women receiving hormone replacement therapy who then stopped fell eventually to the plateau level of bone mineral mass that occurs late in life. Hormone replacement therapy therefore delayed the loss of bone, instead of maintaining a higher than normal level.

A number of studies were undertaken to determine the minimum dose of hormone replacement therapy required to arrest bone loss. A dose of 0.6 mg/day of oral conjugated equine oestrogen[23] or 2 mg/day of oral oestradiol[24] was required to arrest bone loss. Some of the studies using oral hormone replacement therapy showed not only that bone loss could be arrested, but also that a slight increase in bone mineral mass could be achieved. There is also evidence that a greater increase in bone mass can be achieved by percutaneous administration of oestrogen therapy, possibly due to the higher levels of serum oestradiol that can be achieved[25]. It is not yet known how such increases in bone mineral mass will be related, if at all, to increases in bone strength. Trabecular bone is a matrix of bone fibres, the structure of the fibres being related to its strength. A loss of bone mineral can result in a reduction in the connections within the matrix and a loss of strength. An increase in bone mineral may simply increase the width of the bone fibres without restoring the interconnections; in such a situation the strength would not increase.

Ovarian failure is not a sudden event for most women. Oestrogen levels fall gradually before the menopause itself, and symptoms of oestrogen deprivation, such as hot flushes, often begin well before the last menstrual period. This raises the possibility that menopausal bone loss may begin before the last menstrual period, and that the best way of maintaining a woman's bone mass might be to begin oestrogen supplementation before the menopause itself. There is little information about the effectiveness and safety of hormone preparations given at this time in a woman's life, and on the optimum dosage for premenopausal hormone therapy[26].

A Study Group on 'HRT and Osteoporosis', convened at the Royal College of Obstetricians and Gynaecologists in 1990[27], produced a number of conclusions and recommendations, including the following:

(1) Bone loss can be prevented at any stage of osteoporosis, but it is questionable whether skeletal architecture and competence can be restored once lost. Therefore, the emphasis must be on prevention of bone loss by early intervention.

(2) Oestrogen administration is the most effective method currently available for prevention of bone loss in women, although other modalities are available.

(3) Equivalent doses of oestrogen given by any route are equally effective in preventing osteoporosis.

(4) Bone density measurements currently provide the best single estimate of the risk of subsequent fracture, but their role as a screening tool needs evaluation.

(5) The use of hormone replacement therapy in Britain is low at present and it should be more readily available.

(6) Certain groups of women should be considered especially for treatment, particularly those with a premature menopause (natural or surgical).

(7) In order to have an effect on osteoporosis, hormone replacement therapy must be continued for more than 2 years. Studies are required to determine the optimum duration of the treatment.

CONCLUSION

Osteoporosis has a high prevalence, in many countries, which will increase as the proportion of elderly in the population increases. The magnitude of the problem is highest in women, as the menopause increases the rate of bone loss. In women, oestrogen is the most effective treatment for preventing postmenopausal bone loss. To reduce the risk of osteoporotic fractures, oestrogen should be continued for as long as possible after the menopause, perhaps for 10 years or even longer.

There are two approaches for preventing postmenopausal osteoporosis in the population; oestrogen could be given either to all women after the menopause or to a selected high-risk group. The latter approach seems likely to be more acceptable to women and their doctors. However, the identification of women at high risk remains a concern, as bone mineral density measurement has not yet been validated as a predictive technique to identify women at high risk of fractures later in life.

ACKNOWLEDGEMENTS

The authors wish to thank the Medical Research Council, the University of Leeds and the United Leeds Teaching Hospitals NHS Trusts for financial support. We acknowledge the advice and support of the staff of the Leeds Bone Mineralisation Unit: Mr R. Milner, Mr B. Oldroyd, Mrs M. Simpson, Mrs S. Stewart, Mr J. Truscott and Mrs C. Westmacott.

REFERENCES

1. Albright, F., Smith, P.H. and Richardson, A.M. (1941). Postmenopausal osteoporosis. Its clinical features. *J. Am. Med. Assoc.*, **116**, 2465–74
2. Rodin, A., Murby, B., Smith, M.A., Caleffi, M., Fentiman, I., Chapman, M.G. and Fogelman, I. (1990). Premenopausal bone loss in the lumbar spine and neck of femur: a study of 225 Caucasian women. *Bone*, **11**, 1–5
3. Melton, L.J. III (1988). Epidemiology of Fractures. In Riggs, B.L. and Melton, L.J. III (eds.) *Osteoporosis: Etiology, Diagnosis and Management*, pp. 133–53. (New York: Raven Press)
4. Solomon, L. (1968). Osteoporosis and fracture of the femoral neck in the South African Bantu. *J. Bone Jt. Surg.*, **50-B**, 2–13
5. Knowleden, J., Buhr, A.J. and Dunbar, O. (1964). Incidence of fractures in persons over 35 years of age: a report to the MRC Working Party on fractures in the elderly. *Br. J. Prev. Soc. Med.*, **18**, 130–41
6. Boyce, W.J. and Vessey, M.P. (1985). Rising incidence of fracture of the proximal femur. *Lancet*, **1**, 150–1
7. Johnell, O., Nilsson, B., Obrant, K. and Sernbo, I. (1984). Age and sex patterns of hip fracture – changes in 30 years. *Acta Orthop. Scand.*, **55**, 290–2
8. Garroway, W.M., Stauffer, R.N., Kurland, L.T. and O'Fallon, W.M. (1979). Limb fractures in a defined population. II. Orthopaedic treatment and utilization of health care. *Mayo Clin. Proc.*, **54**, 708–13
9. Farmer, M.E., White, L.R., Brody, J.A. and Bailey, K.R. (1984). Race and sex difference in hip fracture incidence. *Am. J. Pub. Health*, **74**, 1374–9
10. Law, M.R., Wald, N.J., Meade, T.W. (1991). Strategies for prevention of osteoporosis and hip fracture. *Br. Med. J.*, **303**, 453–9
11. Tothill, P. (1989). Methods of bone mineral measurement. *Phys. Med. Biol.*, **34**, 543–72

12. Stein, J.A., Hochberg, A.M. and Lazewatsky, L. (1988). Quantitative digital radiography for bone mineral analysis. In Dequeker, J., Geusens, P. and Wahner, H.W. (eds.) *Bone Mineral Measurement by Photon Absorptiometry*, pp. 411–14. (Leuven: Leuven University Press)
13. Horsman, A., Marshall, D.H. and Peacock, M. (1985). A stochastic model of age-related bone loss and fractures. *Clin. Orthop.*, **195**, 207–15
14. Purdie, D.W. and Horsman, A. (1990). Population screening and the prevention of osteoporosis. In Drife, J.O. and Studd, J.W.W. (eds.) *HRT and Osteoporosis. Proceedings of the 22nd Study Group of the Royal College of Obstetricians and Gynaecologists.*, pp. 251–64 (London: Springer–Verlag)
15. Matkovic, V., Kostial, K., Simonovic, I., Buzina, R., Brodarec, A. and Nordin, B.E.C. (1979). Bone status and fracture rates in two regions of Yugoslavia. *Am. J. Clin. Nutr.*, **32**, 540–9
16. Albright, F. (1947). Hormones and human osteogenesis. *Rec. Prog. Horm. Res.*, **1**, 293–353
17. Riggs, B.L. and Melton, L.J. III (1986). Involutional osteoporosis. *N. Engl. J. Med.*, **314**, 1676–86
18. Lindsay, R., Aitken, J.M., Anderson, J.B., Hart, D.M., MacDonald, E.B. and Clarke, A.C. (1976). Long-term prevention of postmenopausal osteoporosis by oestrogen. Evidence for an increased bone mass after delayed onset of oestrogen treatment. *Lancet*, **1**, 1038–41
19. Lindsay, R., MacLean, A., Kraszewski, A., Hart, D.M., Clark, A.C. and Garwood, J. (1978). Bone response to termination of oestrogen treatment. *Lancet*, **1**, 1325–7
20. Nachtigall, L.E., Nachtigall, H., Nachtigall, R.D. and Beckman, M.E. (1979). Estrogen replacement therapy I: a 10-year prospective study in the relationship to osteoporosis. *Obstet. Gynaecol.*, **53**, 277–81
21. Christiansen, C., Christensen, M.S., McNair, P., Hagen, C., Stocklund, K.E. and Transbol, I. (1980). Prevention of early postmenopausal bone loss: controlled 2-year study of 315 normal females. *Eur. J. Clin. Invest.*, **10**, 273–9
22. Christiansen, C., Christensen, M.S. and Transbol, I. (1981). Bone mass in postmenopausal women after withdrawal of oestrogen/gestagen replacement therapy. *Lancet*, **1**, 459–61
23. Genant, H.K., Cann, C.E., Ettinger, B. and Gordan, G.S. (1982). Quantitative computed tomography of vertebral spongiosa: a sensitive method for detecting early bone loss after oophorectomy. *Ann. Intern. Med.*, **97**, 699–705
24. Christiansen, C., Christensen, M.S., Larsen, N.-E. and Transbol, I. (1982). Pathophysiological mechanisms of estrogen effect on bone metabolism. Dose–response relationships in early postmenopausal women. *J. Clin. Endocrinol. Metab.*, **55**, 1124–30
25. Garnett, T., Savvas, M. and Studd, J.W.W. (1990). Reversal of bone loss with percutaneous oestrogens. In Drife, J.O. and Studd, J.W.W. (eds.) *HRT and Osteoporosis. Proceedings of the 22nd Study Group of the Royal College of Obstetricians and Gynaecologists.*, pp. 295–306 (London: Springer–Verlag)
26. Drife, J.O. (1990). Premenopausal therapy. In Drife, J.O. and Studd, J.W.W. (eds.) *HRT and Osteoporosis. Proceedings of the 22nd Study Group of the Royal College of Obstetricians and Gynaecologists.*, pp. 251–7 (London: Springer–Verlag)
27. Drife, J.O. and Studd, J.W.W. (eds.) *HRT and Osteoporosis. Proceedings of the 22nd Study Group of the Royal College of Obstetricians and Gynaecologists.* (London: Springer–Verlag)

11

Hormone replacement therapy and the implications for the oncologist

I. Burn

There is little doubt that the use of hormone replacement therapy can be of great help in alleviating certain unpleasant symptoms which are associated with the climacteric and the menopause. There is good evidence also that the use of hormone replacement therapy is protective against certain types of heart disease in middle-aged women, although there may be other ways of achieving the same benefit more safely. Stopping smoking is one obvious way, and the high incidence of this dangerous habit in young women is to be deprecated. Similarly, the role of hormone replacement therapy in protecting against osteoporosis in elderly women is by no means clear. If such therapy is to have a role, it would seem probable that it would have to be given for many years. This would suggest that, if used for this purpose, it should be given selectively. Accurate methods of prediction of pathological osteoporosis are needed, therefore, and this should be a priority.

The influence of hormone activity on malignant disease has been demonstrated in many organs. Cancers of the adrenal, breast, kidney, ovary, pituitary, prostate, skin and thyroid are examples, and there are others. Sometimes these effects can be exploited to the benefit of the patient. Sometimes the effect is adverse. As long ago as 1975, Smith and his colleagues showed the association between unopposed exogenous oestrogens and endometrial carcinomas, and this would now seem to be irrefutable[1]. Smith reported the risk of endometrial cancer as being 4.5 times greater in women with intact uteri exposed to oestrogen therapy.

The breast poses particular problems, however. Unfortunately, Britain has one of the highest incidences and death rates from breast cancer in the world. Bruning and his colleagues from Holland[2] recorded an age-adjusted death rate in England and Wales from breast cancer, in 1980–81, of 34.3 per 100 000 population, compared with 32.3 in the Netherlands and 6.4 in Japan. Not only is the incidence of the disease very worrying, but its impact on society is a major medical problem. Breast cancer is a particularly unpleasant disease.

ENDOGENOUS HORMONES AND THE BREAST

The breast is an important target for endogenous hormonal activity. The physiology of the breast is highly complex, involving multiple endocrine activity. Imbalance in this activity may lead to a variety of benign mammary disorders. Cystic mastopathy, mastalgia and excessive premenstrual nodularity are examples of benign disorders which represent malfunction of this hormone balance[3]. Oestrogens play a major role in this activity and it is significant that benign mammary disorders of this sort are unusual after the menopause.

HORMONES AND BREAST CANCER

One of the first laboratory studies on the effect of hormones on the human breast cancer *in vitro* demonstrated the stimulatory effect of oestrogen (17β-oestradiol). In only a few instances was there inhibition of the cell cultures[4]. More recently, Williams and Dickerson[5] have summarized the experimental evidence which supports the concept that oestrogens play a significant role in the development and progression of human breast cancer. The evidence is very convincing. Schoental[6], who has studied the effect of oestrogenic agents extensively in animals, maintained that such agents have a dual action. Although they are essential for the adequate functioning of the mammalian body, too little or too much is deleterious.

HIGH-RISK FACTORS

Reference to known high-risk factors for breast cancer shows that many have a hormonal basis. Late menopause, low androgen excretion, nulliparity, late first full-term pregnancy and history of recurrent mammary dysplasia are in this category.

The past history of benign breast disease and subsequent risk of breast cancer has been the subject of numerous reports in the past few years. Dupont and Page[7] report a relative risk of breast cancer of 1.6 in women who have undergone breast biopsy revealing benign proliferative disease. If there is also atypical hyperplasia, the risk rises to 4.4. For women with a family history of breast cancer and atypical hyperplasia on biopsy, the risk is 11.0, a very worrying figure. Dupont & Page[7] also quote the College of American Pathologists consensus on the precancerous nature of fibrocystic disease of the breast. In particular, reference is made to the high risk of atypical hyperplasia (4–5 times) and carcinoma *in situ* (8–10 times).

With regard to aggressive epithelium, there is a risk of this being detected in young women (aged 20–29) who have been using an oral contraceptive for some years, as was reported previously at a conference on the subject of oral contraceptives and breast cancer at the Royal Society of Medicine[8]. Atypical hyperplasia in the breast is rarely seen in young women who have not been taking an oral contraceptive.

HORMONAL TREATMENT OF BREAST CANCER

Much of the treatment of breast cancer, especially of advanced disease, depends upon the manipulation of hormonal activity. The techniques used are well known, and mostly they consist of methods designed to lower oestrogen activity. For younger patients, removal of the ovaries was, at one time, a popular and valuable method of inducing a regression. Other methods, such as the use of androgens and surgical adrenalectomy were also successful because of their anti-oestrogen effect. Nowadays, the agent tamoxifen (Nolvadex ®) has become standard treatment for both younger and menopausal patients. Although the precise way that this agent works – and it can be very effective – remains unclear, it can realistically be regarded as an anti-oestrogen.

Emphasizing the important role of antigens in the behaviour of breast cancer is the relationship between the level of oestrogen receptor activity and the chance of a favourable response to anti-oestrogen therapy. More than any other factor, the levels of intrinsic receptor activity differentiate between responders and non-responders.

HORMONE REPLACEMENT THERAPY

All the evidence concerning the pathogenesis and behaviour of breast cancer indicates that, in the main, oestrogens have an unfavourable role. There must be concern, therefore, over the use of hormone replacement therapy in vulnerable women, especially if the therapy is prolonged unopposed oestrogen. Certain precautions are necessary.

First, a careful history should be taken, with particular reference to high-risk factors for breast cancer. Those women who have a strong family history of breast cancer, who have had their first child after the age of 35 years, or who are nulliparous, are at extra risk for breast cancer. Where there is a history of previous atypical hyperplasia on breast biopsy, then the use of hormone replacement therapy is hard to justify unless the need is exceptional. Where there is previous history of treated cancer of the breast, then hormone replacement therapy should be avoided. It is not just a question of enhancement of existing occult metastases, but of the increased risk of cancer in the remaining breast. Likewise, hormone replacement therapy should be avoided if there is a history of *in situ* carcinoma.

Second, there must be a careful examination of the breasts before any woman starts hormone replacement therapy. This includes thorough clinical examination of the breasts as well as mammography, looking for any evidence of benign or malignant disease.

If there is evidence of existing benign disease of the breast, then hormone replacement therapy should be avoided until the condition has been assessed thoroughly and treated appropriately. The likelihood of hormone replacement therapy aggravating the condition is considerable. It is also clear that patients with a past history of benign mammary disease risk a recurrence of the problem with the use of hormone replacement therapy.

Unfortunately, breast cancer is very common in menopausal women in

Britain. The results of screening for the disease during the past decade indicate the prevalence of occult disease in the community. It is essential, therefore, that every effort is made to ensure that no woman in whom the use of hormone replacement therapy is contemplated already has an occult carcinoma of the breast. Pretreatment mammography is essential, therefore, as well as meticulous clinical examination. If there is any doubt that a lesion is present, then hormone replacement therapy should not be used under any circumstances because of its likely enhancement effect.

As well as its ability to reveal any previously undetected breast cancer, mammography may also show a pattern which is compatible with an increased risk of breast cancer. In these latter patients, also, it is questionable whether the use of hormone replacement therapy is justified.

Third, for those women being treated with hormone replacement therapy, it is essential that arrangements are made for clinical examination of the breasts twice a year, with a mammographic examination every 2 years. It is the responsibility of those prescribing hormone replacement therapy to ensure this. Any evidence of the development of a breast disorder during hormone replacement therapy should result in the immediate reappraisal of its need. If continued study of the relationship of hormone replacement therapy to breast cancer reveals an unacceptable risk, then the entire use of this form of medication must be brought into question, unless given on a highly selective basis.

REFERENCES

1. Smith, D.C., Prentice, R., Thompson, D.J. and Hermann, W.L. (1975). Association of exogenous oestrogens and endometrial carcinoma. *N. Engl. J. Med.*, **293**, 1164–7
2. Bruning, P.F., Bonfrer, J.N.J., Ansink, A., Russell, N.S. and de Jong-Bakker, M. (1988). Why is breast cancer so frequent in the Netherlands? *Eur. J. Surg. Oncol.*, **14**, 115–22
3. Burn, I. (1988). The breast. In Elder, M.J. (ed.) *Reproduction, Obstetrics and Gynaecology*, pp. 221–39. (Edinburgh: Heinemann)
4. Moduszewska, O., Koszarowski, T. and Gorski, C. (1968). The influence of hormones on breast cancer *in vitro* in relation to the clinical course of the disease. In Forrest, A. and Kunkler, P. (eds.) *Prognostic Factors in Breast Cancer*, pp. 347–53. (Edinburgh: Livingstone)
5. Williams, C.M. and Dickerson, J.W.J. (1987). Dietary fat, hormones and breast cancer: the cell membrane as a possible site of interaction of these two risk factors. *Eur. J. Surg. Oncol.*, **13**, 89–104
6. Schoental, R. (1985). Zearaleone, its biological and pathological effects in rodents: implications for humans. In Moss and Frank (eds.) *Proceedings of the 5th Meeting on Mycotoxins in Animal and Human Health*, pp. 62–72. (University of Surrey)
7. Dupont, W.D. and Page, D.L. (1989). Relationship to previous breast disease. In Stoll, B. (ed.) Women at High Risk to Breast Cancer, pp. 47–56. (Kluwer Academic)
8. Burn, I. (1990). General discussion. In Mann, R.D. (ed.) *Oral Contraceptives and Breast Cancer*, pp. 111–12. (Carnforth, UK: Parthenon Publishing)

12

Breast cancer: improved prognosis in hormone users and decreased incidence in oestrogen–progestogen users

R.D. Gambrell, Jr

INTRODUCTION

Women fear breast cancer and rightly so, since carcinoma of the breast will strike one in nine women in the United States. It is the most frequent malignancy in females, accounting for 32% of all cancers[1]. Until 1988, it was also the leading cause of death from cancer in women, causing 18% of all female cancer deaths in the United States. Lung cancer mortality, 22% of all female cancer deaths, is expected to exceed breast cancers deaths in 1992 with 53 000 women dying from this tumour. The American Cancer Society estimates that 180 000 new cases of breast carcinoma will be diagnosed in the United States during 1992 and that 46 000 women will die from this tumour this year. Although the number of breast cancers diagnosed increase every year due to earlier detection by increased use of mammography and the ageing population, the good news is that the percentage increase in number of deaths has steadily declined for the past 4 years, from 4.8% in 1987 to 1.1% in 1991. Mortality from breast cancer varies around the world from a high of 36.0/100 000 in England and Wales to a low of 6.5/100 000 in Ecudador. The mortality from breast cancer in the United States is 27.4/100 000, which ranks 15th in the world.

The frequency of breast cancer increases continuously until very late in the female life-span (Figure 1)[2]. In this respect, the incidence of this malignancy differs from cervical, endometrial and ovarian cancer, which peak by age in the 40s, 50s and 60s, respectively, and then either decline or plateau. The sharpest increase in mammary malignancy incidence occurs between the mid-30s and early 50s, or just before the menopause. The incidence then continues to rise steeply throughout the postmenopausal years, when oestrogen levels are lower but not absent. However, few (if any) postmenopausal women produce any significant amounts of progesterone.

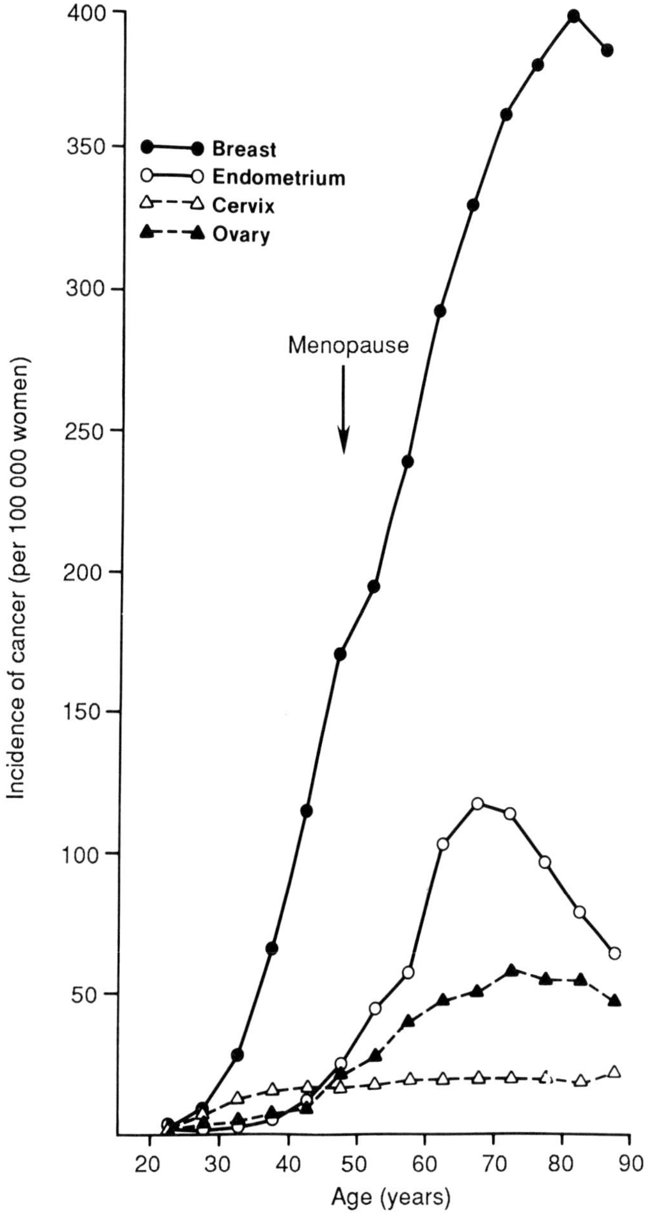

Figure 1 Incidence of breast, endometrial, cervical and ovarian cancer in women by age. (Data from the National Cancer Institute[2], Surveillance, Epidemiology and End Results (SEER), 1981–1985)

IMPROVED PROGNOSIS OF BREAST CANCER IN POSTMENOPAUSAL HORMONE USERS

During the 10-year period from 1972–1981, 461 patients had carcinoma of the breast either diagnosed at Wilford Hall US Air Force Medical Center, or were referred there for therapy. This included 202 premenopausal women (43.8%) and 3 males (0.7%); however, 256 were postmenopausal (55.5%). Hormone use at the time malignancy was diagnosed is listed in Table 1. Of these 256 patients, 63 (24.6%) were using some type of female sex steroid when the breast cancer was diagnosed, including 50 women (19.5%) using unopposed oestrogens and eight (3.1%) who were also using added progestogen. There were three oestrogen vaginal cream users and two patients were being treated with injectable progestogens to relieve vasomotor symptoms secondary to a surgical menopause. There were 21 patients (8.2%) who gave a past history of oestrogen use and seven women (2.7%) who had used oral contraceptives, most of them in the distant past. However, 165 of these 256 postmenopausal women (64.%) had never taken any type of female sex steroid.

Now, with 9 to 18 years of follow-up, 121 of these 256 postmenopausal women with carcinoma of the breast have died, an overall mortality of 47.3% (Table 1). Of the women using some type of hormone when the malignancy was diagnosed, 19 of 63 have expired (30.2%) compared to 85 of the 165 non-hormone users (51.5%). The mortality in the 50 unopposed oestrogen users was 32.0% and only two of the eight oestrogen–progestogen users have died (25.0%); both of the progestogen users are living, after well over 10 years since diagnosis of breast cancer.

Because axillary node status is one of the most reliable prognostic indicators in breast cancer, patients were grouped into the following three groups: negative nodes, one to three positive nodes, and four or more positive nodes[3]. Axillary node status in hormone users at the time of definitive surgery for carcinoma of the breast is listed in Table 2. Of the 256 patients, 117 had negative nodes (45.7%), 50 had one to three positive nodes (19.5%) and 89 (34.8%) had four or more positive nodes (34.8%). In a comparison of the 63 hormone users and the 165 untreated women, 36 of the hormone users had negative nodes (57.1%) while 69 of the non-users also had negative

Table 1 Hormonal therapy at diagnosis and mortality of breast cancer

Therapy group	*Number of patients*	*Number of deaths*	*Mortality (%)*
Total hormone users	63	19	30.2
oestrogen users	50	16	32.0
oestrogen–progestogen users	8	2	25.0
oestrogen vaginal cream users	3	1	33.3
progestogen users	2	0	—
Past history of oestrogen use	21	12	57.1
Past history of oral contraceptive use	7	5	71.4
Non-users	165	85	51.5
Total patients	256	121	47.3

Table 2 Axillary nodes according to hormone therapy at treatment of breast cancer

Therapy group	*Number of patients*	*With negative nodes*		*With 1–3 positive nodes*		*With ≥ 4 positive nodes*	
		Number	(%)	*Number*	(%)	*Number*	(%)
Total hormone users	63	36	(57.1)	11	(17.5)	16	(25.4)
oestrogen users	50	28	(56.0)	9	(18.0)	13	(26.0)
oestrogen–progestogen users	8	5	(62.5)	2	(25.0)	1	(12.5)
oestrogen vaginal cream users	3	1	(33.3)	0	—	2	(66.7)
progestogen users	2	2	(100.0)	0	—	0	—
Past history of oestrogen use	21	10	(47.6)	5	(23.8)	6	(28.6)
Past history of oral contraceptive use	7	2	(28.6)	0	—	5	(71.4)
Non-users	165	69	(41.8)	34	(20.6)	62	(37.6)
Total patients	256	117	(45.7)	50	(19.5)	89	(34.8)

nodes (41.8%), which was statistically significant ($p \leq 0.05$). More of the non-users (37.6%) had four or more positive nodes than either the total hormone users (25.4%) or the subgroup of unopposed oestrogen users (26.0%); however, none of these differences were statistically significant. This clearly indicates that in this patient population, hormone users have earlier detection of their malignancy. This probably reflects both patient awareness as well as rapid reaction to any suspicious lesion by their physician, but are there still other factors involved in the improved prognosis of the hormone users?

Another prognostic indication in survival from breast cancer is the presence of oestradiol and progesterone receptors in cancerous tissue[4]. The presence of both oestrogen and progesterone receptors predicts a 70% chance of favourable response to endocrine manipulation and is related to a longer disease-free interval and decreased mortality. Tumours in 139 of these 256 postmenopausal women were assayed for both oestrogen and progesterone receptors and the results are shown in Table 3. When both the oestrogen receptor and progesterone receptors were positive, 83.3% of these women survived for 9–18 years after surgical treatment for carcinoma of the breast, while 16.7% have expired. When both receptors were negative, only 46.3% are living to date while 53.7% have died. Table 4 indicates the hormone receptor status in the tumours of current users, past users and non-users. More of the current hormone users (64.7%) had tumours positive for both oestrogen and progesterone receptors (ER+/PgR+) than either the past users (43.8%) or non-users (34.8%), which was statistically significant ($p \leq 0.05$). So the presence of progesterone receptors in the mammary cancers of the hormone users seems to be an additional factor that improved their prognosis.

Table 3 Prognosis of breast cancer according to hormone receptors. ER = oestrogen receptor; PgR = progesterone receptor

	Living and well		*Expired*		
Receptors	*Number*	(%)	*Number*	(%)	*Total*
ER+/PgR+	50	(83.3)	10	(16.7)	60
ER+/PgR−	20	(52.6)	18	(47.4)	38
ER−/PgR−	19	(46.3)	22	(53.7)	41
Total patients	89	(64.0)	50	(36.0)	139

Table 4 Oestradiol/progesterone receptors in hormone users vs. non-users. ER = oestrogen receptor; PgR = progesterone receptor

		ER+/PgR+		*EGR+/PgR−*		*ER−/PgR−*	
Therapy group	*Number of patients*	*Number*	(%)	*Number*	(%)	*Number*	(%)
Current users	34	22	(64.7)*	3	(8.8)	9	(26.5)
Past users	16	7	(43.8)	2	(12.5)	7	(43.8)
Non-users	89	31	(34.8)	33	(37.1)	25	(28.1)
Total patients	139	60	(43.2)	38	(27.3)	41	(29.5)

*Current users had significantly higher PgR+ than either the past users or non-users ($p \leq 0.05$)

In the same month the Swedish study was published, purporting to show an increased risk of breast cancer in oestrogen users[5], this same group published another paper, utilizing the same database, where they observed a significantly higher survival rate in breast cancer patients who had received oestrogen treatment[6]. Their report confirmed several earlier studies, with none to the contrary, indicating an improved prognosis for breast cancer developing in oestrogen users. Burch and co-workers were the first, in 1976, to observe a 25% reduction in mortality from breast cancer when this malignancy developed in oestrogen users followed for 15 years[7]. In our original report of the 256 postmenopausal women with breast cancer followed for 2–8 years, the mortality was 22.2% in the 63 hormone users, compared to a death rate of 45.5% in the 165 non-users, which was statistically significant ($p \leq 0.005$)[3]. A study from West Germany observed a 20% reduction in mortality from breast cancer developing in hormone users[8]. In a study from England of 4544 hormone users, the mortality from breast cancer was significantly reduced (relative risk (RR), 0.55; 95% confidence interval (CI), 0.28–0.96)[9]. The Swedish study observed a significant reduction in mortality from mammary malignancy developing in oestrogen users (RR, 0.68; 95% CI, 0.52–0.87)[6]. The lowest risk was in the current users (RR, 0.54; 95% CI, 0.34–0.86). The Nurses' Health Study also observed a reduction in mortality from carcinoma of the breast developing in oestrogen users, although this was not statistically significant (RR, 0.82; 95% CI, 0.64–1.05)[10]. Likewise, the study from Leisure World observed a non-significant reduction in death from breast cancer developing in oestrogen users (RR, 0.81)[11].

REDUCTION IN RISK FOR BREAST CANCER

The role of hormone replacement therapy in reducing the risk of carcinoma of the breast is more controversial. Progestogens are not added to oestrogen replacement to reduce the increased risk from oestrogen therapy, since oestrogen replacement does not increase the risk of breast cancer. Two recent meta-analyses provide strong evidence that menopausal therapy consisting of 0.625 mg daily of conjugated oestrogens does not increase breast cancer risk[12,13]. A third meta-analysis did find a very slight increased risk of breast cancer after 15 years of oestrogen therapy (RR, 1.3; 95% CI, 1.2–2.6)[14]. However, this was based on only 16 of the more than 45 studies that have been published. They rejected several studies for various reasons, including all follow-up studies, and stated in the abstract that the increase in risk was largely due to studies that included premenopausal women or women using oestradiol. Most of the 16 studies they analysed did not extend 15 years. After eliminating studies showing a decreased risk, they mathematically extrapolated the risk each year out to 15 years to arrive finally at the relative risk of 1.3, an assumption shown not to be true[10].

During the 9 years of prospective study at Wilford Hall US Air Force Medical Center, the overall incidence of breast cancer in 5563 postmenopausal women was 141.8/100 000 women per year (Table 5)[15]. The lowest incidence was observed in the oestrogen–progestogen users at 66.8/100 000 per year

Table 5 Incidence of breast cancer at Wilford Hall US Air Force Medical Center: 1975–1983

Therapy group	*Patient-years of observation*	*Patients with cancer*	*Incidence (per 100 000)*
Oestrogen–progestogen users	16 466	11	66.8
Unopposed oestrogen users	19 676	28	142.3
Oestrogen vaginal cream users	4 298	5	116.3
Progestogen users	1 825	3	164.4
Non-users	6 404	22	343.5
Total patients	48 669	69	141.8

(RR, 0.3; 95% CI, 0.1–0.8). However, the incidence of mammary malignancy was not increased in the unopposed oestrogen users but slightly decreased to 142.3/100 000 (RR, 0.7; 95% CI, 0.5–1.1), similar to the findings in many of the case–control studies. The incidence of breast cancer in the progestogen users of 164.4/100 000 was almost that expected (RR, 0.8; 95% CI, 0.5–1.7). The reason for the non-decrease in the progestogen users was that a patient either has to have near-normal endogenous oestrogen production or be using oestrogen therapy to induce progesterone receptors in mammary tissue before the beneficial effect of the added progestogen is observed. There was a significant increase in the incidence of breast cancer in the non-users to 343.5/100 000 (RR, 1.4; 95% CI, 1.1–1.9). This was a biased group of patients, since hormone therapy was withheld from many because of risk factors such as family history of breast cancer, benign breast disease, low parity and previous breast biopsies.

The data from this study are shown graphically, by year, in Figure 2. The most striking feature of this graph is that seven of the 11 oestrogen–progestogen users were diagnosed during the first 4 years of study, with only four additional cancers diagnosed during the last 5 years, including two past users who had been off therapy for up to 6 years. The incidence of breast cancer in the unopposed oestrogen users remained relatively constant throughout the entire 9 years. Overall, the incidence of breast carcinoma increased slightly from 143.4/100 000 in 1975 to a high of 183.8/100 000 during 1978, followed by significant decreases to 104.2/100 000 in 1980 and 110.4/100 000 during 1981, and finally down to 53.9/100 000 in the continuing users during 1983.

The concept of adding progestogens to oestrogen replacement was introduced at Wilford Hall in 1971. Figure 3 compares the number of oestrogen- and oestrogen–progestogen-treated women with the incidence of breast cancer for the 12 years from 1972–1983. With ever-increasing oestrogen use from approximately 1320 patients in 1972 to 3940 oestrogen-treated women during 1975, there was no increase in the incidence of mammary malignancy. The apparent decline in the incidence of breast carcinoma from 189.4/100 000 in 1972 to 143.4/100 000 during 1976 was not statistically significant. However, with ever-increasing progestogen usage from approximately 9.1% of the oestrogen users in 1972 to 61.1% of the oestrogen users in 1983, a significant decrease in the incidence of breast cancer occurred in the 9th and 10th years of study, from 183.8/100 000 in 1978 to 104.3/100 000 in 1980 and

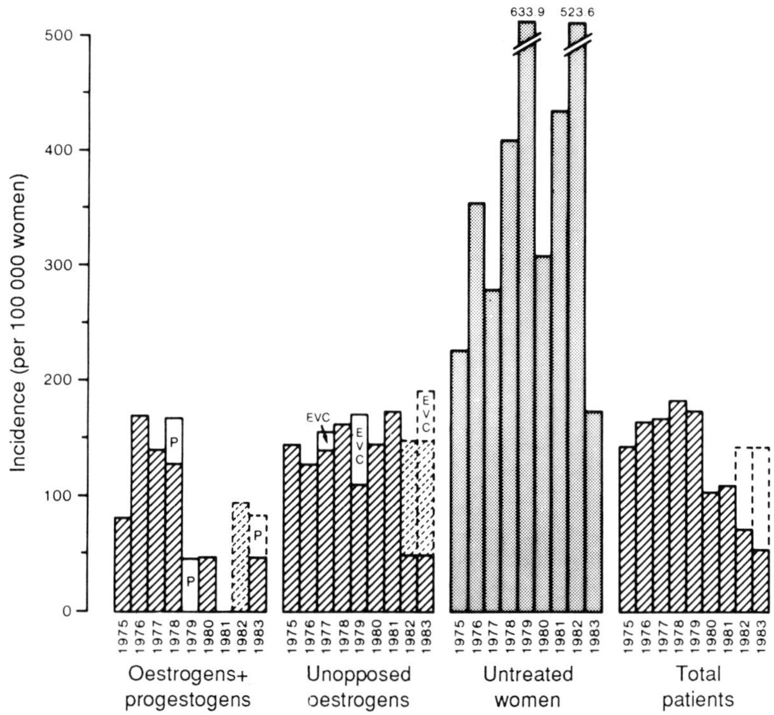

Figure 2 Incidence of breast cancer by year in hormone users compared with that in the untreated women. P = progestogen users; EVC = oestrogen vaginal cream users; solid lines indicate current users and dotted lines former users. (Reproduced from Gambrell[15] with permission of the publisher)

110.4/100 000 during 1981, and finally down to 53.9/100 000 women in the continuing users during 1983.

Table 6 shows the relative risk for breast cancer in 1087 women treated with hormone replacement for the 12 years from 1978–1990. The incidence rates used for calculation are from the Surveillance, Epidemiology and End Results National Cancer Institute data from 1981–1985[2]. There were six cases of breast cancer and all had received oestrogen–progestogen therapy. However, only three of these patients had progestogen added to their oestrogen replacement for more than 5 years. With six cases observed compared to an expected 27, the relative risk for breast cancer in the hormone users was 0.22.

Of the five studies evaluating oestrogen–progestogen use and breast cancer, the three long-term studies of 10–12 years observed significantly decreased risks, while the two shorter-term case–control studies found non-significant increased risks[3,5,8,16,17]. In the New York study there were four breast cancers in the 84 placebo users followed for 10 years with none in the 84 oestrogen–progestogen users, which was statistically significant ($p \leq 0.05$)[16]. In the study from Germany, the incidence of mammary malignancy in the

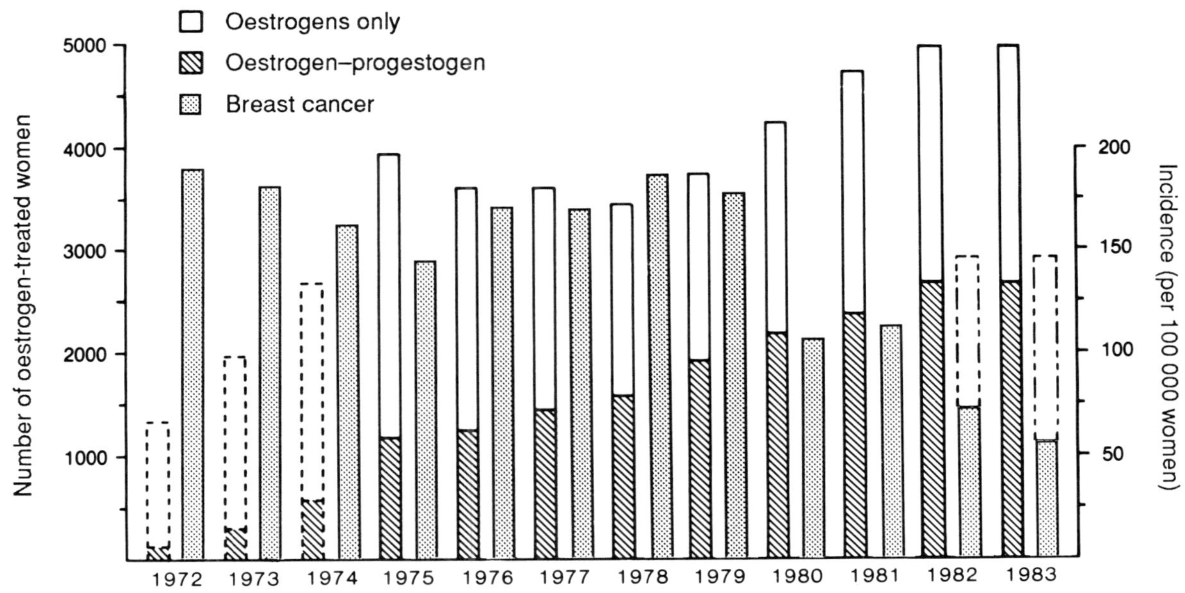

Figure 3 Comparison of the number of oestrogen and oestrogen–progestogen-treated women with the incidence of breast cancer from 1972 to 1983. Dotted lines (1972–1974) indicate estimated data from computerized pharmacy records; solid lines show data from prospective and follow-up studies; broken lines (1982 and 1983) indicate former users. (Reproduced from Gambrell[15] with permission of the publisher)

Table 6 Relative risk of breast cancer in hormone users at the Medical College of Georgia: 1978–1990

Age-range	*Patient-years of observation*	*Incidence* per* 100 000	*Expected cases*	*Observed cases*	*Relative risk*
20–24	276	1.1	0.003	0	0
25–29	252	8.4	0.02	0	0
30–34	432	27.5	0.66	0	0
35–39	996	66.0	1.14	0	0
40–44	1 680	114.6	1.93	0	0
45–49	2 016	169.8	3.42	0	0
50–54	2 064	194.6	4.02	1	0.25
55–59	2 028	244.3	4.95	1	0.20
60–64	1 512	292.2	4.42	1	0.23
65–69	708	331.5	2.35	3	1.28
70–74	660	363.3	2.39	0	0
75–79	204	380.2	0.78	0	0
80–84	192	397.3	0.76	0	0
> 85	24	386.1	0.09	0	0
Total	13 044		26.93	6	0.22

*SEER: 1981–1985

oestrogen–progestogen users (109/100 000) was significantly lower ($p \leq 0.05$) when compared to the non-users (154/100 000)[8]. There was also a slight reduction of breast cancer in the unopposed oestrogen users followed for 10 years (123/100 000). Both the Swedish and Danish studies found non-significantly increased risk of breast carcinoma in oestrogen–progestogen users (RR, 4.4; 95% CI, 0.9–22.4[5] and RR, 1.36; 95% CI, 0.98–1.87[17]). The Swedish study was based on only ten patients with 6–9 years of oestrogen–progestogen use and the methodology employed has been widely criticized[18–21]. It was not until the 9th and 10th years of ever-increasing addition of progestogens to oestrogen replacement that a decreased incidence of breast cancer was observed in the Wilford Hall studies (Figure 3).

FACTORS RELATED TO THE RISK OF BREAST CANCER

Carcinoma of the breast is not primarily a hormonal disorder but is more related to genetic predisposition, such as a family history of breast cancer, especially a mother or sister, and to a lesser extent, a grandmother or an aunt. It is also related to diet, such as high fat and low fibre intake. Smoking and alcohol use may also increase the risk of this malignancy, as does age. Fragments of information are now beginning to fall into place to show some of the hormonal relationships to breast carcinoma. Hormones or hormonal deficiency may serve as cofactors or predisposing factors, perhaps even promoting agents, since at least four studies have shown an increased risk of breast cancer in women with long-term progesterone deficiency[22–25]. Megestrol acetate, a C-21 progestogen, is used to treat metastatic breast cancer in the United States. Comparative trials between tamoxifen and medroxyprogesterone acetate indicate that progestogens are just as effective as the anti-oestrogen tamoxifen in the treatment of metastatic breast cancer[26]. One of the most effective therapies for Stage IV metastatic carcinoma of the breast at the M.D. Anderson Cancer Center is a combination of oestrogen and progestogens[27]. Seven days of oestrogen are given to enhance progesterone receptors in mammary cancer cells followed by 21 days of high-dosage medroxyprogesterone acetate in repeated cycles. The objective remission response was 56.7% for up to 6 years with a medium duration of 22 months. Yet it is ironic that this progestogen, as well as all other progestogens except megestrol acetate, remain listed as contraindicated in women with breast cancer in the United States.

In our Wilford Hall US Air Force Medical Center studies, no reduction in the incidence of breast cancer was observed in the progestogen users (164.4/100 000), only in the oestrogen–progestogen users (66.8/100 000) (Table 5). The reasons for this were that a patient has either to be producing normal endogenous oestrogen or using oestrogen therapy to induce progesterone receptors in mammary tissue before the beneficial effect of progestogen is manifested. Oral contraceptives significantly reduce the incidence of benign breast disease. This has been shown in multiple studies, and the longer the duration of birth control pill use, the greater the reduction in benign breast disease. Both oral contraceptives and progestogens reverse both intraductal hyperplasia and atypia of the breast in the majority of patients and reduce the expected incidence of invasive carcinoma[28]. Progesterone protects against hyperstimulation of the breast by down-regulation of oestrogen receptor levels, increasing intracellular metabolism of oestrogen, and reducing mitosis while inducing epithelial differentiation.

If the ever-increasing incidence of breast cancer by age is closely examined (Figure 1), the role of female sex steroids becomes clarified. The greatest increase in breast cancer by age is between the late 30s and early 50s. What happens at this time in women's lives is declining production of oestrogen from the ovaries as menopause is approached. More important is the fact that more women become anovulatory in the late premenopausal years, resulting in an abrupt cessation of cyclic progesterone levels present throughout the reproductive years. The incidence of breast cancer continues to increase until very late in the postmenopausal years when oestrogen levels are lower but not absent. However, few postmenopausal women, if any, produce progesterone. If unopposed oestrogens were strongly related to carcinoma of the breast, the incidence of this malignancy would peak in the 50s and 60s and decline thereafter, as does the incidence of endometrial cancer. Whatever the role of female sex steroids as cofactors, predisposing factors or promoters for carcinoma of the breast, progesterone deficiency seems to be one of the many factors in this multifactorial disorder.

SUMMARY AND CONCLUSIONS

Our data indicate that when breast cancer develops in hormone users, they have an improved prognosis. This was due not only to earlier detection because of closer surveillance but also because significantly more hormone users had both positive oestrogen and progesterone receptors in their tumours. This confirms seven previous studies, with none to the contrary, that there is an improved survival from breast cancer developing in hormone users[3,6–11]. Whenever oestrogen replacement is prescribed, progestogens should be added for 10–13 days each month, even in women who have had a hysterectomy. This is confirmed by the long-term prospective studies of 9 years or more, which observed significantly reduced risks of breast cancer in oestrogen–progestogen users[8,15,16], while the shorter-term case–control studies found non-significant increased risks[5,17].

REFERENCES

1. American Cancer Society (1991). Cancer statistics, 1991. *Ca–A Cancer J. Clinic.*, **41**, 19–36
2. *Annual Cancer Statistics Review* (1987). NIH Publication No. 88-2789, p.III 36 (Bethesda: National Institutes of Health)
3. Gambrell, R.D., Jr (1984). Proposal to decrease the risk and improve the prognosis of breast cancer. *Am. J. Obstet. Gynecol.*, **150**, 119–32
4. Clarke, G.M., McGuire, W.L., Hubay, C.A., Pearson, O.H. and Marshall, J.S. (1983). Progesterone receptor as a prognostic factor in Stage II breast cancer. *N. Engl. J. Med.*, **309**, 1343–7
5. Bergkvist, L., Adami, H.-O., Persson, I., Hoover, R. and Schairer, C. (1989). The risk of breast cancer after estrogen and estrogen–progestin replacement. *N. Engl. J. Med.*, **321**, 293–7
6. Bergkvist, L., Adami, H.-O., Persson, I., Bergstrom, R. and Krusemo, B. (1989). Prognosis after breast cancer diagnosis in women exposed to estrogen and estrogen–progestogen replacement therapy. *Am. J. Epidemiol.*, **130**, 221–8
7. Burch, J.C., Byrd, B.F., Jr and Vaughn, W.K. (1976). Results of estrogen treatment in one thousand hysterectomized women for 14,318 years. In van Keep, P.A., Greenblatt, R.B. and Albeaux-Fernet, M. (eds.) *Consensus on Menopause Research*, pp.164–9. (Lancaster: MTP Press Ltd)
8. Lauritzen, C. and Meier, F. (1984). Risks of endometrial and mammary cancer morbidity and mortality in long-term oestrogen treatment. In van Henendael, H., van Henedael, B., Riphagen, F.E., Gorssens, L. and van der Pas, H. (eds.) *Climacteric – An Update*, pp.207–16. (Lancaster, England: MTP Press Ltd)
9. Hunt, K., Vessey, M., MacPherson, K. and Coleman, M. (1987). Long-term surveillance of mortality and cancer incidence in women receiving hormone replacement therapy. *Br. J. Obstet. Gynecol.*, **94**, 620–35
10. Colditz, G.A., Stampfer, M.J., Willett, W.C., Hennekens, C.H., Rosner, B. and Speizer, F.E. (1990). Prospective study of estrogen replacement therapy and risk of breast cancer in postmenopausal women. *J. Am. Med. Assoc.*, **264**, 2648–53
11. Henderson, B.E., Paganini-Hill, A. and Ross, R.K. (1991). Decreased mortality in users of estrogen replacement therapy. *Arch. Intern. Med.*, **151**, 75–8
12. Armstrong, B.K. (1988). Oestrogen therapy after the menopause – boon or bane? *Med. J. Aust.*, **148**, 213–4
13. Dupont, W.D. and Page, D.L. (1991). Menopausal estrogen therapy and breast cancer. *Arch. Int. Med.*, **151**, 67–72
14. Steinberg, K.K., Thacker, S.B., Smith, S.J., Stroupe, D.F., Zack, M.M., Flanders, W.D. and Berkelman, R.L. (1991). A meta-analysis of the effect of estrogen replacement therapy on the risk of breast cancer. *J. Am. Med. Assoc.*, **265**, 1985–90
15. Gambrell, R.D., Jr (1986). Role of progestogens in the prevention of breast cancer. *Maturitas*, **8**, 169–76
16. Nachtigall, L.E., Nachtigall, R.H., Nachtigall, R.B. and Beckman, E.M. (1979). Estrogen replacement: II. A prospective study in the relationship to carcinoma and cardiovascular and metabolic problems. *Obstet. Gynecol.*, **54**, 74–9

17. Ewertz, M. (1988). Influence of noncontraceptive exogenous and endogenous sex hormones on breast cancer risk in Denmark. *Int. J. Cancer*, **42**, 832–8
18. Speroff, L. (1990). Breast cancer and postmenopausal hormone therapy. *Contemp. Obstet. Gynecol.*, **71**, 71–82
19. Cutler, W.B. (1990). Hormone replacement therapy and the risk of breast cancer. *Infect. Surg.*, **9**, 10–13
20. Gambrell, R.D., Jr (1990). Editorial: Estrogen therapy and breast cancer. *Int. J. Fertil.*, **35**, 202–4
21. Barrett-Conner, E. (1989). Editorial: Postmenopausal estrogen replacement and breast cancer. *N. Engl. J. Med.*, **321**, 319–20
22. Coulan, C.B. and Annegers, J.F. (1983). Chronic anovulation may increase postmenopausal breast cancer risk. *J. Am. Med. Assoc.*, **249**, 445–7
23. Cowan, L.D., Gordis, L., Tonascia, J.A. and Jones, G.S. (1981). Breast cancer incidence in women with a history of progesterone deficiency. *Am. J. Epidemiol.*, **114**, 209–17
24. Mauvis-Jarvis, P., Sitruk-Ware, R. and Kutten, F. (1982). Luteal phase defect and breast cancer genesis. *Breast Cancer Res. Treat.*, **2**, 139–47
25. Ron, E., Lunenfeld, B., Menczer, J., Blumstein, T., Katz, L., Oesner, G. and Serr. D. (1987). Cancer incidence in a cohort of infertile women. *Am. J. Epidemiol.*, **125**, 780–90
26. Buzdar, A.U. (1988). Progestins in cancer treatment. In Stoll, B.A. (ed.) *Endocrine Management of Cancer*, pp.1–15. (Basel: Karger)
27. Hortobagyi, G.N., Hug, V., Buzdar, A.U. *et al.* (1989). Sequential cyclic combined hormone therapy for metastatic breast cancer. *Cancer*, **64**, 1002–6
28. Voherr, H. (1986). Oral contraceptives and hormone replacement therapy: are progestogens and progestins breast mitogens? *Am. J. Obstet. Gynecol.*, **155**, 1140–2

General discussion III

(*Chairman: Sir David Innes Williams*)

Sir David Innes Williams Could Dr La Vecchia please tell us for how long most Italian women take HRT when they are in that shorter-term group of the study Dr La Vecchia presented? Is it months or years?

Dr C. La Vecchia Two-thirds of the cases and more than two-thirds of the controls took oestrogens for less than 3 years, and about half the cases for less than 1 year.

Prof. M. Elstein There was a brief allusion to exercise in Prof. Smith's ultimate summary, but no data were given on the effects of sustained exercise on the preservation of bone mineral density. Are there any data, and what implications can be drawn from them?

Prof. M. Smith I purposely did not include any data because the subject of this conference is the association with hormone replacement therapy. To my knowledge, there are quite a lot of data – and even more opinions – on the subject. There has been a lot of very good animal data showing that small amounts of stress on bone will maintain or increase the level of bone mineral.

I cannot give a clear answer because I am not aware of the existence of high quality epidemiological data on women; most of the studies that are available fail to overcome the difficulty of assessing the level of exercise. There are a number of smaller studies, but there has not been a series of definitive studies that have shown us the amount of exercise which is really required to prevent a certain bone loss.

Prof. Elstein Would this excellent audience of epidemiologists be able to cast doubt on the validity of the data from South Africa comparing privileged Whites with Bantu and showing striking differences between them. I would venture an opinion, if I may, that a significant factor in these differences might be exercise, rather than the racial one.

Prof. Smith Quite possibly. The racial factor is quite clear in the populations in the USA, for example, where the exercise factor is likely to be similar between the White and the Black population. I am quoting here the work that has been done in places like Washington, looking at populations. I am not aware of the social class effect. They were not looking at heavy manual labourers in one racial group and not in the other.

Mr H.H. Hamed Regarding the effect of exercise on the maintenance of bone, could we extrapolate from the work done on committed female athletes and rowers who, as is well known, develop amenorrhoea? These women develop significant bone loss, and their vigorous exercise is not sufficient to maintain their normal bone mineral content compared with normally menstruating women.

Prof. Smith I would be wary about drawing conclusions from exceptional groups like that. There may well be an abnormal situation in professional athletes, in terms of either bone mass or body composition. The data from a number of workers have shown a beneficial effect of exercise. The questions are: what level of exercise is necessary to maintain bone? and what type of exercise is most appropriate? I am not aware of reliable data to say what is the minimum level of exercise. There are data to suggest that sensible exercise has a beneficial effect, but I cannot relate that to what level of exercise is correlated to a certain level of bone loss in a normal population. In short, I am aware of studies that have looked at the bone mineral in amenorrhoea but not of any that have related the amenorrhoea to the exercise.

Mr Hamed There have been two studies recently and one was on female rowers with vigorous exercise. The exercise did not compensate for diminished oestrogen levels, and their bone mineral content was definitely lower than in a comparable normal group.

Prof. Smith It may not be possible for the exercise to eliminate it. My concern is about drawing conclusions from exceptional people doing very unusual things.

Mr M. Pugh Professor Smith showed that testosterone gave a benefit in bone construction. In a woman who has had a carcinoma of the breast and therefore cannot take oestrogens, would there be merit in anticipating, or trying to prevent, osteoporosis by using a low-dose testosterone implant as a long-term measure?

Prof. J. Drife The kind of dosage that it is possible to give a woman to provide the psychological benefits without masculinization and hirsutism is low. I do not know whether enough is understood about the dosage threshold on bone to know whether it would be of benefit.

Prof. R.E. Mansel We are talking about giving HRT to people at age 45 but if the impact, in terms of fractures, comes 15 or 20 years later then all of these women will have to be dosed for a very long time. Is it thought that women will take a prophylactic regimen for so long? There is always the problem of compliance with prophylaxis when the benefit is somewhere out in the future and does not affect the individual patient in a way that can be recognized.

Prof. Smith This is a sociological type of question. It depends particularly upon the woman's awareness of the risks of osteoporosis. The National

Osteoporosis Society has tended to increase awareness amongst the population of the risks of osteoporosis. It is correct that the fracture incidence tends to increase, in terms of numbers, around 65 or 70. If prophylactic therapy delays any increase until so late in life that it does not become a problem, or the likelihood of suffering from it is less, it is then a question of the benefits against the risks.

Dr P.E. Belchetz I see a great number of patients and I do not think there is a problem. First, many women see their mothers 20 years on and do not want to get like that. This is a very powerful incentive. Secondly, it does not have to be taken for 20 years. After 10 years there may well be some benefit which, as Prof. Smith showed, then dissipates at the same rate as it would in an untreated person. However, that extra bone mineral is already there, so I think it is clear that benefit can be bought, and many women find an incentive to begin this therapy at the perimenopause.

Mr R. Badwe I entirely agree with Mr Burn regarding the importance of mammography as a safety measure in postmenopausal patients who have been on hormone replacement therapy. I would take the argument a little further. It has been said that 50 is the age limit for differentiating whether or not mammography is effective. The population below the age of 50 (in whom this screening method of diagnosis has not been shown to be very effective in improving survival) and the population beyond the age of 50 (in whom it has been shown to be effective) have an essential difference in terms of the presence or absence of circulating hormones. Fifty is just an age at which we are trying to segregate the presence or absence of hormones, but patients who are on hormone replacement have circulating hormones. Would Mr Burn agree in their case that, as far as mammography detection is concerned, they are similar to those less than 50 years of age? If that is so, how effective will mammography be as a safety measure in patients who have been on hormone replacement?

Mr I. Burn Mammography is a very valuable technique, as I hope I indicated, but it is fallible and, as you say, more fallible in the younger woman than in the truly menopausal patient. Nevertheless, if a woman under 50 is placed on HRT for seemingly very good reasons – which is now happening in women even before they reach the menopause – I would certainly include a mammogram as part of the follow-up programme of surveillance in the way that I have indicated. Having said that, I still regard the clinical examination as the most important aspect of patient care. I do not think mammography should be used in place of clinical examination. We must always be aware of the still unproven risk of too great a use of mammography as itself acting as a carcinogen. The Medical Research Council tried, about 20 years ago, to get some idea about the safety levels of radiation from mammography in the average female breast over a lifetime. I think they came to the conclusion that the absolute upper limit of delivery of radiation to the breast that could be permitted was 80 rad. That is a lot of mammograms these days, but like many of these things we are often wise after the event, are we not? I would not want any patient of mine to have up to 80 rad to a single breast from mammograms, yet I see patients who are going through various clinics and having mammograms at regular intervals. It is not too difficult to reach that target dose. If we start adding mammography in screening for HRT, it will provide quite a dosage of radiation to the breast.

Prof. C.E.D. Chilvers I was very interested in Mr Burn's view that HRT should be avoided in a woman with a previous mastectomy. I can quite see why, but nevertheless this seems to be a problem. Women who are unhappy about having a breast cancer then get even more unhappy because they go through the menopause and have problems. What is the strength of the evidence that HRT is particularly dangerous for them? In this country a randomized trial has recently started looking at the effects of HRT on ovarian cancer.

Mr Burn There is documented evidence of a stimulatory effect of oestrogen on existing carcinoma, both experimental and in clinical experience, some of which I have shown today. Stilboestrol was used for treatment of advanced breast cancer until the advent of tamoxifen, mainly in women over the age of 65, but it was not unusual for it to be given to younger postmenopausal women. The alternative was androgens, which were very unpleasant. Certainly, there was enhancement not infrequently, with metastatic disease actively aggravated so that the treatment had to be stopped very quickly.

There is no doubt that oestrogens can stimulate existing cancer. Unfortunately, any woman who has had breast cancer runs the risk of there being cells in hibernation. The actual event of seeing metastatic disease from breast cancer treated many years ago is not common but does occur.

The other problem is the residual breast. If a woman has had a carcinoma in one breast, the likelihood of developing a carcinoma in the remaining breast is 3–5 times the normal risk, so there is already a major risk factor. This would seem to me a very good reason for being extremely cautious about possibly adding to that risk, even if the factor being added is not great. This is my opinion. I would not wish to see women who have had breast cancer treated with HRT unless there is an overwhelming reason.

Prof. R.E. Mansel I must agree. For instance, autopsy studies show that a silent duct carcinoma *in situ* (DCIS) may exist in 15–20% of women who are totally asymptomatic. To put it another way, we do not know the effect of oestrogen on *in situ* cancer of the breast – there are no data. In fact, we are now starting a trial in which we are proposing to treat it with anti-oestrogens, so it becomes totally illogical to say let us treat the population and see what can be done for DCIS treated with oestrogen.

If the surveillance programme that Mr Burn suggests is adopted then I think that the cost of this has to be put into the cost–benefit analysis. People talk about giving HRT as if that is the end of the matter. What about the repeated mammography, visits, clinical examinations and so on, all of which cost money? Do you not think they should be included in the equation?

Mr Burn If I might comment on Dr Gambrell's paper, I would have no hesitation in supporting, in certain circumstances, the concept of the usefulness of oestrogens as a protective mechanism, for example against osteoporosis. The thing that still concerns me is the vulnerability of certain subgroups (which I think Dr Gambrell hinted at). These are the ones about whom I would be particularly concerned in the surveillance programme of women on these agents. I still think they may prove to be at higher risk than is justified.

Dr L. Rosenberg In the first two studies discussed, the oestrogen users had a much better survival rate than the non-users, but no information was presented on the respective ages of the groups that were compared, or the age at menopause, which is known to be the strongest predictor of oestrogen use and a very important risk factor. I think Dr Gambrell's oestrogen users would have had an early age at menopause, and therefore would have been at decreased risk to start with. Is there an analysis that took these factors into account?

Dr R.D. Gambrell Several factors were analysed, including the age of treatment and obesity. Unfortunately, we did not have all the risk factors for breast cancer because the study started as a study of endometrial cancer. The non-users were an older group of women, but not statistically significantly older. I am not sure whether we looked at the age of menopause in the two groups.

Dr E.C.G. Grant Mr Studd has been promoting hormone replacement therapy in this country. He has suggested that the rise in endometrial cancer at the menopause was one of the reasons for giving HRT. The British data are quite different; they show that ovarian, endometrial and cervical (apart from *in situ* cancers) rise slowly to age 60, being fairly steady at 60, 70 and 80. I published the comparisons in the *Journal of Hospital Medicine* . The peak level in the UK in 1961 for breast cancer for the oldest women (the incidence rises straight up) was 175, and by 1981 it had increased 36% to 240. The American figure was 370, and today Dr Gambrell has given a peak of up to 386... [*Dr Gambrell agreed*]. The Chief Medical Officer in the UK is very concerned about the rise in breast cancers, liver disease, suicides and cervical cancer in young women.

My own theory is that older women may be reacting to hormones in food or in the environment, or to mycotoxins, and need only a very small amount of oestrogen to stimulate breast cancer.

Dr Gambrell I cannot comment on that. I presented the National Cancer Institute surveillance, epidemiology and end-result reporting (SEER) data. I do not know why there would be differences.

Prof. N.S. Weiss The likely explanation for the difference in the shape of the age–incidence curve of endometrial cancer in the USA and the UK could relate to the much heavier use of unopposed oestrogens in the USA, particularly at the ages – the early 50s – where a sharp peak in incidence is seen.

Dr D.W. Kaufman I was interested in the comparison of the effects of different groups of oestrogen and progestogen combinations on breast cancer cells. There were four groups: untreated, oestrogen, oestrogen plus tamoxifen, and with the addition of progestogen. The control group with no hormones had an equally good effect in terms of DNA synthesis, and the best effect in terms of the resting state, which I interpret as suggesting that perhaps no hormones are better. What is your view?

Dr Gambrell For breast cancer cells in tissue culture, there was the control group, the baseline, and then it showed the effects, of oestradiol, oestradiol plus tamoxifen, and oestradiol plus 17α-dihydroequilin. The study shows that the conjugated oestrogen, 17α-dihydroequilin, is equally as anti-carcinogenic as tamoxifen.

Dr Kaufman But I think it also shows that the treatment groups were all below the baseline of no hormones... [*Dr Gambrell assented*].

Prof. Mansel Dr Gambrell quoted Voherr[1] showing an anti-mitogenic effect of progestogens on normal human epithelial cells in the breast. How can the experiment be explained, and what is the evidence for that effect? [*Dr Gambrell* I am not familiar with the experiment]. Our group has looked at normal human breast implanted in an euthymic mouse. Despite everybody feeling that progestogen will have an effect which might be the same as in the endometrium, it has no effect on normal human breast, whereas oestradiol has the expected stimulatory effect. In fact, it does not oppose oestrogen in that model. The MCF7 is not a normal cell, and we cannot extrapolate from it. But if we take normal human breast cells, an effect of progesterone cannot be shown. [*Dr Gambrell* What is the point?] You are showing a protective effect, saying it is anti-mitogenic and will oppose the oestradiol effect – but in practice, it does not.

Dr Gambrell How, then, does it reverse atypia? [*Prof. Mansel* I do not believe it does] That was biopsy proven.

Prof. Mansel It was a very small number of series. The mechanism has never been explained. I would like to know what it is, but unfortunately nobody knows.

Dr B.S. Hulka I would like to address the issue of the 7, 8 or 9 years that might be expected before progesterone, or any hormone for that matter, would be expected to have an effect, beneficial or adverse. If these hormones were given at a time when the cell has its first mutational event, and we wait for proliferation to occur, I suppose it might take some years. But since all women are very likely to have initiated cells in their breasts and their cells will be in various phases of proliferating already, I see no reason for it to take 8 or 9 years before progesterone, oestrogen and other biological agents to be manifest in clinical breast cancer.

Prof. Weiss We have to be hesitant, as Prof. Adami cautioned in Session 2, when looking at studies of mortality rates from breast cancer between users and non-users of oestrogens. There is a heavy potential for selection bias if, at the outset of such a comparison, women with existing breast cancer are not excluded from the studies. To my knowledge, in at least some of the studies that you described to us, such exclusion of prevalent breast cancer was not done, and those studies have a lot of potential for bias.

REFERENCES

1. Voherr, H. (1986). Oral contraception and hormone replacement therapy: are progestogens and progestins breast mitogens? (Letter to the Editor). *Am. J. Obstet. Gynecol.*, **155**, 1140

13

North Carolina studies of oestrogens, oestrogen receptors and breast cancer

B.S. Hulka and J.M. Schildkraut

INTRODUCTION

In the late 1970s, several members of the University of North Carolina, Departments of Epidemiology and Biostatistics, and Duke University, Department of Community and Family Medicine, conducted a case–control study of breast cancer patients and two control groups in North Carolina. One goal was to evaluate the role of exogenous hormones, particularly oestrogen replacement therapy, in breast cancer occurrence. Furthermore, because of an interest in studying a possible biological mechanism for this postulated relationship, we became engaged in the study of oestrogen receptors in breast tumour tissue[1]. These studies followed soon after a similar study of endometrial cancer, and in fact, studies of the two cancers shared a community control group[2]. The first publication from the breast cancer study bearing on the oestrogen hypothesis appeared in 1982[3]. Subsequent publications reported on alcohol and smoking effects[4], oestrogen receptors in breast tumour tissue[5], and the effects of oral contraceptives[6].

In preparation for the current meeting, we have expanded the earlier analyses in a number of ways:

(1) Additional potential confounders have been added to the logistic regression models in an attempt to improve the validity of the odds ratios;

(2) A separate analysis for women with a surgical menopause was performed;

(3) Additional stratified analyses were done to identify the effects of oestrogens combined with other exogenous exposures or endogenous characteristics; and

(4) The data on oestrogen receptors in breast tumour tissue were revisited, which stimulated a review of the literature on the relationship of oestrogens to their receptors in mammary tissue cells.

Findings that were previously observed have not changed substantially, but new analyses have produced some thought-provoking observations. What is most notable, however, is how we view these findings. In the last decade, a major thrust of epidemiological methods has been to advance our capability to do credible studies addressing weak associations. Concurrently, we have witnessed increasing reliance on epidemiological data for use in public health policy and clinical medicine. These factors necessarily influence both how we analyse and interpret epidemiological data.

METHODS

Methods for this study have been reported elsewhere[3] and only a few of the more critical features will be noted here. Case subjects were all newly-diagnosed, histologically-confirmed breast cancer patients admitted to three hospitals in North Carolina between April, 1977 and December, 1978. One hospital is a major referral centre; the other two are community hospitals. Two control groups were recruited, one from the same hospital as the cases and the other from a probability sample of community residences.

Two hospital controls were matched to each case on race, 5-year age-group, approximate date of admission, and hospital. All admissions were potential controls with the exception of those admitted for gynaecological or breast diseases. Interviews were conducted by study personnel during the hospital stay of the cases and the hospital controls. Refusal rates were low, less than 10% of eligible cases and controls.

Community controls were identified through a two-stage probability sampling procedure, based on 52 counties in North Carolina, including the major referral areas for the tertiary care hospital and the two community hospitals. In sampled households, women aged 30 and above were eligible for the study; 12% of eligible subjects either refused or were unable to complete the interviews that were conducted by study personnel in the subjects' homes.

Questionnaires were extensively pilot-tested, and interviewer training sessions were conducted before and during data collection. Photographic displays of commonly used oestrogens and oral contraceptives were supplied to respondents. Specialized data-management procedures for collecting data on oestrogens and oral contraceptives were instituted. After coding and key punching, our strategy was to computer-generate a chronology of all hormone data by calendar time and age for each individual, omitting identification of case or control status. Duration of use was accumulated for different oestrogen products and the 'usual' oestrogen (based primarily on duration of use) was established for analysis purposes. A procedure was also established, and has been reported, for classifying hormones of uncertain composition, a particular problem for injectable hormones[3].

Oestrogen use was defined as 6 months or more of accumulated use. This decision was retained from our earlier analysis when review of the oestrogen data revealed that less than 6 months of use was usually sporadic and only for 1–2 months. Although analyses were done in which oestrogen use of less than 6 months was a separate category, in the current presentation subjects with these brief exposures have been included as non-users.

Oestrogen receptor assays were performed at Duke University Medical Center. The technique of tumour tissue collection and the methods for cytosol preparation for the sucrose density gradient assay have been described[7]. Tissues were washed in buffer immediately after excision. Cryostat-prepared sections were made of each tissue specimen to confirm the presence of carcinoma. The quantity of oestrogen receptor present in each specimen was determined from the amount of diethylstilboestrol-inhibitable 8S binding species.

Odds ratios, as estimates of the relative risk, were used to measure the association between oestrogen use and breast cancer occurrence. Odds ratios and 95% confidence intervals were calculated from parameter estimates in unconditional logistic regression models, using the LOGIST procedures of SAS[8]. Matching was not retained in the analysis. Possible confounders included in the models were age at diagnosis or interview (continuous variable), history of gall-bladder disease, biopsy for benign breast disease, first-degree relative with breast cancer, nulliparity, and education (less than high school vs. high school or more). These selections were based on potential confounding in the data set, review of the literature on risk factors for disease and exposure, and confounder choices made by other authors.

RESULTS

Table 1 shows the number of subjects in each group, percentage of oestrogen users, age at menopause, age at diagnosis/interview, mean education and percentage of Caucasian subjects. Among naturally postmenopausal subjects, more cases (26%) had used oestrogens than controls, about 18% in both groups, whereas among the surgically menopausal, the case group was less likely to have used oestrogens (31.8%) than the controls (40–42%).

Data are presented separately for naturally and surgically postmenopausal women in Tables 2 and 3, respectively. Table 2 shows small elevations in the odds ratios in most categories of each variable describing oestrogen use patterns. In Table 3, almost all the odds ratios are less than unity. Logistic

Table 1 Characteristics of naturally and surgically postmenopausal women

	Natural			*Surgical*		
		Controls			*Controls*	
	Cases	*Community*	*Hospital*	*Cases*	*Community*	*Hospital*
Numbers	152	620	309	44	222	136
Oestrogen users* (%)	26.3	18.1	18.4	31.8	40.1	41.9
Age at diagnosis or interview (mean)	64.8	63.2	65.2	54.0	51.2	51.8
Age at menopause† (mean)	47.0	46.5	45.0‡	39.5	40.0	37.6
Years of school (mean)	10.6	9.4‡	9.3‡	11.5	10.4‡	10.9
Caucasian (%)	78.0	74.0	73.0	77.3	74.8	89.0

*6 months or more of use; †missing data on five cases, 18 community controls, eight hospital controls; ‡differs from cases, $p \leq 0.05$

Table 2 Risk estimates for breast cancer in relation to oestrogen-use characteristics: naturally postmenopausal women

	Cases	Community controls			Hospital controls		
Use characteristics	*Number*	*Number*	*Odds ratio*†	*95% CI*	*Number*	*Odds ratio*†	*95% CI*
Non-users*	112	508	1.0		252	1.0	
Users	40	112	1.7	(1.1–2.6)	57	1.6	(1.0–2.7)
Duration (years)							
0.5–3	23	57	1.8	(1.0–3.0)	21	2.6	(1.4–5.1)
4–9	11	37	1.3	(0.6–2.6)	17	1.5	(0.7–3.5)
10+	6	16	1.5	(0.6–4.0)	19	0.7	(0.3–1.8)
unknown	0	2			0		
Time since first use (years)							
0.5–4	5	22	1.3	(0.5–3.5)	6	1.7	(0.5–6.0)
5–9	14	31	2.3	(1.2–4.7)	10	2.8	(1.2–6.8)
10–14	9	21	1.8	(0.8–4.3)	15	1.5	(0.6–3.6)
15+	12	38	1.4	(0.7–2.8)	24	1.3	(0.6–2.8)
unknown	0	0			2		
Time since last use (years)							
0–1	15	46	1.5	(0.8–2.9)	25	1.3	(0.6–2.6)
2–5	9	22	2.2	(1.0–5.0)	6	3.3	(1.1–9.8)
6+	16	44	1.7	(0.9–3.1)	24	1.8	(0.9–3.7)
unknown	0	0			2		
Dose (mg)							
≤ 0.625	12	32	1.8	(0.9–3.6)	74	1.8	(0.8–4.1)
> 0.625	9	45	0.9	(0.4–2.0)	28	0.7	(0.3–1.6)
injection	12	13			8		
unknown	7	22			7		
Mode							
continuous	13	34	1.7	(0.9–3.5)	25	1.2	(0.6–2.5)
monthly	10	58	0.8	(0.4–1.7)	19	1.1	(0.5–2.5)
other	3	6	2.6	(0.6–10.9)	4	1.6	(0.4–7.7)
injection	12	13	4.7	(1.0–10.8)	8	4.3	(1.6–11.3)
unknown	2	1			1		

*Includes use of < 6 months duration; †controlling for age, education, gall-bladder disease, benign breast disease, breast cancer in first-degree relative, nulliparity; CI = confidence interval

Table 3 Risk estimates for breast cancer in relation to oestrogen-use characteristics: surgically postmenopausal women

	Cases	*Community controls*			*Hospital controls*		
Use characteristics	*Number*	*Number*	*Odds ratio*†	*95% CI*	*Number*	*Odds ratio*†	*95% CI*
	30	133	1.0		79	1.0	
Users	14	89	0.7	(0.4–1.5)	57	0.6	(0.3–1.3)
Duration (years)							
0.5–3	5	46	0.5	(0.2–1.4)	27	0.5	(0.2–1.3)
4–9	2	26	0.4	(0.1–1.8)	21	0.3	(0.1–1.2)
10+	7	17	2.0	(0.7–5.5)	8	2.5	(0.7–8.8)
unknown	0	0			1		
Time since first use (years)							
0.5–4	3	33	0.4	(0.1–1.5)	15	0.5	(0.2–1.3)
5–9	1	20	0.3	(0.0–2.8)	19	0.1	(0.0–1.1)
10–14	3	17	0.8	(0.2–3.2)	8	1.3	(0.3–6.8)
15+	7	19	1.4	(0.5–4.1)	15	1.0	(0.9–7.7)
unknown	0	0			0		
Time since last use (years)							
0–1	10	57	0.8	(0.4–1.9)	33	0.8	(0.3–2.0)
1–5	1	14	0.3	(0.0–2.9)	10	0.2	(0.0–2.0)
6+	3	17	0.7	(0.2–2.7)	14	0.5	(0.1–1.9)
unknown	0	1			0		
Dose (mg)							
≤ 0.625	2	19	0.4	(0.1–1.9)	10	0.7	(0.1–4.2)
> 0.625	6	51	0.6	(0.2–1.6)	33	0.4	(0.1–1.2)
injection	3	9			8		
unknown	3	10			6		
Mode							
continuous	9	35	1.6	(0.6–3.8)	29	0.7	(0.3–1.8)
monthly	2	36	0.3	(0.1–1.3)	15	0.5	(0.1–2.6)
other	0	6			4		
injection	3	9	1.7	(0.4–7.1)	8	0.9	(0.2–4.2)
unknown	0	3			1		

*Includes use of < 6 months duration; †controlling for age, education, gall-bladder disease, benign breast disease, breast cancer in first-degree relative, nulliparity; CI = confidence interval

regression models including an interaction term for type of menopause and oestrogen use substantiated the visual impression of interaction in the full data set. The ratio of the odds ratios for breast cancer risk from oestrogen use in naturally postmenopausal women relative to surgically postmenopausal women was 2.5 (1.11–5.77) with community controls and 2.9 (1.20–6.96) with hospital controls. For this reason analyses are presented separately for naturally and surgically postmenopausal women.

Consider first the naturally postmenopausal women in Table 2. The odds ratios for ever-use are 1.7 with community controls and 1.6 with hospital controls. The pattern of odds ratios for duration, latency and recency are similar in magnitude, whether the contrast is with hospital or community controls. Odds ratios are generally elevated for all categories of each variable. Odds ratio elevations approaching 2 or more are noted for: (1) use duration of 3 years or less; (2) time since first use of 5–9 years; (3) time since last use of 2–5 years; and (4) for injectable oestrogens. The lower boundary of the 95% confidence interval for most of these odds ratios is greater than 1.

A different pattern of odds ratios appears in Table 3. Among women with a surgical menopause, oestrogen use appears to reduce the risk of breast cancer. Odds ratios are mostly less than 1, although duration of use of 10+ years shows an elevation. Risk estimates are imprecise, as evidenced by the broad 95% confidence intervals, all of which overlap unity.

The women represented in Table 3 include a mixture of subjects, most of whom had had a hysterectomy, but only about half of whom had also had a bilateral oophorectomy. Thus, although the women are classified as surgically postmenopausal (menses ceased following surgery), many did retain ovarian function. Overall, surgically postmenopausal women were about 7 years younger at time of menopause than women who had undergone a natural menopause (Table 1).

Tables 4 and 5 focus on the effect of combinations of exposures, including oestrogens, in naturally postmenopausal women. They illustrate particular endogenous characteristics or life-style behaviours which may alter the risk of breast cancer in the presence of oestrogen replacement therapy.

Table 4 shows the influence of oestrogen on breast cancer risk for naturally postmenopausal women who have a history of biopsy for benign breast disease, a family history of breast cancer in a first-degree relative, and a late age at menopause (50 years or greater). Consider, firstly, women with biopsy for benign breast disease. Oestrogen use in these women appears to add to their breast cancer risk, which is already elevated because of the benign breast disease. Odds ratios for oestrogen use among women with prior biopsy for benign breast disease are 3.5 (community controls) and 2.2 (hospital controls) relative to women without prior biopsy who do not use oestrogen. Family history may interact with oestrogen use to increase breast cancer risk, although the large odds ratios for oestrogen use among those with a first-degree relative with breast cancer are based on very small numbers in our data.

Age at menopause groupings are divided at age 50 because 25% of the community control subjects experienced menopause above that age. Women aged 50 or above at the time of menopause have a higher breast cancer risk

Table 4 Analyses of oestrogen use and breast cancer in naturally postmenopausal women: biopsy for benign breast disease, breast cancer in first-degree relative, age at menopause

	Cases	Community controls			Hospital controls		
Use characteristics	*Number*	*Number*	*Odds ratio**	*95% CI*	*Number*	*Odds ratio**	*95% CI*
Benign breast disease							
No							
oestrogen use							
no	96	470	1.0		232	1.0	
yes	33	102	1.7	(1.0–2.7)	49	1.7	(1.0–2.9)
Yes							
oestrogen use							
no	16	38	1.8	(1.0–3.5)	20	1.6	(0.8–3.4)
yes	7	10	3.5	(1.3–2.3)	8	2.2	(0.7–6.4)
Breast cancer in first-degree relative							
No							
oestrogen use							
no	103	472	1.0		234	1.0	
yes	36	110	1.6	(1.0–2.4)	56	1.5	(0.9–2.5)
Yes							
oestrogen use							
no	9	36	1.0	(0.5–2.3)	18	1.0	(0.4–2.4)
yes	4	2	8.0	(1.4–46.4)	1	8.7	(0.9–81.3)
Age at menopause							
<50							
oestrogen use							
no	70	314	1.0		166	1.0	
yes	22	78	1.3	(0.7–2.3)	45	1.2	(0.6–2.2)
≥ 50							
oestrogen use							
no	38	176	0.9	(0.6–1.4)	78	1.1	(0.7–1.8)
yes	17	34	2.3	(1.2–4.4)	12	3.3	(1.5–7.6)
Missing	5	18			8		

*Controlling for age, education, gall-bladder disease, benign breast disease, breast cancer in first-degree relative, nulliparity; CI = confidence interval

Table 5 Analysis of oestrogen use and breast cancer in naturally postmenopausal women: alcohol use and cigarette smoking

	Cases	*Community controls*			*Hospital controls*		
Use characteristics	*Number*	*Number*	*Odds ratio**	*95% CI*	*Number*	*Odds ratio**	*95% CI*
Alcohol use							
Past or never oestrogen use							
no	80	432	1.0		205	1.0	
yes	28	85	2.0	(1.2–3.3)	39	2.0	(1.1–3.5)
Current alcohol user oestrogen use							
no	31	74	2.3	(1.4–3.9)	45	1.7	(1.0–3.0)
yes	12	26	2.6	(1.2–5.7)	18	1.8	(0.8–4.2)
Cigarette smoking							
Past or never oestrogen use							
no	96	45	1.0		202	1.0	
yes	35	84	1.9	(1.1–3.0)	44	1.7	(1.0–3.0)
Current smoker oestrogen use							
no	16	93	0.7	(0.4–1.3)	50	0.6	(0.3–1.2)
yes	5	28	0.7	(0.3–2.0)	13	0.7	(0.2–2.1)

*Controlling for age, education, gall-bladder disease, benign breast disease, breast cancer in first-degree relative, nulliparity; CI = confidence interval

when using oestrogen than women with a younger age at menopause. In the former group, odds ratios are 2.3 (community controls) and 3.3 (hospital controls) with lower limits of the confidence intervals above unity.

Table 5 shows risks associated with oestrogen use by alcohol consumption and cigarette smoking among naturally postmenopausal women. With respect to alcohol consumption, 'never-drinkers' and past drinkers who use oestrogens exhibit odds ratios of 2.0 with either community or hospital controls; lower boundaries of the confidence intervals exceed 1. Current consumers of alcohol are at increased breast cancer risk irrespective of oestrogen use[4].

Our prior analyses revealed some reduction in breast cancer risk among current smokers[4]. Data in Table 5 suggest that this finding persists for oestrogen users as well as non-users. Current non-smokers experience some risk elevation with oestrogen use (odds ratio = 1.9 for community controls and 1.7 for hospital controls).

Table 6 addresses the relationship between oestrogen use and oestrogen receptor presence in breast tumour tissue. Median oestrogen receptor values for each of several oestrogen use characteristics are presented separately for cases with natural and surgical menopause. The analysis is restricted to women < 70 years of age at diagnosis, because of the high receptor content in tumours from older White women and the low likelihood of their having used oestrogens due to secular changes in oestrogen prescribing patterns[5]. For naturally menopausal cases, median oestrogen receptor values do not distinguish oestrogen users from non-users. Based on the small number of cases who had undergone surgical menopause and who also had receptor data, the suggestion appears of lower oestrogen receptor values among oestrogen users. Values for oestrogen receptor content are plotted in relation to type of menopause and oestrogen use in Figure 1.

Logistic regression analyses were performed using separate models for cases with natural and surgical menopause. Oestrogen use (dichotomous) and age (continuous) were the predictor variables. The odds ratio for having an oestrogen receptor-positive tumour in relation to oestrogen use was 1.57 (95% confidence interval (CI) , 0.58–4.26) for naturally menopausal women, and 0.27 (95% CI, 0.05–1.41) for surgically menopausal women. A single logistic regression model, including an interaction term for type of menopause and oestrogen use, produced results that were comparable to those from the separate models.

DISCUSSION

The main observations in this study are the elevated breast cancer risk estimates for naturally postmenopausal women who use oestrogen replacement therapy. Odds ratios are 1.6 (95% CI, 1.0–2.7) for hospital controls and 1.7 (95% CI, 1.1–2.6) for community controls with oestrogen use of 6 months or more. Odds ratios were generally elevated irrespective of duration of use, time since first use or time since last use. As reported previously, injectable oestrogens used for 6 months or more incur greater risks than

Table 6 Median oestrogen receptor content in relation to characteristics of oestrogen use for naturally and surgically postmenopausal women < 70 years of age

	Natural menopause			*Surgical menopause*		
Characteristics of oestrogen use	*n*	*Median oestrogen receptor*	*Interquartile range*	*n*	*Median oestrogen receptor*	*Interquartile range*
Ever-use						
no	69	36.2	88.6	24	39.2	93.9
yes	29	32.4	88.8	10	15.2	44.6
Duration (years)						
0.5–4	18	41.1	163.0	3	2.4	18.5
5+	11	20.5	28.3	7	22.0	104.9
Recency						
0–1	13	11.5	31.7	8	15.2	86.0
2+	16	56.0	154.4	2	12.2	19.6
Latency						
0.5–10	21	30.3	73.3	4	15.2	21.2
11+	8	58.1	152.0	6	12.2	150.5
Dose*						
low	10	35.3	86.6	2	144.6	284.4
high	7	32.4	67.6	5	11.3	21.1
missing	12			3		

*Low dose was ⩽ 0.625 mg and high dose was > 0.625 mg conjugated oestrogens

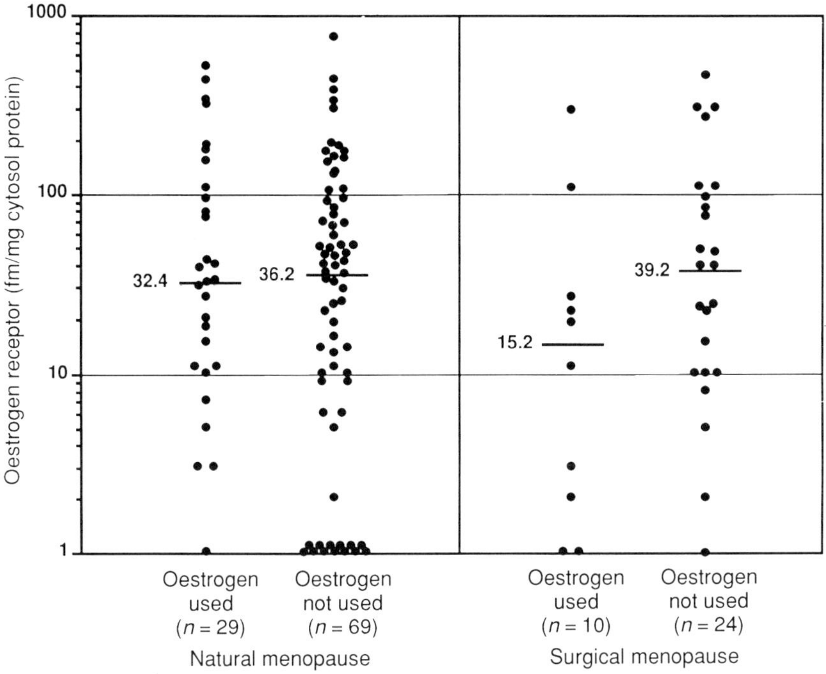

Figure 1 Oestrogen receptor concentration in breast tumour tissue in relation to type of menopause and oestrogen use. Bars indicate median values

orally administered products (odds ratio ~ 4)[3]. The timing of these elevated risks is not consistent with a recent meta-analysis[9] and review[10], both of which suggested that long-term oestrogen use (10–15 years) was required to increase breast cancer risks to 1.3 or 1.5 at most.

The current findings are more consistent with the observations from animal models and *in vitro* systems, in which oestrogens appear to exhibit promotional activity, causing cell proliferation, but not genotoxicity[11]. If oestrogen effects in model systems are extrapolated to human carcinogenesis, a role for oestrogen in tumour promotion and progression of cells with previously damaged genetic material would be expected. These phenomena could take place in a much shorter time-frame than that required for genotoxic agents, which cause mutations, to produce clinically manifest cancer.

The short time-frame suggested by these data is also consistent with genetic susceptibility in a few individuals, the expression of which is enhanced by oestrogen administration. The problem is to identify the relevant biological marker or genetic alteration that would distinguish the small subgroup susceptible to oestrogens. Our usual epidemiological information on cancer history in family members is not sufficiently specific, since there is genetic heterogeneity underlying susceptibility and many cancers, even in the first-degree relatives of cases, are sporadic.

Family history information is useful, however. In the Centers for Disease Control meta-analysis, oestrogen administration in the presence of a positive family history increases risk of breast cancer disproportionately[9]. From a clinical perspective, positive family history in a first-degree relative may be a contraindication to prescribing oestrogen.

The elevation in breast cancer risk associated with oestrogen use appeared to be greater for women with a prior biopsy for benign breast disease than for those without a prior biopsy, as was also noted in the Centers for Disease Control meta-analysis[9]. However, interview information on prior biopsy is a weak proxy for the information we would like to have on the actual histological findings from a biopsy. Hyperplasias and atypical hyperplasias are the primary lesions associated with increased breast cancer risk and the majority of biopsies identify lesions of no import[12,13]. Thus, the variable, prior biopsy for benign breast disease, involves extensive misclassification with respect to the histological information of interest. Given the extent of mammographic screening during the 1980s, and the resulting increase in biopsies, one could also expect that the positive predictive value of biopsy for any histologically significant lesion has dropped. Introduction of mammography has caused secular changes in both the indications for and the significance of biopsy. To evaluate oestrogen effects on precursor lesions requires histological data. Although two large historical prospective studies have been reported, the results with respect to oestrogen use are inconsistent[12,14].

The possible interaction of oestrogen with late age at menopause has been reported by other authors[15–17] as well as in the current study. Women with a late age at natural menopause experience additional years of endogenous oestrogen exposure with or without regular cycling and endogenous progesterone. How this would affect their response to postmenopausal oestrogen administration is not known.

Some aspect of cigarette smoking appears to reduce endogenous oestrogens. In premenopausal women, smokers exhibit lower urinary oestrogens in the luteal phase of the menstrual cycle than non-smokers[18]. In postmenopausal women administered various does of oestrogens or placebo in a double-blind fashion, serum concentrations of oestrone and oestradiol are lower in smokers than in non-smokers[19]. A possible mechanism for these differences relates to hepatic metabolism of oestrogens. A metabolic pathway for oestrogens with increased 2-hydroxylation, forming a metabolic product with little oestrogenic activity, has been shown to be more extensive in smokers than in non-smokers[20]. To the extent that decreasing tissue exposure to biologically active oestrogens decreases breast cancer risk, smokers might be expected to have lower risks even in the presence of exogenously administered oestrogens. Our study did not have adequate power to address this issue formally, but the odds ratios shown were in a direction consistent with this expectation.

Other authors have shown an increased risk of breast cancer among smokers, most notably among those who start smoking early in life[21]. These observations are not inconsistent with the reduction in risk noted in our study. Tobacco smoke contains many carcinogens – initiators, promoters and complete carcinogens. It is most likely that different chemical constituents function through different mechanisms of action at different periods of life.

In many epidemiological studies, and in a recent meta-analysis, alcohol consumption increased breast cancer risk[22]. This finding was also observed in our data, irrespective of oestrogen consumption. Only the non-drinkers exhibited an increased breast cancer risk from exogenous oestrogen. These findings are not consistent with the recent report from the Nurses' Health Study in which the increased risk of breast cancer from oestrogen use was concentrated among women who consumed alcohol[23].

The possibility of differing oestrogen effects by type of menopause was also raised by the current analysis. Breast cancer risk appeared to be decreased in response to oestrogen use among women with a surgical menopause, as defined by cessation of menstruation. This finding is not consistent with most other studies, except for that of LaVecchia and colleagues[16]. The surgical menopause group included women with bilateral oophorectomy, unilateral oophorectomy, and retention of both ovaries. However, even retention of both ovaries does not assure normal ovarian function after hysterectomy. Hysterectomy alone can disturb ovarian blood supply with subsequent alteration of hormone production and release[24]. Furthermore, selective factors may influence the type of surgical procedure performed and the use of replacement oestrogens. The proportion of hysterectomies in which both ovaries are removed has increased during the past 25 years and is also higher in women who are near the age of natural menopause[25]. Since the group of women with a surgical menopause is heterogeneous with respect to endogenous sex steroid hormone production and availability to tissues, the effect of adding exogenous oestrogens is difficult to anticipate.

We should also recognize the limitations of epidemiological interview data in classifying ovarian status among women who have had a hysterectomy. Misclassification can occur because women are not fully informed about the removal of ovaries at the time of hysterectomy. Furthermore, among women who are menstruating at the time of hysterectomy without bilateral oophorectomy, the actual age at cessation of ovarian function cannot be readily determined.

In our previous report, we noted that oestrogen receptor presence was positively associated with old age of patients and negatively associated with Black racial group[5]. In both the past and present analysis oestrogen receptor status showed no association with oestrogen use patterns, although a larger sample of tissues from women who had used oestrogens near the time of breast cancer diagnosis might lead to a different conclusion. What is also missing from this study is a theoretical foundation that would help us to predict what the associations might be. For this reason, we undertook a literature review on the functional interrelationship of oestrogen receptor and oestrogens in breast tissue.

Most authors agree that oestrogens induce their own receptors and also progesterone receptors. Progesterone down-regulates oestrogen receptor formation. Synthesis of oestrogen receptor and progesterone receptor by mammary cancer cells is considered to be a manifestation of biochemical differentiation[26]. Oestrogen receptor content is significantly higher in malignant breast tissue than in normal cells[27]; dysplasias and adenomas also exhibit elevated oestrogen receptor levels[28–30].

Oestrogen receptor has been identified in normal breast tissue obtained by needle biopsy. Markopoulous and colleagues applied immunocytological techniques with monoclonal antibody to normal breast tissue of premenopausal women and found oestrogen receptor-positive cells in the follicular phase but not the luteal phase of the menstrual cycle[31]. Oestrogen receptor content was higher in European than in non-European women, and in obese than in non-obese women. Oestrogen receptor content was also noted to be highly correlated with progesterone receptor content[27]. In breast tissues from eight normal postmenopausal women, six were oestrogen receptor-positive[31].

These authors also studied oestrogen receptor content in breast tumour tissue from premenopausal women[31]. Whether the tissues were oestrogen receptor-positive or -negative, they were consistent throughout the menstrual cycle. Cells either synthesized oestrogen receptor continuously or did not express it, despite large fluctuations in serum oestrogens. In neoplastic cells hormonal control of receptor mechanisms is no longer intact.

Oestrogen receptor contains specific binding sites both for oestrogen and for DNA in the cell nucleus. The DNA itself contains specific acceptor sites for the oestrogen receptor complex. Oestrogen binds with cytosolic oestrogen receptor (or nuclear oestrogen receptor) and the complex migrates to the cell nucleus where it binds to a specific region of chromatin near target genes[32]. Receptors alter the transcriptional activity of these target genes by binding with enhancer elements of target gene promoters, resulting in the production of specific proteins, including growth factors[33]. In human breast cancer cell systems, oestrogens enhance RNA transcriptional activity. Oestradiol activates oestrogen and epithelial growth factor receptor genes, and *myc*, *ras* and *fos* oncogenes[34,35]

In malignant breast tissue, oestrogen receptor may be in either an activated or inactivated form. Activation occurs after oestrogen receptor binds to oestrogen, resulting in a receptor complex that can bind DNA and initiate transcriptional activity. The presence of activated oestrogen receptor is a good prognostic indicator in breast cancer, and is also associated with high progesterone receptor levels and creatinine kinase activity in the tumour cells[36].

Studies on the relationship between oestrogen levels in serum and tissue, and concentration of cellular oestrogen receptors have produced variable results. Drafta and colleagues found high levels of circulating oestradiol associated with high cytosol oestrone and oestradiol in tumour cells, and elevated oestrogen receptor content in tumours from postmenopausal women[37]. On the other hand, Mehta and co-workers did not find an association between oestradiol concentration in tissue and oestrogen receptor status of the tumour[38]. Most authors have reported no correlation between oestrogen levels in serum and breast tumour tissue, although the absolute levels of oestrogen in breast tissue is an order of magnitude greater than in plasma[38,39]. Furthermore, oestradiol concentration is about the same in malignant cells from pre- and postmenopausal patients despite the large differences in serum oestrogens, particularly oestradiol[38].

Both normal and malignant mammary cells synthesize and metabolize oestrogens. In tumour tissue the interconversion between oestrone and oestradiol greatly favours the formation of oestradiol, resulting in an elevated ratio of oestradiol–oestrone[40]. One of the actions of progesterone is to increase enzymatic activity of 17β-hydroxysteroid dehydrogenase, which is responsible for converting oestradiol to oestrone[41]. Thus, progesterone may limit the formation of oestradiol, the pivotal oestrogen in neoplasia.

From this information one might infer that additional oestrogens, whether from endogenous or exogenous sources, would increase serum and tissue levels, enhance oestrogen receptor formation, nuclear binding, growth factor production and cellular proliferation[42,43]. In normal cells there are multiple regulatory controls on this cascade of events; in breast cancer cells these controls have gone awry. Figure 2 illustrates the processes related to oestrogen and its receptor in a normal cell and Figure 3 shows theoretical alterations that may occur in cancer cells. Suppression or enhancement of the depicted pathways may be part of the carcinogenic process. In the regulation of breast tissue growth and functional activity, oestrogens and progestins are major determinants, but other hormones play a significant role: prolactin, growth hormone, insulin, glucocorticoids, vitamin D and A, and probably others. Breast tissue in culture requires multiple hormonal factors to allow growth, and some of these undoubtedly influence the development of human breast cancer *in vivo*. Our current effort to portray oestrogen effects on breast cells is rudimentary and represents only one piece among multiple, complex interactions. The point of this effort, however, is to

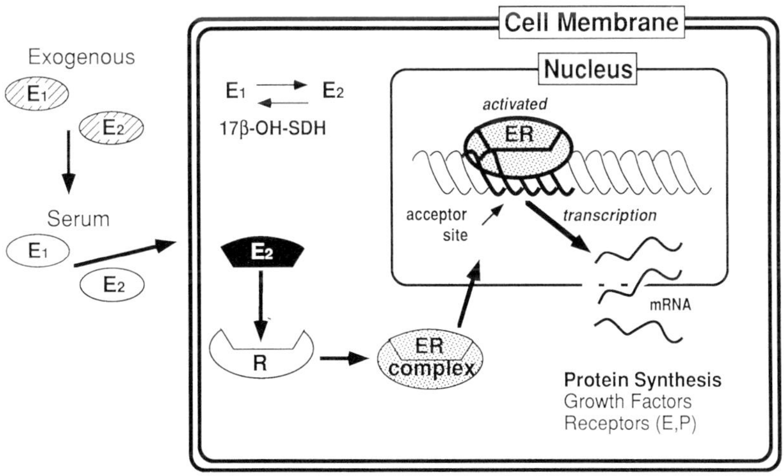

Figure 2 Oestrogen and oestrogen receptors in the normal breast epithelial cell. E_1 = oestrone; E_2 = oestradiol; 17β-OH-SDH = 17β-hydroxysteroid dehydrogenase; ER = oestrogen receptor; E = oestrogen; P = progesterone; R = receptor

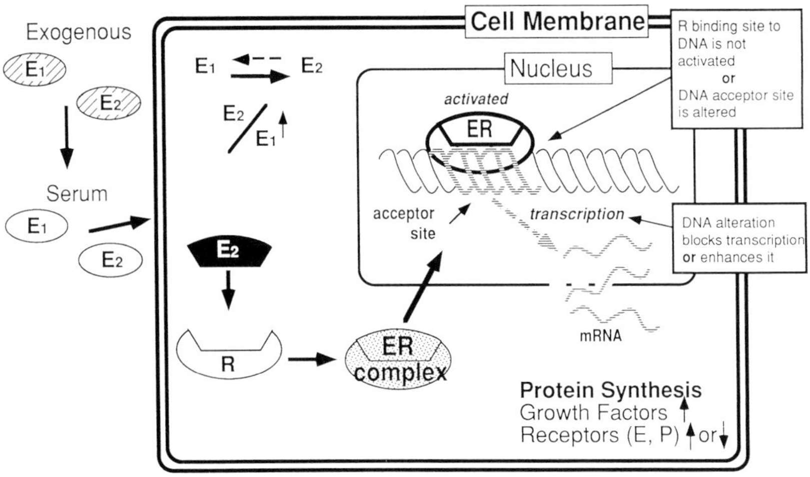

Figure 3 Oestrogen and oestrogen rceptors in the malignant breast cell. E_1 = oestrone; E_2 = oestradiol; R = receptor; ER = oestrogen receptor; E = oestrogen; P = progesterone; R = receptor

reinforce the principle of inter-relating epidemiological data with information from the laboratory and clinical sciences in order to advance knowledge about disease processes.

ACKNOWLEDGEMENTS

We acknowledge the significant contributions of Ms Virginia Reid for her persistence in tracking down references and her gracious co-operation in typing numerous versions of this manuscript.

REFERENCES

1. McCarty, K.S., Silva, J.S., Cox, E.B., Leight, G.S., Wells, S.A. and McCarty, K.S. (1983). Relationship of age and menopausal status to estrogen receptor content in primary carcinoma of the breast. *Ann. Surg.*, **197**, 123–7
2. Hulka, B.S., Fowler, W.C., Kaufman, D.G., Grimson, R.C., Greenberg, B.G., Hogue, C.J.R., Berger, G.S. and Pulliam, C.C. (1980). Estrogen and endometrial cancer: cases and two control groups from North Carolina. *Am. J. Obstet. Gynecol.*, **137**, 92–101
3. Hulka, B.S., Chambless, L.E., Deubner, D.C. and Wilkinson, W.E. (1982). Breast cancer and estrogen replacement therapy. *Am. J. Obstet. Gynecol.*, **143**, 638–44
4. O'Connell, D.L., Hulka, B.S., Chambless, L.E., Wilkinson, W.E. and Deubner, D.C. (1987). Cigarette smoking, alcohol consumption, and breast cancer risk. *J. Natl. Cancer Inst.*, **78**, 229–34
5. Hulka, B.S., Chambless, L.E., Wilkinson, W.E., Deubner, D.C. McCarty, K.S., Sr and McCarty, K.S., Jr. (1984). Hormonal and personal effects on estrogen receptors in breast cancer. *Am. J. Epidemiol.*, **119**, 692–704
6. Schildkraut, J.M., Hulka, B.S. and Wilkinson, W.E. (1990). Oral contraceptives and breast cancer: a case–control study with hospital and community controls. *Obstet. Gynecol.*, **76**, 395
7. McCarty, K.S. Jr., Barton, T.K., Fetter, B.F., Creasman, W.T. and McCarty, K.S., Sr (1979).

Correlations of estrogen and progesterone receptors with histologic differentiation in endometrial adenocarcinoma. *Am. J. Pathol.*, **96**, 171–82
8. Harrell, F.E., Jr (1986). The Logist Procedure. In Hastings, R.P. (ed.) *SUGI Supplementary Library User's Guide, Version* 5, pp. 269–93. (Cary, NC: SAS Institute, Inc.)
9. Steinberg, K.K., Thacker, S.B., Smith, S.J., Stroup, D.F., Zack, M.M., Flanders, W.D. and Berkelman, R.L. (1991). A meta-analysis of the effect of estrogen replacement therapy on the risk of breast cancer. *J. Am. Med. Assoc.*, **265**, 1985–90
10. Hulka, B.S. (1990). Hormone replacement therapy and the risk of breast cancer. *Ca–A Cancer J. Clin.*, **40**, 289–96
11. Weinstein, I.B. (1980). Studies on the mechanism of action of tumor promoters and their relevance to mammary carcinogenesis. In McGrath C.M., Brennan, M.J. and Rich, M.A. (eds.) *Cell Biology of Breast Cancer*. (New York: Academic Press)
12. Dupont, W.D., Page, D.L., Rogers, L.W. and Parl, F.F. (1989). Influence of exogenous estrogens proliferative breast disease and other variables on breast cancer risk. *Cancer*, **63**, 948–57
13. Carter, C.L., Corle, D.K., Micozzi, M.S., Schatzkin, A. and Taylor, P.R. (1988). A prospective study of the development of breast cancer in 16,692 women with benign breast disease. *Am. J. Epidemiol.*, **128**, 467–77
14. Thomas, D.B., Persing, J.P. and Hutchinson, W.B. (1982). Exogenous estrogens and other risk factors for breast cancer in women with benign breast diseases. *J. Natl. Cancer Inst.*, **69**, 1017–25
15. Ewertz, M. (1988). Influence of non-contraceptive exogenous and endogenous sex hormones on breast cancer risk in Denmark. *Int. J. Cancer*, **42**, 832–8
16. La Vecchia, C., DeCarli, A., Parazzini, F., Gentile, A., Liberati, C. and Franceschi, S. (1986). Non-contraceptive oestrogens and the risk of breast cancer in women. *Int. J. Cancer*, **38**, 853–8
17. Mills, P.K., Beeson, W.L., Phillips, R.L. and Fraser, G.E. (1989). Prospective study of exogenous hormone use and breast cancer in Seventh-day Adventists. *Cancer*, **64**, 591–7
18. McMahon, B., Trichopoulos, D., Cole, P. and Brown, J. (1982). Cigarette smoking and urinary estrogens. *N. Engl. J. Med.*, **307**, 1062–5
19. Jensen, J., Christiansen, C. and Rodbro, P. (1985). Cigarette smoking, serum estrogens and bone loss during hormone replacement therapy early after menopause. *N. Engl. J. Med.*, **313**, 973–5
20. Michnovicz, J.J., Hershcopf, R.J., Naganuma, H., Bradlow, H.L. and Fishman, J. (1986). Increased 2-hydroxylation of estradiol as a possible mechanism for the anti-estrogenic effect of cigarette smoking. *N. Engl. J. Med.*, **315**, 1305–9
21. Palmer, J.R., Rosenberg, L., Clarke, E.A., Stolley, P.D., Warshauer, M.E., Zaube, A.G. and Shapiro, S. (1991). Breast cancer and cigarette smoking: an hypothesis. *Am. J. Epidemiol.*, **134**, 1–13
22. Longnecker, M.P., Berlin, J.A., Orza, M.J. and Chalmers, T.C. (1988). A meta-analysis of alcohol consumption in relation to risk of breast cancer. *J. Am. Med. Assoc.*, **260**, 652–6
23. Colditz, G.A., Stampfer, M.J., Willett, W.C., Hennekens, C.H., Rosner, B. and Speizer, F.E. (1990). Prospective study of estrogen replacement therapy and risk of breast cancer in postmenopausal women. *J. Am. Med. Assoc.*, **264**, 2648–53
24. Kaiser, R., Kusche, M. and Wurz, H. (1989). Hormone levels in women after hysterectomy. *Arch. Gynecol. Obstet.*, **244**, 169–73
25. Pokras, R. and Hufnagel, V.G. (1987). Hysterectomy in the United States, 1965–1984. *National Center for Health Statistics*, Washington. US Government Printing Office 1987, DHHS publication no. (PHS)87-1753, (Vital and Health Statistics, series 13, no. 92)
26. Mossler, J.A., McCarty, K.S., Jr and Johnston, W.W. (1981). The correlation of cytologic grade and steroid receptor content in effusions of metastatic breast carcinoma. *Acta Cytol.*, **25**, 653–8
27. Ricketts, D., Turnbull, L., Ryall, G., Bakhshi, R., Rawson, N.S.B., Gazet, J.-C., Nolan, C. and Coombes, R.C. (1991). Estrogen and progesterone receptors in the normal female breast. *Cancer Res.*, **51**, 1817–22
28. Balakrishnan, A., Yang, J., Beattie, C.W. Das-Gupta, T.K. and Nandi, S. (1987). Estrogen receptor in dissociated and cultured human breast fibroadenoma epithelial cells. *Cancer Lett.*, **34**, 233–42

29. Giani, C., D'Amore, E., Delarue, J.C., Mouriesse, H., May-Levin, F., Sancho-Garnier, H., Breccia, M. and Contesso, G. (1986). Estrogen and progesterone receptors in benign breast tumors and lesions: relationship with histological and cytological features. *Int. J. Cancer*, **37**, 7–10
30. Brentani, M.M., Franco, E.L., Oshima, C.T. and Pacheco, M.M. (1986). Androgen, estrogen and progesterone receptor levels in malignant and benign breast tumors: a multivariate analysis approach. *Int. J. Cancer*, **38**, 637–42
31. Markopoulous, C., Berker, U., Wilson, P., Gazet, J.C. and Coombes, R.C. (1988). Oestrogen receptor content of normal breast cells and breast carcinomas throughout the menstrual cycle. *Br. Med. J.*, **296**, 1349–51
32. Hansen, J.C., Welshons, W.V. and Gorski, J. (1988). Toward a more unified model of steroid hormone receptor structure and function. In Sheridan, P. and Blum, K. (eds.) *Steroid Receptors and Disease*, pp. 3–22 (New York: Marcel Dekker, Inc.)
33. Gronemeyer, H., Green, S., Kumar, V., Jeltsch, J.M., and Chambon, P. (1988). Structure and function of the estrogen receptor and other members of the nuclear receptor family. In Sheridan, P. and Blum, K. (eds.) *Steroid Receptors and Disease*, pp. 97–112 (New York: Marcel Dekker, Inc.)
34. Dotzlaw, H., Miller, T., Karvelas, J. and Murphy, L.C. (1990). Epidermal gowth factor gene expression in human breast cancer biopsy samples: relationship to estrogen and progesterone receptor gene expression. *Cancer Res.*, **50**, 4204–8
35. Murayama, Y., Kurata, S. and Michim, Y. (1988). Regulation of human estrogen receptor gene, epidermal growth factor receptor gene, and oncogenes by estrogen and antiestrogen in MCF-7 breast cancer cells. *Cancer Det. Prev.*, **13**, 103–7
36. White, J.O., Herschman, M.J., Parmar, G., Philipson, K.A., Elder, M.G., Habib, N.A. and Wood, C.B. (1987). Activated oestrogen receptor in human breast cancer: clinical and biochemical correlates. *Br. J. Surg.*, **74**, 588–90
37. Drafta, D., Priscu, A., Neacsu, E., Gangura, M., Schindler, A.E., Stroe, E., Anghel, C. and Panaitescu, G. (1983). Estradiol and progesterone receptor levels in human breast cancer in relation to cytosol and plasma estrogen level. *J. Steroid Biochem.*, **18**, 459–63
38. Mehta, R.R., Valcourt, L., Graves, J., Green, R. and Das Gupta, T.K. (1987). Subcellular concentrations of estrone, estradiol, androstenedione and 17β-hydroxysteroid dehydrogenase (17β-OH-SDH) activity in malignant and non-malignant human breast tissues. *Int. J. Cancer*, **40**, 305–8
39. Van Landeghem, A.A.J., Poortman, J., Nabuurs, M. and Thijssen, J.H.H. (1985). Endogenous concentration and subcellular distribution of estrogens in normal and malignant human breast tissue. *Cancer Res.*, **45**, 2900–6
40. Bonney, R.C., Reed, M.J., Beranek, P.A., Ghilchik, M.W. and James, V.H.T. (1986). Metabolism of [^{3}H]oestradiol *in vivo* by normal breast and tumour tissue in postmenopausal women. *J. Steroid Biochem.*, **24**, 361–4
41. Mauvais-Jarvis, P., Kutenn, F. and Gompel, A. (1987). Antiestrogen action of progesterone in breast tissue. *Hormone Res.*, **28**, 212–18
42. Workshop report from the Division of Cancer Etiology, National Cancer Institute, National Institutes of Health. Current perspectives and future trends in hormonal carcinogenesis. (1991). *Cancer Res.*, **51**, 3626–9
43. Stanford, J.L., Szklo, M. and Brinton, L.A. (1986). Estrogen receptors and breast cancer. *Epidemiol. Rev.*, **8**, 42–59

14

Oestrogen replacement therapy and breast cancer: new results from the Slone Epidemiology Unit's Case–Control Surveillance Study

D.W. Kaufman, J.R. Palmer, L. Rosenberg and S. Shapiro

INTRODUCTION

In the United States and Europe, breast cancer is the most common malignancy in women, and exogenous oestrogens taken by postmenopausal women for hormone replacement are among the most commonly used drugs. The possibility of even a modest increase in the risk of breast cancer among users is of substantial concern, and it is not surprising that this issue has been the subject of many epidemiological studies[1–29]. Although it is now clear that there is little (if any) overall excess risk, there have been inconsistent elevations in various subgroups[1,2,5–7,9,11,15,17–19,21,24,26,27]. Some studies have suggested that the risk is increased after long durations of use[9,14,21,24]. Most studies have had insufficient data to evaluate long-term use or they have yielded equivocal or negative results.

In 1984, we published the results of a large case–control investigation based on our ongoing case–control surveillance study, in which there was no increase in the risk of breast cancer overall among users of conjugated or other non-contraceptive oestrogens[13]; there was also no increase in risk after long durations of conjugated oestrogen use, after use in the distant past, or among subgroups of users. In addition, the data were compatible with a reduced risk in one subgroup of postmenopausal women whose use ended in the distant past. Here we report the results of a new analysis, based on data collected since the previous investigation.

METHODS

Case–control surveillance has been conducted by the Slone Epidemiology Unit of Boston University School of Medicine since 1976[30]. Specially trained

Material used in this chapter has previously been published in Kaufman, D.W. *et al.* (1991) *Am. J. Epidemiol.*, **134**, 1375–85 and is reproduced here with permission nurses stationed in hospitals in major metropolitan areas, primarily in the eastern United States, interview patients with various cancers and with a wide variety of other conditions. Information is obtained on demographic factors (e.g. age, years of education), habits (e.g. cigarette smoking, alcohol consumption), relevant medical history (e.g. family history of cancer, history of major illnesses), and medication use. The medication history is obtained by asking about indications for use. For each drug, details of the timing, duration, and frequency of use are obtained for each episode. In addition, for conjugated oestrogens, the dose is recorded; photographs of conjugated oestrogen pills are used to assist recall. Details of the patients' diagnoses are obtained from the hospital record after discharge.

As noted above, the present analysis is confined to subjects enrolled since our previous investigation[13]. All included cases and controls were interviewed from January, 1980 through September, 1988, in hospitals in Boston, New York City, Philadelphia, Baltimore, Tucson, San Francisco, and London, Ontario. Of the patients approached for interview, 4% refused to participate.

Cases

These were postmenopausal women aged 40–69 years with breast cancer diagnosed not more than 6 months previously and with no concurrent or previous cancer; there were a total of 1686 cases.

Controls

These were postmenopausal women aged 40–69 years with malignant and non-malignant conditions judged to be unrelated to oestrogen use. There were 1120 cancer controls, including patients with colorectal cancer (550 patients), malignant melanoma (200), and various other cancers (e.g. Hodgkin's disease, stomach, kidney, leukaemia – a total of 370 patients) diagnosed within the 6 months of admission, and with no other concurrent or previous cancer. Women with female cancers were not eligible. There were 957 non-cancer controls, including patients admitted for trauma (422), acute infections (124), disc disorders (108), and various other conditions (e.g. bowel obstruction, pyelonephritis – a total of 303), and no history of cancer. Women with non-malignant gynaecological conditions were not eligible. Thus, the total control series comprised 2077 women.

Classification of non-contraceptive oestrogen use

The main focus of the analysis was on oestrogen use that began at least 18 months before admission, because more recently initiated use could have begun after the onset of breast cancer or of the control conditions, and hence might not have been aetiologically relevant. Cases and controls were further subdivided according to whether they took unopposed oestrogens (no

Table 1 Oestrogen use among cancer and non-cancer controls according to diagnosis. Rates of use are standardized to the overall age-distribution of the control series

	Cancer controls (1120)		*Non-cancer controls* (957)	
Oestrogen use	*Number*	(%)	*Number*	(%)
Never used oestrogens	869	(78)	751	(79)
Unopposed, for replacement	191	(17)	160	(17)
Unopposed, for other indications	36	(3)	23	(2)
Opposed by progestogens	7	(1)	9	(1)
Any use that began ≤ 18 months before interview	17	(2)	14	(1)

concurrent use of progestogens) as replacement therapy, unopposed oestrogens for other indications (regulation of menstrual periods, pregnancy maintenance, suppression of lactation, and breast conditions), or opposed oestrogens (concurrent progestogen use of at least 1 month's duration). Vaginal oestrogen preparations were not considered.

Table 1 shows oestrogen use separately among the cancer and non-cancer controls, with rates standardized to the overall age-distribution of the control series. The rates in the two groups of controls were closely similar and the controls were combined into a single group for all analyses.

Data analysis

Relative risks and 95% confidence intervals were estimated for various categories of oestrogen use, with never-use of non-contraceptive oestrogens as the reference category. Age and type of menopause (natural, due to hysterectomy with retention of at least one ovary, due to bilateral oophorectomy) were taken into account by the Mantel–Haenszel procedure[31]. Confidence limits for these 'stratified' estimates were calculated by the method of Miettinen[32]. To take into account confounding by numerous factors simultaneously, multiple logistic regression was used[33]. In addition to categories of oestrogen use, the factors included in the multivariate models were age, age at menarche, age at first pregnancy, parity, age at menopause, type of menopause, family history of breast cancer, history of cystic breast disease, race, religion, years of education, body mass index, oral contraceptive use, alcohol consumption, year of interview, and geographic region.

RESULTS

As shown in Table 2, most subjects who took oestrogens did so as unopposed replacement therapy (18% of cases and 17% of controls). The overall stratified relative risk estimate was 1.2 (95% confidence interval 1.0–1.4), and for use of at least 15 years, it was 0.9 (0.5–1.9; based on 16 cases and 25 controls). Unopposed oestrogens were used by 3% of both cases and controls for indications other than replacement, giving a stratified relative risk estimate of 1.0 (0.7–1.4). Opposed oestrogens were used by 1% of each

Table 2 Oestrogen use among 1686 cases of breast cancer and 2077 controls

Oestrogen use	*Cases*	*Controls*	*Stratified relative risk estimate*(95% confidence interval)*	*Multivariate relative risk estimate (95% confidence interval)*
Never used oestrogens	1293	1620	1.0†	1.0†
Unopposed, for replacement	311	351	1.2 (1.0–1.4)	1.1 (0.9–1.4)
conjugated oestrogens only	215	227	1.3 (1.0–1.6)	1.2 (1.0–1.6)
other oestrogens only	15	16	1.3 (0.6–2.8)	1.2 (0.6–2.7)
unknown type of oestrogen only	49	77	0.8 (0.6–1.2)	0.8 (0.5–1.2)
more than one type of oestrogen	32	31	1.4 (0.8–2.3)	1.3 (0.8–2.4)
Unopposed, for other indications‡	47	59	1.0 (0.7–1.4)	1.0 (0.6–1.5)
Opposed by progestogens	22	16	1.7 (0.9–3.3)	1.7 (0.9–3.6)
Ever use that first began ≤ 18 months before admission	13	31	—	—

*Adjusted for decade of age and type of menopause by the Mantel–Haenszel procedure; †reference category; ‡6 cases and 2 controls also took oestrogens for replacement

group, with an overall stratified estimate of 1.7 (0.9–3.3), and an estimate of 1.5 (0.7–3.3) for use of at least 1 year (16 cases, 12 controls). In all instances, the stratified and multivariate estimates were closely similar; only stratified estimates are presented in the remainder of this report.

Among the women who took oestrogens for replacement, the relative risk estimates for users of conjugated oestrogens, other named oestrogens, unspecified oestrogens, and more than one type were all close to 1.0 (Table 2). No specific non-conjugated oestrogen was taken by more than six cases or controls, and relative risks were not estimated for individual compounds. Because conjugated oestrogens accounted for over 90% of named compounds, users of unspecified oestrogens were considered to be conjugated oestrogen users in all further comparisons presented. When the analysis was confined to identified conjugated oestrogens, the results were similar (data not shown).

Table 3 shows the use of conjugated oestrogens for replacement according to duration of use. Relative risk estimates ranged from 0.9 to 1.4; there was no pattern of increased risk. For use that lasted 15 or more years, the relative risk estimate was 0.9 (0.4–1.9).

Table 4 shows the use of conjugated oestrogens for replacement according to the time elapsed since last use. Again, there was no pattern of increased risk. In particular, the estimate for use ending within 1 year of admission (current use) was 1.1 (0.7–1.6); the estimate for current use of at least 5 years' duration (based on 37 exposed cases and 44 exposed controls) was 1.3 (0.8–2.1). The estimate for use that ended 5–9 years before admission was 1.5 (1.0–2.2), but the estimates for use that ended in the distant past were close to 1.0. In particular, for use that ended at least 20 years before admission, the estimate was 0.9 (0.5–1.6). For use of at least 5 years' duration that ended at least 10 years before admission (8 cases, 19 controls), the relative risk estimate was 0.6 (0.2–1.3).

In our previous analysis[13], a significant inverse association was observed

Table 3 Duration of use of conjugated oestrogens for replacement among cases of breast cancer and controls; first used at least 18 months before admission, not opposed by progestogens; includes unknown oestrogens. Ten cases and seven controls had taken both conjugated and unknown oestrogens

Duration of use (years)	*Cases*	*Controls*	*Stratified relative risk estimate*(95% confidence interval)*
Never used oestrogens	1293	1620	1.0†
< 1	95	92	1.3 (1.0–1.8)
1–4	85	96	1.2 (0.9–1.6)
5–9	38	40	1.4 (0.9–2.2)
10–14	30	42	1.0 (0.6–1.6)
≥ 15	13	20	0.9 (0.4–1.9)
Unknown	13	21	—

*Adjusted for decade of age and type of menopause by the Mantel–Haenszel procedure; †reference category

Table 4 Elapsed time since last use of conjugated oestrogens for replacement among cases of breast cancer and controls; first used at least 18 months before admission, not opposed by progestogens; includes unknown oestrogens

Time since last use (years)	*Cases*	*Controls*	*Stratified relative risk estimate*(95% confidence interval)*
Never used oestrogens	1293	1620	1.0†
< 1	47	65	1.1 (0.7–1.6)
1–2	22	21	1.3 (0.8–2.4)
3–4	17	31	0.8 (0.4–1.4)
5–9	67	58	1.5 (1.0–2.2)
10–14	51	48	1.4 (0.9–2.1)
15–19	30	37	1.1 (0.6–1.7)
≥ 20	22	31	0.9 (0.5–1.6)
Unknown	18	20	—

*Adjusted for age and type of menopause by the Mantel–Haenszel procedure; †reference category

for women whose use ended at least 10 years before admission, and whose menopause was due to bilateral oophorectomy (Table 5). For comparison, a similar analysis of the present data was conducted. The age-adjusted relative risk estimates for those whose menopause was natural (57 exposed cases, 53 exposed controls), due to hysterectomy (24 cases, 20 controls), or due to bilateral oophorectomy (22 cases, 43 controls) were 1.3 (0.9–1.9), 1.6 (0.9–3.1), and 0.7 (0.4–1.3), respectively.

Table 6 shows the use of conjugated oestrogens for replacement for at least 5 years according to dose. For those who used the drug at a dose of less than 1.25 mg, the relative risk estimate was 0.8 (0.4–1.5); most of these

Table 5 Salient results from a previous case–control surveillance study of 1610 cases of breast cancer and 1606 controls

Category of oestrogen use	*Relative risk estimate (95% confidence interval)*
Conjugated oestrogens first taken ≥ 18 months before admission	0.9 (0.7–1.1)
Other oestrogens first taken ≥ 18 months before admission	0.8 (0.6–1.1)
Conjugated oestrogens taken for ≥ 10 years	
natural menopause	1.3 (0.6–2.8)
menopause due to hysterectomy	0.3 (0.1–1.0)
menopause due to bilateral oophorectomy	0.5 (0.2–1.0)
Last use of conjugated oestrogens ≥ 10 years before admission	
natural menopause	0.5 (0.3–1.1)
menopause due to hysterectomy	0.6 (0.2–1.9)
menopause due to bilateral oophorectomy	0.3 (0.1–0.8)
Conjugated oestrogen dose ≥ 1.25 mg for ≥ 5 years	0.4–0.7*
Conjugated oestrogens taken for ≥ 5 years according to risk factors for breast cancer	0.1–1.4†

*Range of estimates according to type of menopause; †range of estimates according to category

Table 6 Dose of conjugated oestrogens taken for at least 5 years for replacement among cases of breast cancer and controls; first used at least 18 months before admission, not opposed by progestogens; does not include unknown oestrogens

Dose (mg)	*Cases*	*Controls*	*Stratified relative risk estimate*(95% confidence interval)*
Never used oestrogens	1293	1620	1.0†
< 1.25	15	25	0.8 (0.4–1.5)
≥ 1.25	26	34	1.2 (0.7–2.0)
Mixed doses‡	9	9	1.6 (0.6–4.0)
Unknown dose	20	26	—

*Adjusted for age and type of menopause by the Mantel–Haenszel procedure; †reference category; ‡doses were taken in both categories

(12 cases, 20 controls) took 0.625 mg. For those who took higher doses (mainly 1.25 mg) the estimate was 1.2 (0.7–2.0).

To evaluate the effect of conjugated oestrogens in subgroups, the subjects were stratified according to various risk factors for breast cancer, including age, age at menarche, age at first pregnancy, parity, oral contraceptive use, age at menopause, type of menopause, history of cystic breast disease, family history of breast cancer, and body mass index. Table 7 gives relative risk estimates for women in these subgroups who had taken conjugated oestrogens for at least 5 years, compared to never-users. Most estimates were close to 1.0. The only estimate that was statistically significant was 2.2 (1.1–4.6), for

Table 7 Conjugated oestrogen use for at least 5 years for replacement among cases of breast cancer and controls according to various factors; first used at least 18 months before admission, not opposed by progestogens; includes unknown oestrogens

Factor	*Cases* *Use ≥ 5 years/ never-use*	*Controls* *Use ≥ 5 years/ never-use*	*Stratified relative risk estimate*(95% confidence interval)*
Age (years)			
40–49	2/ 110	13/ 180	0.4 (0.1–2.0)†
50–59	31/ 557	37/ 586	1.1 (0.6–1.8)†
60–69	48/ 613	49/ 809	1.3 (0.8–1.9)†
Age at menarche (years)			
< 15	70/1152	85/1381	1.1 (0.8–1.6)
≥ 15	11/ 141	17/ 239	1.2 (0.5–2.8)
Age at first pregnancy (years)			
< 25	28/ 568	55/ 800	1.5 (0.8–3.1)
≥ 25	30/ 504	29/ 542	0.9 (0.5–1.5)
Parity			
0	24/ 250	21/ 281	1.3 (0.7–2.6)
1–2	32/ 579	43/ 612	0.9 (0.5–1.4)
≥ 3	25/ 457	37/ 711	1.3 (0.7–2.2)
Oral contraceptive use			
yes	9/ 161	11/ 208	1.1 (0.4–3.1)
no	72/1132	91/1412	1.1 (0.8–1.6)
Age at menopause (years)			
< 40	14/ 191	37/ 329	0.8 (0.4–1.5)
40–49	36/ 469	41/ 610	1.1 (0.7–1.8)
≥ 50	28/ 588	24/ 599	1.2 (0.7–2.2)
Type of menopause			
natural	28/ 957	26/1123	1.3 (0.8–2.2)‡
due to hysterectomy	12/ 221	27/ 317	0.6 (0.3–1.2)‡
due to bilateral oophorectomy	41/ 115	49/ 179	1.3 (0.8–2.2)‡
History of cystic breast disease			
yes	20/ 243	10/ 140	1.2 (0.5–2.8)
no	61/1050	92/1480	1.1 (0.7–1.5)
Family history of breast cancer			
yes	18/ 195	9/ 113	1.7 (0.6–4.5)
no	63/1098	93/1507	1.0 (0.7–1.4)
Body mass index (wt/ht^2)			
≤ 20	19/ 154	20/ 314	2.2 (1.1–4.6)
21–28	52/ 796	64/ 933	1.1 (0.7–1.6)
≥ 29	9/ 324	18/ 325	0.6 (0.2–1.3)

*Relative to never-use in each category; adjusted for age and type of menopause by the Mantel–Haenszel procedure; †adjusted for type of menopause; ‡adjusted for age

women whose body mass index was less than 21. Further stratification yielded too few women with an appreciably lower body mass index for informative analysis. The relative risk estimates in other subgroups ranged from 0.4 to 1.7.

DISCUSSION

In this new analysis of recently collected data from our case–control surveillance study, we found no evidence of an elevation in the risk of breast cancer for most categories of replacement oestrogen use. The bulk of the data concerned conjugated oestrogens not opposed with progestogens; for users of these drugs, there was no trend of increasing risk with increasing dose or duration of use, and a doubling could be excluded for use lasting at least 15 years. There was also no evidence of an increase in risk for current use, after latent intervals as long as 20 years, after long-term use at high doses, and among subgroups defined according to known risk factors for breast cancer; again, for most categories a doubling in risk could be excluded. The only statistically significant positive association was a relative risk estimate of 2.2 for 5 or more years of use among women with a relatively low body mass index. There may be some biological credibility for this finding because postmenopausal women with low body mass produce less endogenous oestrogen[34], and may have a lower baseline risk of breast cancer[34–36]. However, given the large number of comparisons, the association may well be a chance one.

There were few subjects who had used oestrogens other than conjugated oestrogens, and it was not possible to estimate the risk of breast cancer among users of specific drugs. However, there was no overall evidence that the risk was elevated. There was also little information on the use of opposed oestrogens: there was no significant association, but the upper confidence limit was consistent with as much as a threefold increase in risk.

As with all epidemiological studies, it is necessary to consider whether the present results could have been affected by methodological problems. Selection of cases conditional on oestrogen use was unlikely, given the inevitability of diagnosis and hospital admission. The control diagnoses were selected to be unrelated to oestrogen use, and rates of use were reassuringly similar between controls with cancer and those with non-malignant conditions. The overall refusal rate was low. Thus, selection bias does not appear to be a plausible explanation for the results. Information bias cannot be ruled out, since the hypothesis was known. However, if a systematic reporting bias were operating, it would probably have led to spurious positive associations, since the cases would have been more likely than the controls to remember and report the details of their oestrogen use.

Another concern was the possibility that oestrogen use might have been initiated after the onset of breast cancer or, alternatively, some of the control conditions. To minimize that possibility, the analysis was focused on use that began at least 18 months before admission (1 year before the earliest cancer diagnosis).

Confounding was controlled in the analysis. The results based on multivariate analysis (in which known and possible risk factors for breast cancer were taken into account) were similar to those based on stratification for age and type of menopause. It remains possible that the results were confounded by factors for which allowance was not made.

The general absence of association in the present study is similar to the findings of our previous investigation, which was based on 1610 cases and

1606 non-cancer controls[13]. The salient results from that analysis are summarized in Table 5. Overall, the relative risk estimate for conjugated oestrogen use was 0.9, with an upper 95% confidence limit of 1.1; the estimate for non-conjugated oestrogen use was 0.8, also with an upper bound of 1.1. Most of the analyses were confined to postmenopausal women; the relative risk estimates for use of conjugated oestrogens for at least 10 years ranged from 0.3 to 1.3 according to type of menopause, and the estimates for last use at least 10 years before admission ranged from 0.3 to 0.6. The estimate of 0.3, for women whose menopause was due to bilateral oophorectomy, was significantly lower than 1.0. This contrasts with an estimate of 0.7, with an upper bound of 1.3, from the present analysis. Estimates for use of relatively high-dose conjugated oestrogens for at least 5 years ranged from 0.4 to 0.7 according to type of menopause. Finally, the relative risk estimates for use of at least 5 years' duration by subgroups of postmenopausal women defined according to various risk factors for breast cancer (family history of breast cancer, history of benign breast disease, age at first pregnancy, parity, and age at menopause) ranged from 0.1 to 1.4 among the categories.

While the results of the two studies are similar in terms of the basic lack of positive association, in the present investigation we did not observe the preponderance of relative risk estimates below 1.0 noted in the earlier analysis. In particular, we did not replicate the significant inverse association with conjugated oestrogens taken in the distant past among women with a menopause due to bilateral oophorectomy. Given the similarity of the methods, the reasons for the discrepancy are not clear. The only important methodological difference was that cancer controls were included in the present study, but the similarity in the rates of oestrogen use between cancer and non-cancer controls rules out the inclusion of cancer controls as an explanation. It is not plausible that the different periods of data collection (1976–81 vs. 1980–88) could account for the difference. The most reasonable conclusion is that the earlier inverse association was a statistical fluke.

There have been many other studies[1–29], of both the case–control and follow-up type, on the relation of exogenous oestrogen use to the risk of breast cancer, and it is beyond the scope of this presentation to comment on all of them in detail. Most have shown no overall effect of oestrogen use. In three studies[15,19,26], there were modest but statistically significant increases in risk that ranged from 60 to 80%. There have also been increases in risk reported in various subgroups of women classified according to risk factors for breast cancer[1–7,9,11,15,17–19,24,26]. The elevated relative risk estimates have generally been based on small numbers, and there has not been any consistent pattern of association across studies.

What is of greater concern is that data from four studies[9,14,21,24] have suggested that the risk may be increased for long durations of oestrogen use. One study[9] was based on relatively small numbers of users. Another[14] was large, but the cases and controls were derived from a breast cancer screening programme, and it is possible that women with symptoms of breast cancer who were also long-standing oestrogen users may have been more likely to participate in the programme than other women. The other two studies[21,24] were conducted in Scandinavia, and most of the data concerned non-conjugated oestrogens. Thus, the results may not be directly comparable with those of the present study and others conducted in the United States, where conjugated oestrogens are by far the most prevalent type. Both of the Scandinavian studies also had elevated relative risk estimates for oestrogen therapy opposed by progestogens, but these were not statistically significant, and they contrast with the results of a follow-up study[28] and small clinical trial[29], which were consistent with a reduced risk for opposed therapy.

Among other large case–control studies, there was no statistically significant association with long-term use in our own Toronto Breast Cancer Study, the results of which are also being presented here, or in the Cancer and Steroid Hormone (CASH) study[20]; however, in both studies the relative risk point estimates were somewhat elevated. In neither study did the risk appear to be increased in the subgroups that have been previously reported.

Finally, two recent follow-up studies[26,27] have shown modest elevations in risk for current users, of the order of 36–70%, and the investigators have proposed that their findings are compatible with a promotional effect. In both studies, the selective diagnosis of breast cancer among current or recent oestrogen users could have contributed to the associations. In addition, the biological plausibility of the findings is reduced by the apparent elevation in the risk for exposure lasting less than 1 year, and by the lack of duration or dose–response effects. By contrast, there was no association with current use in the Cancer and Steroid Hormone study, where the data were sufficient to exclude a 30% increase in risk for current users[20]. Neither was there evidence of an increase in risk for current conjugated oestrogen users in the present study, although the upper confidence limit was insufficient to exclude the recent findings.

Based on present results and those of other large epidemiological studies, we conclude that unopposed conjugated oestrogens taken for hormone replacement do not increase the risk of breast cancer appreciably. The possibility remains open that the risk is modestly increased after very long durations of use, and that opposed therapy, and other non-contraceptive oestrogens, increase the risk. Further studies should focus on the latter questions.

ACKNOWLEDGEMENTS

This work was supported by contracts 223-76-3016, 233-80-3001, 226-82-0007 and co-operative agreements U01 FD01222 and FD-U-000082 from the Food and Drug Administration. Additional support was provided by contracts and grants N01-CP-71029, N01-CB-74099, and R37-CA-45762 from the National Cancer Institute. The Slone Epidemiology Unit has also received support from Hoffman–LaRoche Inc., Nutley, NJ; CIBA–GEIGY Corporation, Summit, NJ; Hoechst AG, Frankfurt, Germany; McNeil Pharmaceutical, Spring House, PA; Merrell Dow Pharmaceuticals, Inc., Cincinnati, OH; Ortho Pharmaceuticals Corporation, Raritan, NJ; and Sterling Drug, Inc., New York, NY. The material is derived in part from a paper published in the American Journal of Epidemiology (Kaufman, D.W., Palmer, J.R., de Mouzon, J., Rosenberg, L., Stolley, P.D., Warshauer, E.,

Zauber, A.G. and Shapiro, S. (1991) Estrogen replacement therapy and the risk of breast cancer: results from the case–control surveillance study. *Am. J. Epidemiol.*, **134**, 1375–85.

The authors are indebted to the many physicians who allowed us to interview their patients, the nurse-interviewers who collected the data, Marguerite Angeloni for co-ordinating the study, and Leonard Gaetano for assistance with data management. The following hospitals participated in this study: Boston: Beth Israel Hospital, Mt. Auburn Hospital, Newton–Wellesley Hospital, Sancta Maria Hospital, Tufts New England Medical Center; New York: Brookhaven Memorial Hospital, Lenox Hill Hospital, Memorial Sloan–Kettering Cancer Center, New York Hospital; Philadelphia: American Oncologic Hospital, Crozier Chester Medical Center, Hahnemann University Hospital, Hospital of the Medical College of Pennsylvania, Hospital of the University of Pennsylvania, Lankenau Hospital, Montgomery Hospital, Pennsylvania Hospital, Presbyterian Hospital, Thomas Jefferson University Hospital; Baltimore: Johns Hopkins University Hospital; Tucson: University of Arizona Health Science Center; Kansas City: Kansas University Medical Center; San Francisco: University of California, San Francisco Moffitt Hospital; London, Ontario: St. Joseph's Hospital.

REFERENCES

1. Casagrande, J., Gerkins, V., Henderson, B.E., Mack, T. and Pike, M.C. (1976). Brief communication: Exogenous estrogens and breast cancer in women with natural menopause. *J. Natl. Cancer Inst.*, **56**, 839–41
2. Hoover, R., Gray, L.A., Cole, P. and MacMahon, B. (1976). Menopausal estrogens and breast cancer. *N. Engl. J. Med.*, **295**, 401–5
3. Sartwell, P.E., Arthes, F.G. and Tonascia, J.A. (1977). Exogenous hormones, reproductive history, and breast cancer. *J. Natl. Cancer Inst.*, **59**, 1589–92
4. Brinton, L.A., Williams, R.R., Hoover, R.N., Stegens, N.L., Feinleib, M. and Fraumeni, J.F., Jr (1979). Breast cancer risk factors among screening program participants. *J. Natl. Cancer Inst.*, **62**, 37–44
5. Ross, R.K., Paganini-Hill, A., Gerkins, V.R., Mack, T.M., Pfeffer, R., Arthur, M. and Henderson, B.E. (1980). A case–control study of menopausal estrogen therapy and breast cancer. *J. Am. Med. Assoc.*, **243**, 1635–9
6. Jick, H., Walker, A.M., Watkins, R.N., D'Ewart, D.C., Hunter, J.R., Danford, A., Madsen, S., Dinan, J. and Rothman, K.J. (1980). Replacement estrogens and breast cancer. *Am. J. Epidemiol.*, **112**, 586–94
7. Brinton, L.A., Hoover, R.N., Szklo, M. and Fraumeni, J.F., Jr (1981). Menopausal estrogen use and risk of breast cancer. *Cancer*, **47**, 2517–22
8. Kelsey, J.L., Fischer, D.B., Holford, T.R., LiVolsi, V.A., Mostow, E.D., Goldenberg, I.S. and White, C. (1981). Exogenous estrogens and other factors in the epidemiology of breast cancer. *J. Natl. Cancer Inst.*, **67**, 327–33
9. Hoover, R., Glass, A., Finkle, W.D., Azevedo, D. and Milne, K. (1981). Conjugated estrogens and breast cancer risk in women. *J. Natl. Cancer Inst.*, **67**, 815–20
10. Lawson, D.H., Jick, H., Hunter, J.R. and Madsen, S. (1981). Exogenous estrogens and breast cancer. *Am. J. Epidemiol.*, **114**, 710–13
11. Hulka, B.S., Chambless, L.E., Deubner, D.C. and Wilkinson, W.E. (1982). Breast cancer and estrogen replacement therapy. *Am. J. Obstet. Gynecol.*, **143**, 638–44
12. Hiatt, R.A., Bawol, R., Friedman, G.D. and Hoover, R. (1984). Exogenous estrogen and breast cancer after bilateral oophorectomy. *Cancer*, **54**, 139–44
13. Kaufman, D.W., Miller, D.R., Rosenberg, L., Helmrich, M.S., Stolley, P., Schottenfeld, D. and Shapiro, S. (1984). Non-contraceptive estrogen use and the risk of breast cancer. *J. Am. Med. Assoc.*, **252**, 63–7

14. Brinton, L.A., Hoover, R. and Fraumeni, J.F., Jr (1986). Menopausal oestrogens and breast cancer risk: an expanded case–control study. *Br. J. Cancer*, **54**, 825–32
15. La Vecchia, C., Decarli, A., Parazzini, F., Gentile, A., Liberati, C. and Franceschi, S. (1986). Non-contraceptive oestrogens and the risk of breast cancer in women. *Int. J. Cancer*, **38**, 853–8
16. McDonald, J.A., Weiss, N.S., Daling, J.R., Francis, A.M. and Polissar, L. (1986). Menopausal estrogen use and the risk of breast cancer. *Breast Cancer Res. Treat.*, **7**, 193–9
17. Nomura, A.M.Y., Kolonel, L.N., Hirohata, T. and Lee, J. (1986). The association of replacement estrogens with breast cancer. *Int. J. Cancer*, **37**, 49–53
18. Buring, J.E., Hennekens, C.H., Lipnick, R.J., Willett, W., Stampfer, M.J., Rosner, B., Peto, R. and Speizer, F.E. (1987). A prospective cohort study of postmenopausal hormone use and risk of breast cancer in US women. *Am. J. Epidemiol.*, **125**, 939–47
19. Hunt, K., Vessey, M., McPherson, K. and Coleman, M. (1987). Long-term surveillance of mortality and cancer incidence in women receiving hormone replacement therapy. *Br. J. Obstet. Gynecol.*, **94**, 620–35
20. Wingo, P.A., Layde, P.M., Lee, N.C., Rubin, G. and Ory, H.W. (1987). The risk of breast cancer in postmenopausal women who have used estrogen replacement therapy. *J. Am. Med. Assoc.*, **257**, 209–15
21. Bergkvist, L., Adami, H.-O., Persson, I., Hoover, R. and Schairer, C. (1989). The risk of breast cancer after estrogen and estrogen–progestin replacement. *N. Engl. J. Med.*, **321**, 293–7
22. Thomas, D.B., Persing, J.P. and Hutchinson, W.B. (1982). Exogenous estrogens and other risk factors for breast cancer in women with benign breast diseases. *J. Natl. Cancer Inst.*, **69**, 1017–23
23. Rohan, T.E. and McMichael, A.J. (1988). Non-contraceptive exogenous oestrogen therapy and breast cancer. *Med. J. Aust.*, **148**, 217–21
24. Ewertz, M. (1988). Influence of non-contraceptive exogenous and endogenous sex hormones on breast cancer risk in Denmark. *Int. J. Cancer*, **42**, 832–8
25. Dupont, W.D., Page, D.L., Rogers, L.W. and Parl, F.F. (1989). Influence of exogenous estrogens, proliferative breast disease, and other variables on breast cancer risk. *Cancer*, **63**, 948–57
26. Mills, P.K., Beeson, W.L., Phillips, R.L. and Fraser, G.E. (1989). Prospective study of exogenous hormone use and breast cancer in Seventh-day Adventists. *Cancer*, **64**, 591–7
27. Colditz, G.A., Stampfer, M.J., Willett, W.C., Hennekens, C.H., Rosner, B. and Speizer, F.E. (1990). Prospective study of estrogen replacement therapy and risk of breast cancer in postmenopausal women. *J. Am. Med. Assoc.*, **264**, 2648–53
28. Gambrell, R.D., Jr, Maier, R.C. and Sanders, B.I. (1983). Decreased incidence of breast cancer in postmenopausal estrogen–progestogen users. *Obstet. Gynecol.*, **62**, 435–43
29. Nachtigall, L.E., Nachtigall, R.H., Nachtigall, R.D. and Beckman, E.M. (1979). Estrogen replacement therapy. II. A prospective study in the relationship to carcinoma and cardiovascular and metabolic problems. *Obstet. Gynecol.*, **54**, 74–9
30. Slone, D., Shapiro, S. and Miettinen, O.S. (1977). Case–control surveillance of serious illnesses attributable to ambulatory drug use. In Colombo, F., Shapiro, S., Slone, D. and Tognoni, G. (eds.) *Epidemiological Evaluation of Drugs*, pp. 59–82. (Amsterdam: Elsevier North-Holland Inc.)
31. Mantel, H. and Haenszel, W. (1959). Statistical aspects of the analysis of data from retrospective studies. *J. Natl. Cancer Inst.*, **22**, 719–48
32. Miettinen, O.S. (1976). Estimability and estimation in case referent studies. *Am. J. Epidemiol.*, **103**, 226–35
33. Schlesselman, J.J. (1982). *Case–Control Studies: Design, Conduct, Analysis.* (New York: Oxford University Press)
34. Key, T.J.A. and Pike, M.C. (1988). The role of estrogens and progestogens in the epidemiology and prevention of breast cancer. *Eur. J. Cancer Clin. Oncol.*, **24**, 29–43
35. Kelsey, J.L. (1979). A review of the epidemiology of human breast cancer. *Epidemiol. Rev.*, **1**, 74–109
36. Helmrich, S.P., Shapiro, S., Rosenberg, L., Kaufman, D.W., Bain, C., Miettinen, O.S., Stolley, P.D., Rosenshein, N.B., Knapp, R.C., Leavitt, T., Schottenfeld, D., Engle, R. and Levy, M. (1983). Risk factors for breast cancer. *Am. J. Epidemiol.*, **117**, 35–45

15

Hormone replacement therapy and breast cancer: overview of the University of Oxford studies

M.P. Vessey, K. Hunt and K. McPherson

INTRODUCTION

In 1977 the Medical Research Council Working Group on Hormone Replacement Therapy decided to support our proposal that a cohort study should be done of women attending specialist menopause clinics in the United Kingdom. In this paper we describe the methods used in our study and summarize the main results with regard to breast cancer to have emerged so far in the two published reports, Hunt *et al.* (1987)[1] and Hunt *et al.* (1990)[2].

THE STUDY OF HUNT *et al.* (1987)

Methods

Recruitment to the study, which had both a retrospective and a prospective component, began in 1978 after the co-operation of the staff at 21 menopause clinics had been obtained. To be eligible for recruitment a woman had to be a current user of hormone replacement therapy attending one of the participating clinics and in addition had to have had at least 1 year's continuous treatment. At recruitment, information was obtained about each woman's obstetrical, gynaecological and past medical history. In addition, information was recorded about some social and physical characteristics and a detailed hormone replacement therapy history was documented up to the date of recruitment.

Up to the end of 1982 4544 women were recruited to the study and a postal questionnaire was sent to 4387 of these in 1983. The response rate to the questionnaire was almost 80%. The main purpose of the questionnaire was to elicit information on hormone replacement therapy use since entry

This brief paper cites some of the results from two published articles: Hunt, K. *et al.* (1987)[1] and Hunt, K. *et al.* (1990)[2], with permission to the study and to enquire about major morbidity. In addition it was used to complete missing baseline data.

From the above it will be apparent that several means of identifying cancers among the women in the study were available to us from four sources, as follows:

(1) National Health Service Central Registries (all the women are flagged in these registries);

(2) Hospital and clinic notes where there was occasion to review them;

(3) Notifications provided directly by doctors working in some clinics; and

(4) Self-reported information on the postal questionnaires.

Each notification of a death or of a cancer was followed up through the relevant doctor to confirm the diagnosis and to complete treatment details. In addition, a more detailed follow-up was undertaken for cancers of the breast; thus, an attempt was made to stage the breast cancers at the time of diagnosis from clinical notes using the tumour–node–metastases (TNM) system.

Subjects

The present analysis is limited to the 4544 women entering the study before the end of 1982. Most of these women were aged 45–54 years at recruitment (60%) and at first use of hormone replacement therapy (63%), about 6% had never been married and nearly 20% had never given birth. Distributions by parity and by age at first term birth were broadly similar to those in the population at large but women in the cohort tended to be of a higher social class than women in general (46% in social classes 1 or 2; the corresponding figure from the 1971 census is 23%). Smoking patterns were unremarkable.

Almost 36% of the women had already undergone hysterectomy at first use of hormone replacement therapy, some two to two-and-a-half times the proportion in the British population. Of the women with intact uteri, approximately equal numbers were either naturally postmenopausal or were pre- or perimenopausal at their first use of hormone replacement therapy. Past oral contraceptive use was infrequent among women in the cohort; thus only 24% recorded some use.

Complete hormone replacement therapy histories up to the closure date for the analysis of the data (June, 1984) were available for only 70% of the women in the cohort. Details of treatment up to the recruitment date were, of course, known for all 4544 women but are of limited value. Of the 3198 women for whom complete histories were available, 51% had taken hormone replacement therapy for more than 5 years and the average duration of use per woman was 67 months.

One striking feature about our study is the great variety of hormone replacement therapy preparations and combinations of preparations which have been used by the participants; indeed over 175 different treatments are included in the survey coding schedule. Table 1 provides data on the ten most commonly used regimens, although considered together these constitute only 71% of all use. Premarin® taken alone accounted for only 17% of hormone replacement therapy use, a finding in marked contrast to the figures in North American studies.

One important way in which hormone replacement therapy regimens can be grouped is according to whether or not oestrogen is opposed by a progestogen. Women with intact uteri had received, on average, 21.3 months of unopposed therapy and 39.2 months of opposed therapy. By contrast, women who had already undergone hysterectomy and bilateral salpingo-oophorectomy at entry to the study had received an average 66.4 and 8.6 months of unopposed and opposed treatment, respectively. Women who retained at least one ovary at hysterectomy were intermediate between the other two groups on these measures of hormone replacement therapy use.

We did not code either the number of days for which progestogens were given in each cycle or the dose of progestogens; indeed these data were often unknown. It is safe to say, however, that most of the opposed therapy received by women in our study was much less progestogenic than that which is generally given today.

RESULTS

Mortality

Twelve deaths from breast cancer were observed in comparison with a figure of 21.9 expected from national rates, giving a mortality ratio of 0.55 with 95% confidence limits of 0.28–0.96.

Table 1 The ten most commonly used preparations among 3198 women

*Preparation**	*Total duration of use* (months)	*Average duration of use per woman* (months)
1. Premarin	35 976	11.2
2. Premarin + norethisterone	23 167	7.2
3. Premarin + Neogest	20 406	6.4
4. Harmogen	12 854	4.0
5. Ethinyloestradiol	11 537	3.6
6. Progynova	10 952	3.4
7. Mestranol	10 901	3.4
8. Oestradiol and testosterone implant + norethisterone	9306	2.9
9. Cyclo-Progynova	8744	2.7
10. Oestradiol and testosterone implant	8077	2.5

*Premarin® = conjugated equine oestrogens 0.625 mg, 1.25 mg or 2.5 mg (Ayerst); Neogest® = norgestrel 75 μg (Schering); Harmogen® = piperazine oestrone sulphate 1.5 mg (Abbot); Progynova® = oestradiol valerate 1 mg or 2 mg (Schering); Cyclo-Progynova® = oestradiol valerate 1 mg (11 tablets) and oestradiol valerate 1 mg plus levonorgestrel 0.25 mg (10 tablets) (Schering)

Morbidity

The incidence of breast cancer was found to be significantly elevated in comparison with cancer registry rates (50 cases observed, 31.38 expected; morbidity ratio 1.59; 95% confidence limits, 1.18–2.10). There was also evidence of a non-significant positive trend in ratio with interval since first use of hormone replacement therapy.

Adjustment of the ratios for social class had little effect, but there was some evidence that diagnosis might have been accelerated amongst women using hormone replacement therapy, perhaps as a result of increased surveillance. Thus, of the 40 breast cancers we were able to stage, 27 (68%) were in clinical stage 1 at diagnosis, a much higher proportion than that reported by many other authors. However, 15 of the 27 stage 1 cancers were T2, all 50 cancers were invasive, there was no difference in the proportion of stage 1 cancers when current users of hormone replacement therapy were compared with ex-users, and few if any of the women with breast cancer had been diagnosed as a consequence of screening by mammography.

To explore the findings further we undertook a case–control within cohort analysis using two controls per case matched for age, and including four additional breast cancer cases diagnosed after the closure date.

When comparisons were made between the cases and controls, it was found that the cases tended to be of lower parity and to be slightly older when they first gave birth than the controls, although neither difference was statistically significant. Unexpectedly, cases were more likely to have had a prior hysterectomy (with or without bilateral salpingo-oophorectomy) than the controls, a finding that was also apparent when the data were analysed on a cohort basis.

Comparisons of overall duration of use are shown in Table 2 for the 53 cases and 97 controls for whom complete data were available. There is some evidence that the cases had longer overall durations of treatment than the controls, although the relation is not entirely straightforward. Most marked differences are seen in the tails of the distribution. Distributions showing use of opposed and unopposed hormone replacement therapy separately did not contribute much.

A multivariate analysis was undertaken in an attempt to disentangle the effects of duration of use and of ovarian and uterine status. In this analysis the duration of treatment was divided into four groups: 12–30, 31–48, 49–72 and 73+ months; these groupings were chosen by dividing the numbers of

Table 2 Comparisons of use of hormone replacement therapy between breast cancer cases and controls

	Overall duration of treatment (months)					
	12–24	*25–48*	*49–72*	*73–96*	*97+*	*Total*
Cases	2	23	16	2	10	53
Controls	23	33	18	14	9	97
Total	25	56	34	16	19	150

χ^2 for trend = 3.38 (not significant)

subjects under study as nearly as possible into quartiles. The analysis was conducted on 48 matched sets.

A number of different models were fitted to the data, all of which gave broadly comparable results. The figures shown in Table 3 may be taken as representative. Increased relative risks of breast cancer are apparent for women with hysterectomy with or without bilateral salpingo-oophorectomy in comparison with women with intact uteri. Likewise, increased relative risks of breast cancer are apparent for women taking hormone replacement therapy for durations longer than 30 months in comparison with those with shorter durations of use. The substantial magnitude of the relative risks associated with prolonged hormone replacement therapy use is, of course, a reflection of the small number of cases of breast cancer with short durations of use. As expected, the adjusted relative risks are generally appreciably smaller than the crude relative risks. Nonetheless, all the relative risks remain substantially in excess of unity, indicating that the effect of duration of hormone replacement therapy use is only partially explained by the effect of type of menopause and vice versa.

Durations of use of unopposed and opposed hormone replacement therapy were also fitted into various models, both singly and together. These analyses were no more illuminating than those shown in Table 3 and no obvious patterns emerged.

One further way in which use of hormone replacement therapy was considered in the case–control analysis was to compare the average duration of use of particular preparations and combinations (Table 4). It is unwise to draw firm conclusions from such an analysis on the basis of small numbers of subjects but ethinyloestradiol was taken much more extensively by the cases than by the controls. Use of this steroid was largely concentrated

Table 3 Risk of breast cancer by uterine and ovarian status and by duration of hormone replacement therapy (95% confidence limits in parentheses). Note: the substantial magnitude of the relative risks associated with prolonged hormone replacement therapy use is a reflection of the small number of cases of breast cancer with short durations of use (see Table 2)

Variable	*Relative risk (unadjusted)*	*Relative risk (adjusted)*
No hysterectomy	1.0	1.0
Hysterectomy without bilateral salpingo-oophorectomy	3.4 (1.4–8.4)	2.9 (1.1–7.5)
Hysterectomy with bilateral salpingo-oophorectomy at age (years)		
under 40	7.1 (0.6–89.8)	2.2 (0.1–34.3)
40–44	2.4 (0.5–11.1)	1.9 (0.4–9.1)
45–49	2.0 (0.2–17.5)	1.3 (0.1–12.9)
over 49	2.3 (0.5–10.7)	2.7 (0.5–15.1)
Hormone replacement therapy (months)		
12–30	1.0	1.0
31–48	5.2 (1.8–15.6)	4.8 (1.5–15.6)
49–72	6.1 (1.8–20.4)	5.3 (1.4–20.2)
73 +	4.8 (1.3–17.0)	3.6 (0.9–15.0)

Table 4 Use of ten most commonly taken hormone replacement therapy preparations by women with breast cancer and matched controls. (See footnote to Table 1 for details of preparations)

	Women with breast cancer ($n = 53$)				*Matched controls* ($n = 97$)			
Preparation	*Total duration of use* (months)	*Average duration of use* (months)	*Number of users*	*Average duration per user* (months)	*Total duration of use* (months)	*Average duration of use* (months)	*Number of users*	*Average duration per user* (months)
1. Premarin	777	14.7	24	32.4	834	8.6	37	22.5
2. Premarin + norethisterone	223	4.2	6	37.2	634	6.5	19	33.4
3. Premarin + Neogest	319	6.0	13	24.5	265	2.7	15	17.7
4. Harmogen	286	5.4	13	22.0	336	3.5	23	14.6
5. Ethinyloestradiol	705	13.3	18	39.2	141	1.5	12	11.8
6. Progynova	151	2.8	8	18.9	234	2.4	20	11.7
7. Mestranol	170	3.2	2	85.0	217	2.2	2	108.5
8. Oestradiol and testosterone implant + norethisterone	23	0.4	1	23.0	174	1.8	6	29.0
9. Cyclo-Progynova	60	1.1	9	6.7	112	1.2	8	14.0
10. Oestradiol and testosterone implant	0	—	0	—	178	1.8	6	29.7

among hysterectomized women and particularly among those who retained their ovaries. Only three cases are known to have taken daily doses of ethinyloestradiol in excess of 50 μg.

THE STUDY OF HUNT *et al.* (1990)

A further analysis of the cohort study was undertaken, covering deaths only from July, 1984 to December, 1988. Unfortunately, no new data on use of treatment were obtained for this exercise so the analyses that could be undertaken were essentially very simple ones.

During the interval of July, 1984 to December, 1988 there were 19 breast cancer deaths, while 19.05 were expected at national rates, giving a mortality ratio of 1.0 with 95% confidence limits of 0.55–1.45. This mortality ratio is strikingly higher than the ratio of 0.55 obtained during the first analysis. Furthermore, there was quite strong evidence, when the data for all 31 breast cancer deaths were put together, of an increasing trend in mortality ratio with years since first exposure to hormone replacement therapy (Table 5). This trend still does not reach statistical significance, however.

DISCUSSION

In our first report we suggested that a plausible interpretation for the significantly elevated incidence of breast cancer observed in the face of significantly low mortality from the disease was that women with clinically recognizable breast cancer, and those at high risk of the disease, had been deemed not to be suitable candidates for long-term hormone replacement therapy and had therefore been selected out of the cohort. In such circumstances one might also have expected a low incidence of the disease as well as low mortality if hormone replacement therapy had no harmful effects. As this was not what we observed, we suggested that breast cancer mortality would rise, in due course. It is of considerable interest that such a rise is already apparent in our second report. This is slightly worrying since we judged that a small part of the elevated incidence seen might have been attributable to diagnostic surveillance bias, as the staging distribution of the

Table 5 Breast cancer mortality in the cohort by interval since first exposure to hormone replacement therapy

Years since first exposure to hormone replacement therapy	*Number of deaths (breast cancer)*			
	Observed	*Expected*	*Ratio of observed/expected*	*95% confidence interval*
0–4	3	7.94	0.38	0.00–1.07
5–9	13	17.60	0.74	0.27–1.21
10+	15	15.43	0.97	0.47–1.47
Total	31	40.97	0.76	0.45–1.06

χ^2 for trend = 2.41 (not significant)

incident tumours was relatively favourable. Of the 19 additional breast cancer deaths in the second analysis, 11 were known to us as incident cases in the first analysis. The suggestion that breast cancer mortality may increase with increasing intervals since first exposure to hormone replacement therapy is consistent with an adverse effect of hormone replacement therapy on breast cancer which has taken some time to manifest itself in a basically low-risk selected population. The analysis of the incident cases of breast cancer in our first report produced some unexpected results with regard to the relationship between risk and hysterectomy, but nonetheless suggested that there was some elevation in risk in association with increasing duration of hormone replacement therapy use. No difference could be detected between the effects of opposed and unopposed therapy. The analysis examining the association between type of preparation and breast cancer suggested quite strongly that unopposed ethinyloestradiol might be harmful, but to the best of our knowledge this has not been confirmed in any other study.

On balance, the Oxford cohort study adds modest support to the view that a slight increase in breast cancer risk is associated with the use of hormone replacement therapy, but there are clearly many problems with the study with regard to selection for the study cohort, the absence of non-user control subjects, and the use of national mortality and cancer registration data for the computation of expected numbers.

ACKNOWLEDGEMENTS

This study would not have been possible without the kind co-operation of those in the participating clinics, to whom we extend our thanks. We would also like to thank Dr D Yeates, Dr C. Wells, Mrs D. Collinge and Mrs J. Challenger and the staff in the survey section of the National Health Service Central Registries. The Medical Research Council kindly provided financial support.

REFERENCES

1. Hunt, K., Vessey, M.P. and McPherson, K. (1987). Long-term surveillance of mortality and cancer incidence in women receiving hormone replacement therapy. *Br. J. Obstet. Gynaecol.*, **94**, 620–35
2. Hunt, K., Vessey, M.P. and McPherson, K. (1990). Mortality in a cohort of long-term users of hormone replacement therapy: an updated analysis. *Br. J. Obstet. Gynaecol.*, **97**, 1080–6

16

Hormone replacement therapy and risk of breast cancer: a population-based case–control study in Australia

T.E. Rohan

INTRODUCTION

Hormone replacement therapy usually consists of oestrogens given alone, or of oestrogens given in combination with progestogens. Because endogenously produced ovarian hormones influence the development (and progression) of breast cancer[1], there has been considerable concern that their exogenous counterparts might exert similar effects. To date, however, studies of the relationship between hormone replacement therapy and breast cancer (which have been, primarily, studies of conjugated oestrogens and breast cancer) have yielded inconsistent results[2–32]. Thus, case–control studies have variously shown the risk of breast cancer overall (i.e. the risk for ever-users relative to that for never-users) to be increased[15,17,24], unaltered[2,5,7,13,14,18,20,23,25,26,29,30], or decreased[3], while of the cohort studies, most have shown risk to be increased[6,8,21,28,31,32], and the remainder have shown hormone replacement therapy use either to have no effect[4,22,27], or to be associated with reduced risk[10,19]. A recent report[33] from an earlier cohort study[27] showed an increase in risk confined to current users of oestrogen replacement therapy.

As noted previously[24], most of these studies were conducted in North America, and there is a clear need for investigations to be undertaken in other populations. In this regard, the present report describes the results of a population-based case–control study of hormone replacement therapy and breast cancer that was conducted in Adelaide, South Australia. Results from this study have been described elsewhere[34].

SUBJECTS AND METHODS

Study subjects

Women whose histologically-confirmed first diagnosis of breast cancer was reported to the population-based South Australian Central Cancer Registry (notification of cancer diagnoses to the Registry is mandatory) between April, 1982 and July, 1984 were eligible for selection as cases if their age at diagnosis was between 20 and 74 years, if they resided within the Adelaide metropolitan area, and if they were registered on the electoral roll. Of the 559 eligible cases, 15 died before an interview could be arranged, 44 were deemed by the attending surgeon to be unfit for interview, 44 refused to be interviewed, and five were untraceable. Therefore, 451 cases were included in the study, representing a response rate of about 81%.

Controls were women who had no past history of breast cancer, who resided in the Adelaide metropolitan area, and who were registered on the electoral roll (in South Australia, 97.2% of persons eligible to vote are registered[35]). For each case, one control was selected at random from the electoral roll from those women of approximately the same age as that of the case at diagnosis. Thus, 97% of the members of the case–control pairs included in this study had ages within 1 year of each other; the mean age of the included cases was 55.3 years, and that of the included controls was 55.4 years. Because some women either refused to participate or were untraceable, 648 women in total were approached in order to enrol the 451 controls (70.0%) included in the study. Reasons for non-participation were recorded during recruitment of the first 100 controls, for 37 of whom it was necessary to approach more than one potential control. Of the 51 potential controls who did not participate, 39 refused to be interviewed, 11 were untraceable, and one had died. Overall, in 326 instances, the person first approached as a potential control agreed to participate.

Data collection

All potential study subjects were approached initially by a letter which referred non-specifically to a continuing study of life-style and personal factors in relation to various diseases. Study subjects were interviewed in their homes by trained interviewers who administered questionnaires in a standardized manner and whose performance was monitored regularly; interviewers were assigned randomly to case–control pairs. The average interval between case diagnosis and interview was 4.8 months. Each control was interviewed as soon as possible after her corresponding case had been enrolled in the study, and approximately 90% of controls were interviewed within 2 months of their cases. Thus, case–control matching on calendar time was implicit in the conduct of the study.

Sociodemographic and medical information was collected from the study subjects using an interviewer-administered structured questionnaire. The questionnaire sought basic biographical information, personal medical history, family history of cancer, gynaecological history, reproductive history, and history of hormone use. With respect to use of hormone replacement therapy, participants were asked to indicate whether they had ever used it, and if so, to indicate their age at first and last use, the duration of use, and, if possible, the name of the preparation that they had used the most. Cases were instructed to provide answers relating to the period up to the date of diagnosis of their breast cancer.

Data analysis

Although analyses were conducted overall and in the postmenopausal stratum, emphasis in this report is placed on the results for postmenopausal women, since the major reported indication for use of hormone replacement therapy was for the relief of menopausal symptoms. Women were considered to be postmenopausal if they had not experienced a menstrual period within the last 12 months, or if they had undergone a bilateral oophorectomy. In addition, women who had undergone a hysterectomy before the natural cessation of menstruation and who had retained at least one ovary were deemed to be postmenopausal if they were aged 56 years or older (so that they were more than 5 years older than the median age at natural menopause for the controls). On this basis, 281 cases and 288 controls were deemed to be postmenopausal, and among these postmenopausal women there were 262 case–control pairs.

The matched design of the study was taken into account in most of the analyses. For this purpose, the conditional logistic regression model was used to derive odds ratios and associated 95% confidence intervals[36]. Initially, the univariate association of each aspect of hormone replacement therapy with risk of breast cancer was examined. Thereafter, the effects of several potential confounding variables on these associations were adjusted for simultaneously in multiple conditional logistic regression models. The following variables were included in these models as potential confounders: family history of breast cancer; history of bilateral oophorectomy; age at last menstrual period; practice of breast self-examination; and years of education. The inclusion of several other variables in these models – namely, history of benign breast disease, age at first menstrual period, age at first full-term pregnancy, ever-use of oral contraceptives, obesity and history of cigarette smoking – did not change the estimates of association appreciably. Therefore, only the results derived from use of the smaller set of confounders are presented here.

In a final series of analyses, the risk of breast cancer in association with hormone replacement therapy was examined within strata formed by categorizing several risk factors for breast cancer. For these analyses, age-matching was broken because there were only very small numbers of case–control pairs (and in some instances there were none) that were concordant on the stratification criterion of interest, and age-adjusted odds ratios were derived from unconditional logistic regression models[36]. If the estimates of association were biased as a result of not retaining the matching, it is likely that they were biased conservatively[36].

RESULTS

The results of the present study with respect to some of the commonly described risk factors for breast cancer are summarized in Table 1. Risk of breast cancer was increased in association with a history of breast cancer in a first-degree relative, a history of benign breast disease, a relatively late age at menopause, failure to practise breast self-examination (statistically significant), and a post-primary education (an index of social class). There was also a non-uniform increase in risk with increasing age at first full-term pregnancy, and a statistically significant reduction in risk in association with a history of bilateral oophorectomy. Finally, there was also a small increase in risk of breast cancer with obesity and with an early age at menarche (data not shown).

In the total study population, less than 20% of cases and controls reported ever having used hormone replacement therapy (for at least 1 month), and the unadjusted matched odds ratio for ever- vs. never-use was 0.87 (95% confidence interval (CI), 0.62–1.23); after adjustment for potential confounding, the odds ratio associated with ever-use of hormone replacement therapy was 0.88 (95% CI, 0.61–1.27). Although study subjects were not asked whether they were current or past users of hormone replacement therapy, it was possible to determine their status with respect to this variable by comparing age at last use of hormone replacement therapy with current age. However, the question concerning age at last use was introduced only after about 50 case–control pairs had been interviewed; therefore, the latter cases

Table 1 Risk of breast cancer by selected study variables

Variable	*Level*	*Odds ratio (95% confidence interval)*
History of breast cancer in a first-degree relative	no	1.0*
	yes	1.54 (0.94–2.52)
History of benign breast disease	no	1.0*
	yes	1.46 (0.72–2.96)
Age at last menstrual period (years)	≤ 46	1.0*
	47–50	1.31 (0.58–1.18)
	> 50	1.52 (0.98–2.36)
History of bilateral oophorectomy	no	1.0*
	yes	0.50 (0.28–0.88)
Ever practised breast self-examination	yes	1.0*
	no	1.32 (1.02–1.70)
Years of education	≤ 7	1.0*
	8–12	1.37 (0.98–1.93)
	≥ 13	1.12 (0.67–1.86)
Age (years) at first† full-term pregnancy	< 20	1.0*
	20–24	1.45 (0.88–2.40)
	25–29	1.23 (0.74–2.05)
	≥ 30	1.44 (0.79–2.63)
	nulliparous	1.53 (0.85–2.75)

*Reference category; †defined as pregnancy of at least 5 months' duration

and controls were considered to be current users if age at first use of hormone replacement therapy plus total duration of use was equal to their current age (if it was not, the possibility of discontinuous use of hormone replacement therapy up to current age could not be excluded). The majority of ever-users of hormone replacement therapy were past users (Table 2), for whom the risk of breast cancer was about 10% less than that for never-users (adjusted odds ratio 0.89, 95% CI, 0.59–1.33); current users had a statistically non-significant 15% reduction in risk (adjusted odds ratio 0.85, 95% CI, 0.40–1.81).

Since the most commonly reported reason for use of hormone replacement therapy was for the relief of menopausal symptoms, subsequent analyses focused on the relationship between hormone replacement therapy and risk of breast cancer in postmenopausal women. For those who had ever used hormone replacement therapy, risk was slightly lower than that for those who had never used it (Table 3), the adjusted odds ratio being 0.82 (95% CI, 0.50–1.34). Both current and past users of hormone replacement therapy were at slightly decreased risk of breast cancer, but neither of the point estimates of association was statistically significant. Also, although risk of breast cancer decreased with increasing duration of use of hormone replacement therapy, the test for trend was not statistically significant. Risk varied in an irregular and mostly insubstantial manner with age at first use and with years since first use, and women who had last used hormone replacement therapy more than 12 years earlier had a 30% (non-significant) decrease in risk of breast cancer.

Duration of use of hormone replacement therapy is related to years since first use, in that the longer the interval since first use of hormone replacement therapy, the greater the opportunity for an individual to have used it for relatively long periods. Examination of the joint association with risk of breast cancer (in postmenopausal women) of these two variables revealed that, relative to a risk of unity for women who had never used hormone replacement therapy, women who had used it for 2 years or more and had first used it more than 15 years earlier had a 50% increase in risk (odds ratio, 1.54), although the associated 95% confidence interval (0.43–5.45) was very wide. Duration of use of hormone replacement therapy is also related to years since last use, and women who had used it for 2 years or more, and had last used it more than 2 years earlier, had a 40% reduction in risk of breast cancer (odds ratio, 0.60), but this estimate was similarly unstable (95% CI, 0.19–1.90).

To explore the possibility of interactions between use of hormone replacement therapy and risk factors for breast cancer, the risk of breast cancer in association with ever-use of hormone replacement therapy was examined within strata of several risk factors – namely, a history of benign breast disease, a family history of breast cancer in a first-degree relative, parity, and a history of bilateral oophorectomy (Table 4). Ever-use of hormone replacement therapy was associated with increases in risk of breast cancer in women who had a family history of breast cancer or who were nulliparous (both statistically non-significant). Otherwise, apart from the unaltered risk in women who had not had a bilateral oophorectomy, ever-use of hormone

Table 2 Risk of breast cancer in the total study population in association with ever-use, current use, and past use of hormone replacement therapy

Aspect of use	*Number of cases**	*Number of controls*	*Unadjusted odds ratio (95% confidence interval)*	*Adjusted odds ratio (95% confidence interval)*†
Never used	386	356	1.0‡	1.0‡
Ever used	76	85	0.87 (0.62–1.23)	0.88 (0.61–1.27)
Unknown if used	7	10	—	—
Past use	60	64	0.91 (0.63–1.33)	0.89 (0.59–1.33)
Current use	14	19	0.76 (0.38–1.54)	0.85 (0.40–1.81)
Unknown	9	12	—	—

*Matched odds ratio cannot be calculated directly from the (unmatched) distribution of cases and controls; †adjusted for years of education, practise of breast self-examination, history of breast cancer in a first-degree relative, age at last menstrual period, and history of bilateral oophorectomy; ‡reference category

Table 3 Risk of breast cancer in postmenopausal women by various aspects of use of hormone replacement therapy

Aspect of use	*Number of cases**	*Number of controls*	*Unadjusted odds ratio (95% confidence interval)*	*Adjusted odds ratio (95% confidence interval)*[†]
Never used	225	218	1.0[‡]	1.0[‡]
Ever used	50	61	0.88 (0.57–1.37)	0.82 (0.50–1.34)
Unknown	6	9	—	
Past use	41	50	0.93 (0.58–1.48)	0.82 (0.48–1.37)
Current use	7	10	0.73 (0.25–2.13)	0.80 (0.25–2.52)
Unknown	8	10	—	—
Age at first use (years)				
≤ 42	10	19	0.62 (0.26–1.49)	0.65 (0.25–1.71)
43–49	16	20	0.86 (0.41–1.82)	0.89 (0.39–2.04)
≥ 50	24	20	1.22 (0.63–2.37)	0.92 (0.45–1.89)
unknown	6	11	—	—
Duration of use (months)				
< 12	29	25	1.26 (0.68–2.33)	1.08 (0.55–2.11)
12–47	13	21	0.67 (0.31–1.46)	0.63 (0.27–1.44)
≥ 48	6	13	0.46 (0.16–1.34)	0.50 (0.15–1.63)
unknown	8	11	—	—
p for trend			0.175	0.190
Years since first use				
≤ 8	19	19	1.27 (0.53–3.03)	1.10 (0.44–2.70)
9–15	9	19	0.54 (0.24–1.22)	0.44 (0.18–1.09)
≥ 16	22	21	1.10 (0.58–2.08)	1.05 (0.52–2.10)
unknown	6	11	—	—
Years since last use (past users only)				
1–11	22	22	1.22 (0.59–2.54)	1.15 (0.51–2.58)
≥ 12	17	23	0.79 (0.41–1.53)	0.68 (0.33–1.41)
unknown	10	15		

*Matched odds ratio cannot be calculated directly from the (unmatched) distribution of cases and controls; [†]adjusted for years of education, practise of breast self-examination, history of breast cancer in a first-degree relative, age at last menstrual period, and history of bilateral oophorectomy; [‡]reference category

Table 4 Risk of breast cancer in postmenopausal women in association with ever-use of hormone replacement therapy, by levels of breast cancer risk factors

Risk factor	*Level*	*Hormone replacement therapy use** *Cases*	*Controls*	*Odds ratio (95% confidence interval)*†
History of benign breast disease	yes	2/7	4/8	0.57 (0.06–5.82)
	no	46/255	55/261	0.87 (0.55–1.36)
Family history of breast cancer in a first-degree relative	yes	6/28	2/20	2.20 (0.36–13.38)
	no	42/234	58/250	0.78 (0.49–1.23)
Parity	nulliparous	8/41	9/44	1.35 (0.42–4.34)
	parous	40/221	51/226	0.77 (0.48–1.24)
History of bilateral oophorectomy	yes	6/25	20/43	0.30 (0.09–0.94)
	no	42/237	40/227	1.01 (0.69–1.47)

*Number reporting ever-use of hormone replacement therapy/total number in category (excluding unknowns); †expressed relative to a risk of unity for those reporting never-use of hormone replacement therapy and adjusted by unconditional logistic regression for age and, for the first three factors listed in the table, for type of menopause

replacement therapy was associated with reduced risk of breast cancer. The reduction in risk for ever-users of hormone replacement therapy who had undergone a bilateral oophorectomy was statistically significant (odds ratio, 0.30, 95% CI, 0.09–0.94).

Only one-third of cases and controls were able to provide the name and dose of the hormone replacement therapy preparation which they had used the most. Therefore, no attempt was made to estimate the risk of breast cancer associated with use of specific types and dosages of hormone replacement therapy. However, of those study subjects who were able to provide the name of preparation that they had used the most, the majority indicated that they had used some form of oestrogen replacement therapy.

DISCUSSION

The results of this population-based case–control study provide little support for a positive association between use of hormone replacement therapy and risk of breast cancer, either overall, or in postmenopausal women. There was little alteration in the risk of breast cancer for women who had ever used hormone replacement therapy, and in further analyses in postmenopausal women, there were non-uniform (and mostly insubstantial) variations in risk with age at first use and years since first use of hormone replacement therapy, a statistically non-significant trend of decreasing risk with increasing duration of use, and a 30% reduction in risk for women who had last used it at least 12 years earlier. Furthermore, when the risk of breast cancer associated with ever-use of hormone replacement therapy was examined within strata defined by risk factors for breast cancer, the only subgroup with a substantial increase in risk was that of women with a family history of breast cancer, although their increase in risk was not statistically significant. Similarly, although the results of the analyses in which the risk of breast cancer was examined at combined levels of duration of use and years since first or last use of hormone replacement therapy might be interpreted as being consistent with cancer-initiating or cancer-promoting effects, respectively, the wide confidence intervals associated with these estimates suggest that chance is the more likely explanation.

Study of the relationship between hormone replacement therapy and risk of breast cancer poses some special methodological problems. Firstly, there appear to be secular trends in the frquency with which hormone replacement therapy is prescribed[37]. In Australia, for example, there was a 50% increase in sales of oestrogens through retail pharmacies between 1981 and 1987, an increase far in excess of the increase in the number of women in the likely target population[38]. Furthermore, at any one point in time, there appears to be some variation between physicians in their readiness to prescribe hormone replacement therapy, so that the likelihood of a woman being given it will depend to some extent on whom she consults. These considerations will be of importance if they are related to attributes of potential recipients of hormone replacement therapy, which themselves are related to risk of breast cancer. For example, the likelihood of receiving hormone replacement therapy may differ by social class. Indeed, there is empirical evidence to suggest that women with a higher level of education (an index of social class) are more likely to receive oestrogen replacement therapy[39]. Secondly, hormone replacement therapy is prescribed primarily for the treatment of menopausal symptoms, and therefore the opportunity for its use and the extent of its use by a given age will depend partially on the age at which a woman reaches menopause, and also on the type of menopause which she experiences; for example, a woman who has a bilateral oophorectomy at a relatively young age seems particularly likely to be given hormone replacement therapy. This raises the possibility of confounding of the association between hormone replacement therapy and risk of breast cancer by age at and type of menopause, since the latter two variables are related to risk of breast cancer[40].

To some extent, these issues were dealt with in the present study. In addition to being matched with respect to age, cases and controls were matched with respect to calendar time, which would have provided partial control for any secular trends in the frequency of prescribing hormone replacement therapy; any potential confounding introduced by individual physician preferences in prescribing habits is likely to have been accounted for, at least partially, by controlling for social class; also, odds ratios were adjusted for age at menopause and type of menopause, and were also derived within strata defined by type of menopause.

As in most case–control studies, selection bias and recall bias are of some potential concern here. Selection bias would have occurred if hormone replacement therapy users were somehow selectively included in or excluded from the study, and if this occurred differentially between the cases and controls. This bias seems more likely to be a problem in hospital-based assessments of the relationship between hormone replacement therapy use and risk of breast cancer[26] than in population-based case–control studies.

However, it is usually only possible to make indirect assessments of the likelihood of selection bias. Thus, in this study, when sociodemographic and tumour characteristics of the 81% (451/559) of all eligible cases who were actually included in the study were compared with those of the cases who were not included, the differences were not marked. Also, restriction of the analyses in postmenopausal women to the 176 case–control pairs in whom the person who was first approached as a potential control was actually recruited into the study gave results that differed little from those based on all case–control pairs.

It is also possible that the results were influenced by recall bias, since either the cases or the controls (or both) might have overstated or understated their histories of hormone replacement therapy. Although, in the present study, cases were more likely than controls to be able to provide answers concerning use of hormone replacement therapy (that is, they were less likely to claim not to know the answer to a question), the difference was small. Nevertheless, this last observation suggests that the extent of hormone replacement therapy use in the controls might have been underestimated, as a result of which estimates of the magnitude of the association between its use and risk of breast cancer would have been biased conservatively (given the apparent reduction in risk).

The statistical power of this study was somewhat limited by the relatively small number of women who had ever used hormone replacement therapy, of whom only a minority reported relatively long durations of use. Nevertheless, indirect support for the validity of the predominantly negative findings of this study with respect to hormone replacement therapy use is provided by the patterns of risk that were observed in association with the established risk factors for breast cancer. While most of the associations were of moderate strength only, they were generally in accord with those that have been observed previously[40].

The results of three recent meta-analyses suggest that, in aggregate, and despite apparent inconsistencies between studies, there is no evidence that women who have ever used hormone replacement therapy (and, in particular, conjugated oestrogens) are at altered risk of breast cancer[38,41,42]. Attempts to determine whether there is a dose–response relationship between use of hormone replacement therapy and risk of breast cancer, while potentially more informative than an overall comparison of ever-users with never-users, have also yielded inconsistent results. Various indices of dose have been used, including duration of use, average daily dose, and some combination of the two. Of these, duration of use has been used most widely, and risk of breast cancer in association with increasing duration of use has been observed to increase[6,8,11,13,15,24,25,28,31,32], change relatively little[2,17,20,26,27,29,30], or decrease[3,14]. Studies which have examined risk in relation to average daily dose[11,13,20,25,29] and mg months of use[14,29] have mostly shown little evidence of an association. In evaluating these results, it should be noted that many of the studies referred to above were conducted some years ago, so that the women in these studies had had relatively little opportunity for prolonged use of hormone replacement therapy. Of the more recent studies[24–32], more than half[24,25,28,31,32] have provided evidence for a dose–response relationship. Furthermore, a meta-analysis of 16 case–control studies suggested that risk of breast cancer is increased by 30% after 15 years of oestrogen replacement therapy use[42].

In several recent studies, evidence has been sought for a cancer-initiating effect of hormone replacement therapy, by examining the association between years since first use and risk of breast cancer[24–30,32]. Although two[28,32] of these studies showed a positive association, which is consistent with a cancer-initiating effect of hormone replacement therapy, the remainder did not show an association.

As indicated earlier, the results of most studies to date relate primarily to use of conjugated oestrogens. With respect to the use of other types of oestrogen preparations, Hunt and colleagues[28] found some evidence for a positive association between use of unopposed ethinyloestradiol and risk of breast cancer; Bergkvist and co-workers[32] reported a 1.8-fold increase in risk after more than 6 years of use of oestradiol, but found no increase in risk in association with use of conjugated or other types of oestrogens, and several other studies have reported an increase in risk of breast cancer in association with use of diethylstilboestrol[21–23,25].

In the last decade, there has been a tendency to prescribe progestins in combination with oestrogens to counter the adverse effect of unopposed oestrogens on the endometrium[43]. Given that this is a relatively recent innovation, it has not been possible to study the effect of prolonged use of combined oestrogen–progestogen preparations on the risk of breast cancer. Nevertheless, in two recent studies[30,32], risk was increased in association with use of these preparations. Although these results must be viewed as preliminary, they are consistent with the prediction of Key and Pike[1] (based on consideration of hormonal influences on the rate at which mammary epithelium proliferates) that combined hormone replacement therapy will cause an increase in risk of breast cancer at least as great as that of oestrogen replacement therapy alone. In contrast, however, use of combined oestrogen–progestogen preparations was associated with reduced risk of breast cancer in two earlier studies[10,19], but both of these results were based on relatively small numbers of cases.

With respect to the effects of progestins alone, a number of synthetic progestogens (e.g. chlormadinone acetate, megestrel acetate, and medroxyprogesterone acetate) have been observed to produce benign and malignant mammary tumours in beagles[44]. However, there have been relatively few studies of the relationship between these substances and risk of breast cancer in women. Of three recent case–control studies of depot medroxyprogesterone, one[45] showed a positive association, while the remaining two[46,47] showed no overall association. However, in one of the latter studies[47], risk was increased in women diagnosed with breast cancer before the age of 35. Clearly, there is a need for further data before a conclusion can be drawn as to the carcinogenic potential of the synthetic progestogens.

Absence of an effect of hormone replacement therapy overall does not preclude effects within certain subgroups of those who use it. Several studies have shown risk to be increased in women with a history of bilateral oophorectomy[13,15,25,31], while others[24,27,29] have not; similarly, of the studies which have examined the association between hormone replacement therapy and breast cancer in women with a history of natural menopause[24,25,27,29–31], only some[24,25,31] have shown an effect. The results of analyses in subgroups of users defined on the basis of a family history of breast cancer[14,15,17,24,27,30,31] or a history of benign breast disease[6,13,20,24,27,30,31] have also been inconsistent.

There is other evidence which bears on the possibility of a carcinogenic effect of hormone replacement therapy. In particular, animal experiments have shown that the incidence of breast cancer is increased in association with administration of oestrogens[48], and there are case reports of breast cancer in oestrogen-treated male transsexuals[49].

In conclusion, although it is evident that the epidemiological evidence linking hormone replacement therapy with risk of breast cancer is inconsistent and insufficient to allow assertion that the relationship is causal, two aspects of the data currently available provide some basis for concern. The first is the 50–100% increase in risk with prolonged oestrogen replacement therapy use (generally, use of at least 6 years, but in some studies only after 20 years of use) which has been observed in the more recent studies[25,27,29–32], and the second is the apparent increase in risk of breast cancer in association with combined oestrogen–progestogen replacement therapy[30,32]. In making decisions about the advisability of prescribing hormone replacement therapy, however, the possibility of an adverse effect on risk of breast cancer must be weighed against the undoubted benefits to be had from its use, particularly in terms of the relief of the vasomotor symptoms associated with the menopause, and the retardation of postmenopausal bone loss[36].

REFERENCES

1. Key, T.J.A. and Pike, M.C. (1988). The role of oestrogens and progestagens in the epidemiology and prevention of breast cancer. *Eur. J. Cancer Clin. Oncol.*, **24**, 29–43
2. Boston Collaborative Drug Surveillance Program. (1974). Surgically confirmed gallbladder disease, venous thromboembolism and breast tumors in relation to postmenopausal estrogen therapy. *N. Engl. J. Med.*, **290**, 15–19
3. Henderson, B.E., Powell, D., Rosario, I., Keys, C., Hanisch, A., Young, M., Casagrande, J., Gerkins, V. and Pike, M.C. (1974). An epidemiologic study of breast cancer. *J. Natl. Cancer Inst.*, **53**, 609–14
4. Burch, J.C., Byrd, B.F., Jr and Vaughn, W.K. (1975). The effects of long-term estrogen administration to women following hysterectomy. In *Frontiers in Hormone Research. Vol.* 3. *Estrogens in the Post-menopause*, pp. 208–14. (Basel: Karger)
5. Casagrande, J., Gerkins, V., Henderson, B.E., Mack, T. and Pike, M.C. (1977). Exogenous estrogens and breast cancer in women with natural menopause. *J. Natl. Cancer Inst.*, **59**, 1589–92
6. Hoover, R., Gray, L.A., Cole, P. and MacMahon, B. (1976). Menopausal estrogens and breast cancer. *N. Engl. J. Med.*, **295**, 401–5
7. Sartwell, P.E., Arthes, F.G. and Tonascia, J.A. (1977). Exogenous hormones, reproductive history and breast cancer. *J. Natl. Cancer Inst.*, **59**, 1589–92
8. Bibbo, M., Haenszel, W.M., Wied, G.L., Hubby, M. and Herbst, A.L. (1978). A twenty-five year follow-up study of women exposed to diethylstilboestrol during pregnancy. *N. Engl. J. Med.*, **298**, 763–7
9. Thomas, D.B. (1978). Role of exogenous female hormones in altering the risk of benign and malignant neoplasms in humans. *Cancer Res.*, **38**, 3991–4000

10. Nachtigall, L.E., Nachtigall, R.H., Nachtigall, R.D. and Beckman, E.M. (1979). Estrogen replacement therapy II: A prospective study in the relationship to carcinoma and metabolic problems. *Obstet. Gynecol.*, **54**, 74–9
11. Ross, R.K., Paganini-Hill, A., Gerkins, V.R., Mack, T.M., Pfeffer, R., Arthur, M. and Henderson, B.E. (1980). A case–control study of menopausal estrogen therapy and breast cancer. *J. Am. Med. Assoc.*, **243**, 1635–9
12. Jick, H., Walker, A.M., Watkins, R.N., D'Ewart, D.C., Hunter, J.R., Danford, A., Madsen, S., Dinan, B.J. and Rothman, K.J. (1980). Replacement estrogens and breast cancer. *Am. J. Epidemiol.*, **112**, 586–94
13. Brinton, L.A., Hoover, R.N., Szklo, M. and Fraumeni, J.F. (1981). Menopausal estrogen use and risk of breast cancer. *Cancer*, **47**, 2517–22
14. Kelsey, J.L., Fischer, D.B., Holford, T.R., LiVolsi, V.A., Mostow, E.D., Goldenberg, I.S. and White, G. (1981). Exogenous estrogens and other factors in the epidemiology of breast cancer. *J. Natl. Cancer Inst.*, **67**, 327–33
15. Hoover, R., Glass, A., Finkle, W.E., Azevedo, D. and Milne, K. (1981). Conjugated estrogens and breast cancer risk in women. *J. Natl. Cancer Inst.*, **67**, 815–20
16. Lawson, D.H., Jick, H., Hunter, J.R. and Madsen, S. (1981). Exogenous estrogens and breast cancer. *Am. J. Epidemiol.*, **114**, 710–13
17. Hulka, B.S., Chambless, L.E., Deubner, D.C. and Wilkinson, W.E. (1982). Breast cancer and estrogen replacement therapy. *Am. J. Obstet. Gynecol.*, **143**, 638–44
18. Sherman, B., Wallace, R. and Bean, J. (1983). Estrogen use and breast cancer. *Cancer*, **51**, 1527–31
19. Gambrell, R.D., Maier, R.C. and Sanders, B.I. (1983). Decreased incidence of breast cancer in postmenopausal estrogen–progestogen users. *Obstet. Gynecol.*, **62**, 435–43
20. Kaufman, D.W., Miller, D.R., Rosenberg, L., Helmrich, S.P., Stolley, P., Schottenfeld, D. and Shapiro, S. (1984). Non-contraceptive estrogen use and the risk of breast cancer. *J. Am. Med. Assoc.*, **252**, 63–7
21. Greenberg, E.R., Barnes, A.B., Resseguie, L., Barrett, J.A., Burnside, S., Lanza, L.L., Neff, R.K., Stevens, M., Young, R.H. and Colton, T. (1984). Breast cancer in mothers given diethylstilboestrol in pregnancy. *N. Engl. J. Med.*, **311**, 1393–8
22. Hadjimichael, O.C., Meigs, J.W., Falcier, F.W., Thompson, W.D. and Flannery, J. T. (1984). Cancer risk among women exposed to exogenous estrogens during pregnancy. *J. Natl. Cancer Inst.*, **73**, 831–4
23. Hiatt, R.A., Bawol, R., Friedman, G.D. and Hoover, R. (1984). Exogenous estrogen and breast cancer after bilateral oophorectomy. *Cancer*, **54**, 139–44
24. La Vecchia, C., Decarli, A., Parazzini, F., Gentile, A., Liberati, C. and Frenceschi, S. (1986). Non-contraceptive oestrogens and the risk of breast cancer in women. *Br. J. Cancer*, **38**, 853–8
25. Brinton, L.A., Hoover, R., Fraumeni, J.F., Jr (1986). Menopausal oestrogens and breast cancer risk: an expanded case–control study. *Br. J. Cancer*, **54**, 825–32
26. Nomura, A.M.Y., Kolonel, L.N., Hirohata, T. and Lee, J. (1986). The association of replacement estrogens with breast cancer. *Int. J. Cancer*, **37**, 49–53
27. Buring, J.E., Hennekens, C.H., Lipnick, R.J., Willett, W., Stampfer, M.R., Rosner, B., Peto, R. and Speizer, F.E. (1987). A prospective cohort study of postmenopausal hormone use and risk of breast cancer in US women. *Am. J. Epidemiol.*, **125**, 939–47
28. Hunt, K., Vessey, M., McPherson, K. and Coleman, M. (1987). Long-term surveillance of mortality and cancer incidence in women receiving hormone replacement therapy. *Br. J. Obstet. Gynaecol.*, **94**, 620–35
29. Wingo, P.A., Layde, P.M., Lee, N.C., Rubin, G. and Ory, H.W. (1987). The risk of breast cancer in postmenopausal women who have used estrogen replacement therapy. *J. Am. Med. Assoc.*, **257**, 209–15
30. Ewertz, M. (1988). Influence of non-contraceptive exogenous and endogenous sex hormones on breast cancer risk in Denmark. *Int. J. Cancer*, **42**, 832–8
31. Mills, P.K., Beeson, L., Phillips, R.L. and Fraser, G.E. (1989). Prospective study of exogenous hormone use and breast cancer in Seventh-day Adventists. *Cancer*, **64**, 591–7
32. Bergkvist, L., Adami, H.-O., Persson, I., Hoover, R. and Schairer, C. (1989). The risk of breast cancer after estrogen and estrogen–progestin replacement. *N. Engl. J. Med.*, **321**, 293–7

33. Colditz, G.A., Stampfer, M.J., Willett, W.C., Hennekens, C.H., Rosner, B. and Speizer, F.E. (1990). Prospective study of estrogen replacement therapy and risk of breast cancer in postmenopausal women. *J. Am. Med. Assoc.*, **264**, 2648–53
34. Rohan, T.E. and McMichael, A.J. (1988). Non-contraceptive exogenous oestrogen therapy and breast cancer. *Med. J. Aust.*, **148**, 217–21
35. Australian Electoral Office. (1983). A quantitative assessment of electoral enrollment in Australia. (Research report). (Canberra: Australian Electoral Office)
36. Breslow, N.E. and Day, N.E. (1980). *Statistical Methods in Cancer Research. Vol.* 1. *The Analysis of Case–Control Studies.* (Lyon: IARC Scientific Publications)
37. Wilkes, H.C. and Meade, T.W. (1991). Hormone replacement therapy in general practice: a survey of doctors in the MRC's general practice framework. *Br. Med. J.*, **302**, 1317–20
38. Armstrong, B.K. (1988). Oestrogen therapy after the menopause – boon or bane? *Med. J. Aust.*, **148**, 213–14
39. Bergkvist, L., Persson, I., Adami, H.-O. and Schairer, C. (1988). Risk factors for breast and endometrial cancer in a cohort of women treated with menopausal oestrogens. *Int. J. Epidemiol.*, **17**, 732–7
40. Kelsey, J.L. and Berkowitz, G.S. (1988). Breast cancer epidemiology. *Cancer Res.*, **48**, 5615–23
41. Dupont, W.D. and Page, D.L. (1991). Menopausal estrogen replacement therapy and breast cancer. *Arch. Intern. Med.*, **151**, 67–72
42. Steinberg, K.K., Thacker, S.B., Smith, S.J., Stroup, D.F., Zack, M.M., Flanders, W.D. and Berkelman, R.I. (1991). A meta-analysis of the effect of estrogen replacement therapy on the risk of breast cancer. *J. Am. Med. Assoc.*, **265**, 1985–90
43. Barrett-Connor, E. (1989). Postmenopausal estrogen replacement and breast cancer. *N. Engl. J. Med.*, **321**, 319–20
44. World Health Organization. (1982). Facts about injectable contraceptives: memorandum from a WHO meeting. *Bull. WHO*, **60**, 199–210
45. Lee, N.C., Rosero-Bixby, L., Oberle, M.W., Grimaldo, C., Whatley, A.S. and Rovira, E.Z. Pp. 1247–1254 (1987). A case–control study of breast cancer and hormonal contraception in Costa Rica. *J. Natl. Cancer Inst.*, **79**, 1247–54
46. World Health Organization. (1986). Depot-medroxyprogesterone acetate (DMPA) and cancer: memorandum from a WHO meeting. *Bull. WHO*, **64**, 375–82
47. Paul, C., Skegg, D.C.G. and Spears, G.F.S. (1989). Depot medroxyprogesterone (Depo-Provera) and risk of breast cancer. *Br. Med. J.*, **299**, 759–62
48. IARC working group on the evaluation of carcinogenic risk of chemicals to man. (1974). *Vol.* 6. *Sex Hormones.* (Lyon: IARC)
49. Symmers, W.S. (1968). Carcinoma of breast in transsexual individuals after surgical and hormonal interference with the primary and secondary characteristics. *Br. Med. J.*, **2**, 82–5

General discussion IV

(*Chairman: Dr Carlo La Vecchia*)

Dr C. La Vecchia A comprehensive model is needed to test and better understand the process of breast carcinogenesis. Dr Hulka has certainly given some insight in this direction with her very useful model.

Prof. C.E.D. Chilvers Dr Hulka showed a lot of data and subgroup analysis. Am I right in thinking that there were no significant interactions in any of those subgroups?

Dr B.S. Hulka The only statistically significant interaction – putting the interaction term into the model approach – was in type of menopause, natural versus surgical, by oestrogen use. Another interaction term that came close to being statistically significant was the age at menopause and oestrogen use, but in general these were not statistically significant interactions.

Dr La Vecchia The measures of oestrogen receptor levels would suggest that this factor cannot explain the higher survival of breast cancer in women under oestrogen replacement therapy (ERT).

Dr Hulka I do not know if it is known whether ERT increases receptors – it might be expected to, but I am not sure that it does. There are a lot of data showing that breast tumours that have oestrogen receptors (and certainly those that have oestrogen and progesterone receptors) have a better prognosis than tumours without them.

Dr H.P. McEwan I was very interested in Dr Hulka's concept of the oestrogen receptor role. What is its place in clinical practice? She said that it really is an age factor, that there is an increase in oestrogen receptor content with age. Yet, in clinical practice, emphasis is put on whether a tumour is oestrogen receptor-positive or negative. This often influences therapy. It was interesting to hear Dr Hulka say that it is not related to the menopause, and seemed to be the same in users and non-users. Should we scrap the influence of the oestrogen receptor on our practice?

Mr H.H. Hamed The role of oestrogen receptors in the management of breast cancer is now questionable. There are many problems associated with the estimation of the receptors, particularly in relation to the old method of using assays which relied mainly on the free binding sites rather than on the presence or absence of receptor protein. I think, therefore, that in clinical practice there is now less emphasis on the oestrogen receptor levels in the primary management of breast cancer. They may have a more important role in treating recurrent disease.

Prof. W.D. Dupont Could Dr Kaufman speculate on how he would do a clinical trial following women for, say, 15 or more years, of sufficient magnitude to detect the small risks with any degree of reliability.

Dr D.W. Kaufman I am not sure that I would care to speculate on how such a trial could be conducted. It would need to be a very large-scale undertaking, lasting for many years, and it would be very expensive. Perhaps such a trial could not be done. On the other hand, I doubt whether more epidemiological studies of the type that have been conducted, with relative risks in the range of 1.3–1.4, will be conclusive. It does not take a very large or prominent bias to create a relative risk of 1.3. As we all know, it is impossible to rule out bias entirely. Thus, I think the present findings provide a real dilemma.

Dr La Vecchia More than duration and cost, a key problem in clinical trials is compliance.

Prof. S. Shapiro There is one possibility. Under causal assumptions, it may be that if more data are collected – and we are now able to look at 20 or more years of use – an elevation in the risk may be observed. Even then, the relative risk would have to be beyond 1.3 or 1.4 before I would be willing to say that it is not due to bias. There is the general belief that for long durations of use there cannot be bias. If two assumptions are made, the first that for short-term use controls forget more than cases, and the second that cases slightly overestimate and controls slightly underestimate their duration of use, a spurious duration-related effect can readily be observed.

I agree with Dr Kaufman that we need to do a randomized controlled trial. If we want to recommend that people take the drug for 20 years, perhaps we ought to start planning such a trial.

Dr Hulka Would breast cancer be the outcome in this randomized trial? Are you proposing a randomized trial in which the outcome is cancer?

Dr Kaufman My initial reaction is the same as Dr Hulka's, that it is unethical to do a trial in which one of the end-points is cancer. In fact, however, the end-point is total morbidity. Taking the whole picture into account, it is not at all clear that the balance would be negative for hormone replacement therapy. In such a situation the trial is not unethical.

Prof. Shapiro If such a trial were proposed, by the end of the specified number of years there would inevitably be more cases of myocardial infarction. It would be known whether more lives have been saved by preventing myocardial infarction than deaths have been caused by increasing the risk of breast cancer. It would be an entirely ethical study.

Dr U. Lachnit-Fixon I think that a controlled randomized clinical trial is almost impossible in HRT. After a few weeks it would be clear which group the women were in because of the effect of HRT on hot flushes, sweating and so on. Also, how can it be ethical when a woman asks for HRT to give her a placebo? The opposite is also true: if in your opinion it might cause or promote breast cancer, how can you give HRT?

Dr L. Rosenberg I agree with Dr Lachnit-Fixon that such a trial would be unfeasible and impossible. I doubt that enough women could be kept either in the oestrogen or placebo group for 20 years. To involve 300 000 women in this trial would take much of the National Institutes of Health budget. The question is whether it is worth several billion dollars for 20 years to find out if there is a 40% increase in breast cancer incidence. I think the answer will come from an understanding of the basic biology of breast cancer.

Dr M.W. Deitch Another reason why it may be impossible to do such a trial in the USA is the tamoxifen prevention trial that is starting, which will cut down the pool of women available.

Dr La Vecchia Prof. Vessey has addressed two of the major issues under discussion at this meeting: the survival of women with breast cancer under HRT and the possible harmful effect of continued oestradiol.

Dr P.G. Wardle Prof. Vessey commented on the very high proportion of patients who had had a hysterectomy, but not on the surprisingly high proportion of childless women. I think it was 20%, which is an exceptionally high level. Could he comment on this?

Prof. M. Vessey I agree that the childless proportion is rather high, and perhaps I should have stressed it. Interestingly, the rate of childlessness within marriage was fairly accurate, at about 6%. Given this level of childlessness, parity and age at first birth distributions were quite typical of the general population. I expect that some of these women had conditions that interfered with fertility and quite probably led to the hysterectomy, which led in turn to the use of HRT.

Dr Hulka Dr Rohan's choice of the population to include women aged 20 and above would seem to include a lot of women who are potentially not at risk of using hormone replacement therapy. Secondly, was any analysis done for the postmenopausal women with natural menopause only?

Dr T. Rohan As I mentioned, the bulk of the analyses focused on postmenopausal women. The study was designed also for other purposes, which justified the inclusion of younger women. Analysis for natural menopause only was not done.

Dr Hulka It might be interesting to do that analysis, considering that there was a reduction in risk (which may be totally aberrant) for the women who had undergone bilateral oophorectomy.

Dr B.M. Campbell-Brown In Britain, unopposed oestrogen is given to women who have had hysterectomy and bilateral oophorectomy. Therefore, whether or not they have symptoms is irrelevant. The women who appear at a postmenopausal clinic asking for HRT generally have symptoms. Their bodies may have a different response to oestrogens – which they certainly have in terms of their subjective symptoms – and there may indeed be differences in the effect of oestrogens on other tissues, such as breast. This would perhaps account for the difference between those who have opposed and unopposed oestrogens in Britain.

Dr La Vecchia To summarize the session briefly then, Dr Hulka and Dr Rohan presented more detailed analyses available from their data sets, and showed no specific pattern of risk in various subgroups on the interactions considered. Dr Kaufman presented a new, unpublished data set, and again gave a very reassuring picture of the status of hormone replacement therapy. There was also an update on the British cohort study by Prof. Vessey, who emphasized a few issues which I would like to stress for discussion.

Prof. R.E. Mansel Does the data provide information on what we can say to the patient who comes along with a strong family history of breast cancer and asks to commence HRT? As Prof. Vessey, pointed out, there may be a bias in these women, in that those who come forward for discussion of HRT may well be dissuaded because of the concern in the past.

Dr Hulka The bias, if it exists, that women who have a family history (particularly a first-degree relative, or more than one) would not be prescribed HRT, should presumably falsely lower the risk of breast cancer *if* HRT has anything to do with breast cancer occurrence in that group. Many studies have shown some increased breast cancer risk amongst women with a family history of breast cancer who also receive oestrogen replacement therapy (ERT). Although I do not believe that Prof. Dupont showed this in his meta-analysis, the Centers for Disease Control meta-analysis certainly did. From the standpoint of the USA, with the numbers of studies that do show this association, I would be inclined to think that both from the medico-legal standpoint and from that of the best interests of the patient, it might be advisable not to prescribe ERT or HRT for these women.

The real issue, as I see it, is that we need better markers; 'Do you have a first-degree relative, a mother, sister or daughter, who has had breast cancer?' is a weak marker for what we are really interested in. It is surprising that it has shown much at all. We really want to find some subset of those women with a family history who are not only at increased risk of breast cancer, but for whom oestrogens, or oestrogen plus progestins, would be ill-advised.

Dr La Vecchia We should also remember the other open question that Dr Kaufman raised at the end of his talk – the possible importance of a low-risk group. We have already heard that a stronger association with oestrogens is possible among leaner women because they have a low natural level of oestrogens. I would like to know which of the low-risk groups may be of interest from this viewpoint.

Dr Kaufman This brings us back to the question of the feasibility of a clinical trial. I agree that a clinical trial may well not be feasible. Even if it is feasible, it may not be worth spending the money that it would cost, because it would clearly consume phenomenal resources.

Unfortunately, in my opinion, we will not learn more from further epidemiological studies in general populations, such as have been conducted, because we will continue to be plagued with the problem of modest increases in risk where it is not possible to distinguish between bias and causality.

The other possibility, as Dr La Vecchia mentioned, is a study in a low-risk group of women. I would certainly try this first before doing a clinical trial. In a low-risk group of women, higher relative risks might be expected, if indeed anything is going on, and a judgement could more easily be made about whether the findings were likely to be causal or due to bias.

To carry the discussion slightly further, there is also the fact that we saw a relative risk of 2.2 for lean women – postmenopausal women of low body mass index – who had used conjugated oestrogens unopposed for at least 5 years, which is indeed a low-risk group.

In our data there is certainly no consistent suggestion of an elevation of risk among women otherwise at low risk of having breast cancer. This suggests to me that we will not get very far by trying to define low-risk groups within existing studies but rather, if we are going to take this route, that we need a new study in such women – if we can find a population of relatively low-risk women using ERT.

Prof. Vessey Attempts are being made by Tom Meade and his colleagues at St Bartholomew's Hospital to set up a randomized controlled trial in the UK. It is a highly contentious topic because a lot of people think it will not work, but it has been agreed that the Medical Research Council should allow him to determine whether he can do it. He has already done some quite promising pilot work. He is anxious to set up a randomized controlled trial for the very reason stressed by Dr Kaufman; that is, that it is very difficult to interpret small increases and small decreases in risk in anything other than such a trial – and it can be difficult enough even then. It would be very valuable if this attempt were to succeed.

I may say that we have plans for doing another large cohort study because we think that the attempt to do the randomized trial will fail. These plans are temporarily in abeyance while Tom Meade tries to see whether or not a randomized controlled trial is possible.

Prof. Chilvers Is HRT being looked at in this pilot study or will there be randomization between ERT and HRT in women with an intact uterus?

Prof. Vessey Both have been suggested. Tom Meade was keen to compare

HRT and ERT, but most of us thought it would be very difficult to do and less attractive than a trial which compares the appropriate form of therapy – that is, depending upon whether or not a woman has a uterus – with a randomized control group, so that either type of therapy could be administered.

Prof. Shapiro Do the panellists, and perhaps also Prof. Adami, suspect that there is a difference in breast cancer risk for conjugated oestrogens, oestradiol and combined therapy?

Prof. Vessey It is very difficult even to attempt to answer this question. In many ways, we rely on the big American studies, apart from the big Swedish study. The former, even those that are published now, tend to lean most towards Premarin®. I do not know how much of the therapy presented by Dr Kaufman was combined. I am aware that combined therapy is being used in the USA, typically Premarin® plus Provera®.

In the publications that I have seen there are very few studies that include a comparison. There is a study in Denmark from Marianne Ewertz using a variety of different preparations, and this did not come to any clear answer with regard to type of preparation. Our study includes different types of preparation, but there are very few studies that have compared, within the same study, the different sorts of treatment.

Dr Kaufman I agree. I think you summarized the position very well. We clearly want to know if there are differences between formulations, but we do not yet have the necessary information.

Dr Hulka Studies on HRT, and the addition of progestins to Premarin®, are in progress in the USA. They are being undertaken in California and in Washington, by Dr Kaufman's group and others. This then will not remain a mystery for much longer.

Prof. Dupont I would like to take issue with Dr Kaufman's contention that nothing more is to be learnt from observational studies. While it is certainly true that they cannot reliably detect low relative risks of less than 2, the fact remains that we still do not have anywhere near enough information about either long-term or combination ERT and HRT. It is possible that an observational study could demonstrate that, say, therapy for 20 years is associated with a sixfold increase in breast cancer risk. Were that to be true, it would be of great clinical importance. That, in itself, is sufficient justification for collecting more information on long-term usage. We do not need another short-term duration study on unopposed oestrogens, but the further out we go in terms of length of follow-up, the more sparse the data become. It would, therefore, be very valuable to gain more information on these therapies.

Dr Kaufman I think that is probably right in terms of opposed therapy – for many of the studies which have provided information on opposed therapy have included only small numbers of patients. Perhaps I could be persuaded to modify my sweeping statement about that.

I do not agree about duration. For example, the Cancer and Steroid Hormone (CASH) study considered at least 20 years of use. The upper confidence limit on their estimate was 5.8. They certainly were excluding a sixfold increase in risk. The possibility of bias in that study could be argued. As far as duration of use is concerned, my opinion is that we probably will not reach the level of risk in the general population that will let us escape from this dilemma.

Dr Hulka CASH is not an ideal study for HRT (or ERT), in that the women had a maximum age of 54. So for long-term use they included women who had had a hysterectomy or oophorectomy early in life. The study does not provide much information about natural menopause and ERT or HRT use for the majority of women.

We have to ask where epidemiology comes into all this, and what is its place? I agree that more case–control studies, adding a few more thousand cases, does not seem likely to provide much more information. I would like to see more integration of epidemiology with some of the laboratory capability. There is interest in more biological markers and their use in epidemiological studies. What are the markers of exposure to oestrogen and of oestrogen effect? We have talked a little about receptors, though I am not sure how they will behave in non-cancerous or precursor states in relation to oestrogen exposure. We could talk about markers of susceptibility. There have been linkage studies that identify a ‘breast cancer’ locus on chromosome 17p in particular. This is known to be an area very near to oncogenes that have been linked to breast cancer. Oncogenes could be markers of early pathogenesis in breast cancer. We need to consider markers of exposure, of susceptibility and of health effect. I would like to see further epidemiological studies that integrate the principles of epidemiology with some of the newer laboratory capability.

Dr P. Last If we are going to set up new trials, we must ensure that symptomatic women are separated from women who take HRT for other reasons. Perhaps women who take oestrogens and progestogens for symptoms are a different group. There are women who do not have menopausal symptoms who would take HRT to protect against heart disease or bone loss. They are an important subset.

I am not clear how menopause is being defined. The menopause definition used by surgeons, such as no period for 6 months or 1 year, is quite wrong in terms of hysterectomized women. The difference between the natural and the surgical menopause is very important and needs to be emphasized. A woman who has had a hysterectomy and still has functioning ovaries is not postmenopausal in terms of anything.

Is there any thought of giving half a soluble aspirin a day as part of the randomized controlled trial? I am sure this would protect against heart disease as much as HRT.

Professor R.K. Ross Dr Hulka showed a model of hormone-related carcinogenesis of the breast, and suggested that oestradiol was clearly the most potent oestrogen to breast tissue. What sort of circulating levels of oestradiol are achieved with the various commonly used doses of Premarin®? If, say, the age–incidence curve for breast cancer premenopausally is entirely due to oestradiol, would these levels be sufficiently high to make that curve continue unabated postmenopausally? If the oestradiol levels are high enough, we should be able to detect that.

Dr Hulka There are others present who could tell us the actual serum levels of oestradiol produced by Premarin®, and perhaps some of the other oestrogens, in premenopausal and postmenopausal women. But it is not as simple as this. One of the big problems, and why the model is very simplistic, is that many studies show a poor correlation between serum oestrogen, tissue oestrogen and oestrogen receptors in the tissue, so it is more complicated than the model.

Dr G. Colditz The literature, as I know it, is about one paper (a small report, I think from Whitehead's group) that has looked at the levels of oestradiol in women receiving, I think, 0.625 mg oestrogen replacement. The estimate is that about 70% of the premenopausal oestradiol level is achieved with this dose. Further increase in the dose of oestrogen replacement does not raise the oestradiol any higher. This highlights the lack of work done at the level of the biological effect, even in terms of circulating oestradiol among women taking replacement. This is further complicated, at least in the USA, by the almost absent ability to measure oestradiol reliably. Our experience is that the coefficient of variation for oestradiol is about 30% in most laboratories when we send blind replicates to them; this is so even though the published coefficients of variation are of the order of 5%. We need, I believe, to collaborate with the laboratories in order to get them to tighten their methods so that one day it may be possible to interpret laboratory oestradiol levels.

Dr B. Santra I find that there is some evidence of increase in breast cancer due to oestrogen therapy. We give HRT – an oestradiol implant – to women who have had a hysterectomy before the age of 50. I wonder whether we should give them progesterone as well instead of giving oestradiol alone. What is the opinion of the participants?

Prof. Vessey A consensus group in the USA concluded that progestogen should not be given to a woman who had a hysterectomy who required HRT.

Dr Santra However, the West German studies suggest that there is less chance of breast cancer if combined therapy is given.

Dr Hulka One of the groups reviewing this issue in the USA was the Food and Drug Administration (FDA) Advisory Committee on Fertility and

Maternal Health Drugs. Their general recommendation was to use ERT for women who have had their uterus removed and need or want hormone replacement. As Professor Vessey said, there is no need for additional progestin.

Prof. J. Drife To take that one stage further, if a study randomizing women who have had a hysterectomy into opposed and unopposed groups is being contemplated – the study being designed to see what the difference is between two therapies – one of the objections raised might be that it is unethical to give progestins to someone who has had a hysterectomy. Obviously, if a lot of people had that reservation, such a study will not get started. Would the participants go as far as that? I realize that the recommendation, if no randomization is involved, is that oestrogen alone is the correct treatment, but are there enough reservations about progestogen to say that a study including it is unethical?

Prof. Vessey It depends a lot on your views about the effects of added progestogen on the cardiovascular system. If you believe that there is some reduction in benefit from adding the progestogen to the oestrogen, this weighs heavily against progestogen. I am, of course, aware of the recent work which shows that it is possible to identify progestogens and doses that appear to have no adverse effect on any clotting factor or metabolic parameter that can be measured. It is correct to say that there is a lot of opposition to the notion of randomizing these two types of treatment in women without a uterus.

Prof. Drife Is the worry about the progestogen effect really extrapolation from oral contraceptive data, and not actually based on HRT? [*Prof. Vessey assented*]

Dr Campbell-Brown On the practical point of compliance with progestogens, one of the reasons why implants in our practice are confined to women who have had a hysterectomy is because experience has shown that those who have not had a hysterectomy will not comply with taking progestogens because of the side-effects of these drugs. Even using the varieties now available, in the doses shown by Whitehead and his colleagues to protect the endometrium, it is extremely difficult to persuade women to comply, and when they do not comply, there are all the problems of endometrial hyperplasia, atypia and of knowing (or not knowing) what to do next.

17

The risk of breast cancer in postmenopausal women who have used oestrogen replacement therapy

P.A. Wingo, P.M. Layde, N.C. Lee, G. Rubin and H.W. Ory

Non-contraceptive oestrogens were first marketed in the United States in 1942[1]. Since the 1960s, physicians have prescribed them for many women to manage symptoms of menopause and to gradually adjust oestrogen levels among women who have had bilateral oophorectomy[1]. More recently, non-contraceptive oestrogens have been shown to confer a protective effect against osteoporosis and possibly cardiovascular disease in postmenopausal women[1]. In 1983, enough non-contraceptive oestrogens were purchased to treat an estimated 2.3 million postmenopausal women[2].

Such widespread use of non-contraceptive oestrogens or oestrogen replacement therapy requires careful consideration of all potential risks and benefits. In addition to possible effects on osteoporosis and cardiovascular disease, we must consider the influence of oestrogen replacement therapy on breast cancer risk. A positive relationship between breast cancer and oestrogen replacement therapy is biologically plausible and potentially has significant clinical and public health importance. In 1986, more than 123 000 women in the United States are expected to be newly diagnosed with breast cancer and 39 900 women are expected to die of the disease[3]. Overall, most studies indicate that women who have ever used oestrogen replacement therapy do not have an increased risk of breast cancer[4–9]. However, some studies suggest that long-term oestrogen replacement therapy, oestrogen replacement therapy that began in the distant past, or high-dosage oestrogen replacement therapy may increase the risk of breast cancer[8,10–13].

Analyses of the effects of surgical and natural menopause on the relationship between breast cancer and oestrogen replacement therapy have yielded conflicting results. Three studies found that oestrogen replacement therapy appeared to increase the risk of cancer[7,8,14], specifically among naturally menopausal women who were current users of oestrogen replacement therapy or users of injectable oestrogens[7,14]. In contrast, Brinton and colleagues[12]

This article was previously published in *J. Am. Med. Assoc.* (1987), **257**, 209–15 found that risk increased with continued use among women who had undergone bilateral oophorectomy. Other studies reported that risk among ever-users was not altered by type of menopause and presence or absence of ovaries[5,6,10].

We studied the relationship between oestrogen replacement therapy and breast cancer according to type of menopause with data collected during the Cancer and Steroid Hormone Study.

METHODS

The methods for the Cancer and Steroid Hormone Study have been described in detail elsewhere[15]. The study was a large, population-based, case–control study primarily designed to assess the possible association between oral contraceptives and breast, ovarian, and endometrial cancer. The Division of Reproductive Health of the Centers for Disease Control, Atlanta, with support from the Center for Population Research of the National Institute of Child Health and Human Development and the National Cancer Institute, Bethesda, MD, coordinated data collection in eight geographic locations: the metropolitan areas of Atlanta, Detroit, San Francisco, and Seattle; the states of Connecticut, Iowa, and New Mexico; and four urban counties in Utah.

Cases

Cases were identified from women 20–54 years old, living in the eight geographic study locations. Women with histologically confirmed, primary breast cancer were ascertained by the Surveillance, Epidemiology, and End Results Centers of the National Cancer Institute. All women had breast cancer first diagnosed between December 1, 1980 and December 31, 1982. Of the 5896 women who met these criteria for inclusion in the study, 4742 (80%) consented to be interviewed. Women not interviewed included 224 (4%) who refused, 165 (3%) whose physicians refused, 238 (4%) who were deceased or too ill to be interviewed, and 527 (9%) who were unavailable for an interview within 6 months of diagnosis.

Controls

To reflect the general population of the areas from which cases were identified, women 20–54 years old were selected as potential controls according to Waksberg's[16] method of telephoning randomly selected residential telephone numbers in the same eight geographic areas. An appropriate proportion of controls in each 5-year age-group was sampled from the pool of potential controls to match the expected age-distribution of the breast cancer cases. Of the 5698 women sampled, 4754 (83%) consented to be interviewed. Women not interviewed included 679 (12%) who refused, 93 (2%) who did not speak English, and 172 (3%) who either moved from the study area, were too ill to participate, or were unavailable for other reasons.

Exclusions

To focus on oestrogens used for treating symptoms of menopause in this analysis, we excluded 2952 cases (87%) and 2715 controls (87%) who were premenopausal or perimenopausal and 168 cases (5%) and 160 controls (5%) whose type of menopause was unknown. We excluded 128 cases (4%) and 114 controls (4%) who were uncertain if they had ever used oestrogen replacement therapy, and 93 cases (3%) and 120 controls (4%) who used oestrogens before the last menstrual period or 40 years of age (whichever occurred first among women with a surgical menopause), and before 40 years of age among women reporting a natural menopause. We also excluded 32 cases (1%) with an uncertain history of breast cancer. After all exclusions, 1369 cases and 1645 controls remained for analysis.

Interviews

Standard 1-hour interviews were administered to all women in their homes by interviewers trained at a central location. The interview elicited information about reproductive factors, benign breast disease, family history of female cancers, health care utilization, and other factors known to affect breast cancer risk and female hormone use.

Definitions of terms

Index date was defined as the date of diagnosis for cases and date of interview for controls.

Natural menopause was defined as cessation of menstrual periods, reported as stopping naturally at least 6 months before the index date. Women who reported that their last menstrual period occurred before age 40 years were coded as having an unknown menopausal status and were excluded from this analysis. Surgical menopause was defined as cessation of menstrual periods resulting from an operation performed before the index date.

Oestrogen replacement therapy was defined as use of oral or injectable non-contraceptive oestrogens (excluding vaginal creams) for 3 consecutive months or more where no use occurred before (1) the last menstrual period or age 40 years, whichever occurred first among women who reported a surgical menopause; or (2) age 40 years among women who reported a natural menopause. Mg-months was defined as milligrams of oestrogen contained in the specific preparation multiplied by the number of months of use.

Benign breast disease was defined as breast disease diagnosed as benign through biopsy specimen or mastectomy before index date. Family history of breast cancer was defined as a report of breast cancer in a first-degree relative (mother, sister, or daughter) or a second-degree relative (grandmother, mother's sister, or father's sister). Women with both a first- and second-degree family history of breast cancer were categorized as having a first-degree family history.

Analysis

We used two methods to assess potentially confounding variables that might distort an association between oestrogen replacement therapy and breast cancer. First, we used logistic regression to control simultaneously for six risk factors that we *a priori* considered potential confounders[17]. We used likelihood ratio tests to assess the statistical significance of simultaneously including the risk factors and interactions between the exposure to oestrogen replacement therapy and each risk factor in the model. The risk factors included in the model were two continuous variables: age at last menstrual period, and age at index date, and four categorical variables: (1) menopausal status (surgical menopause and zero ovaries, surgical menopause and at least one ovary, natural menopause); (2) age at first full-term pregnancy (never pregnant and pregnant at ages 19 years or younger, 20–29 years, 30 years or older, unknown); (3) history of benign breast disease (yes, no); and (4) family history of breast cancer (none, history in first-degree relative, history in second-degree relative, unknown).

When we tested for the significance of trends among women exposed to oestrogen replacement therapy, we included the exposure in the model as a continuous variable.

Second, using stratification and the Mantel–Haenszel procedure, we assessed the influence of 26 potentially confounding variables[18], including risk factors for breast cancer (e.g. family history of breast cancer, benign breast disease, and parity), indexes of medical care utilization (e.g. self-breast examination and mammography), and determinants of non-contraceptive hormone use (e.g. menopausal status and history of diseases). We identified those variables that, when controlled for individually, yielded an adjusted relative risk estimate appreciably different from the unadjusted estimate. We then controlled for these variables simultaneously, again using the Mantel–Haenszel procedure. Because the results of this technique closely paralleled the results of the logistic regression analysis, only the latter are presented. We present results for three groups of women: those who underwent a surgical menopause and had no ovaries, those with a surgical menopause who had at least one ovary, and those who underwent natural menopause.

RESULTS

Characteristics of the 1369 cases and 1645 controls included in the analysis are shown in Table 1. Compared with controls, postmenopausal women with breast cancer were more likely to be nulliparous, be older at the time of the

Table 1 Characteristics of postmenopausal breast cancer cases and controls

Characteristic	*Percentage of cases* (*n* = 1369)	*Percentage of controls* (*n* = 1645)
Age (years)		
25–39	6.4	5.7
40–44	10.7	9.6
45–49	25.6	30.2
≥ 50	57.3	54.5
total	100.0	100.0
Race		
White	84.1	82.8
Black	10.1	11.4
other/unknown	5.8	5.8
total	100.0	100.0
Parity		
0	13.4	9.0
1–2	34.8	30.7
3–4	36.8	40.1
≥ 5	14.0	19.6
unknown	1.0	0.6
total	100.0	100.0
Age at first full-term pregnancy (years)		
< 20	21.0	26.4
20–24	41.3	41.0
25–29	16.5	16.7
≥ 30	5.0	4.1
nulliparous	13.4	9.0
unknown	2.8	2.8
total	100.0	100.0
Age at menarche (years)		
< 12	23.7	20.8
12–14	64.5	67.1
≥ 15	11.4	11.9
unknown	0.4	0.2
total	100.0	100.0
Type of menopause		
natural	37.2	36.0
surgical	62.8	64.0
total	100.0	100.0
Number of ovaries		
none	21.9	24.8
1	10.9	10.8
2	67.2	64.4
total	100.0	100.0
History of benign breast disease	20.6	13.3
Family history of breast cancer		
none	36.5	43.6
first degree	12.6	6.5
second degree	14.8	13.3
unknown	36.1	36.6
total	100.0	100.0

first full-term pregnancy, have an early menarche, have a history of benign breast disease, and report a first-degree relative who had breast cancer.

Overall, women who had used oestrogen replacement therapy had a risk of breast cancer similar to that of women who were never-users (Table 2). The adjusted relative risk among ever-users was 1.0, with a 95% confidence interval (CI) of 0.9–1.2. Women who reported surgical menopause and had no ovaries appeared to have slightly elevated risks in all oestrogen replacement therapy duration strata. The relative risk of breast cancer among these women who used oestrogens for at least 15 years was 1.7 compared with never-users. Among women who reported a surgical menopause but had at least one intact ovary, the risk estimates were less consistent; among women who experienced a natural menopause, the relative risk of breast cancer for ever-users was 0.8 compared with never-users. No relative risk for ever-users with any type of menopause was significantly different from 1.0. Similarly, the tests for trends of increasing risk with increasing duration of oestrogen replacement therapy were not statistically significant, regardless of type of menopause.

Analyses of latency or time since first use, recency or time since last use, and mg-months of oestrogen replacement therapy produced relative risk estimates similar to the risks shown in Table 2. Tables 3 and 4 present the risk of breast cancer according to latency and recency, respectively. For both measures of exposure and all types of menopause, the tests for trend were not statistically significant, although there was some suggestion of possible trends of increasing risk with increasing latency and recency among women who reported having no ovaries. Table 5 presents relative risks of breast cancer according to mg-months of oestrogen replacement therapy. Because greater than 90% of all oral oestrogen replacement therapy involves the Premarin® brand of conjugated oestrogens[2], we restricted use in Table 5 to oral conjugated oestrogens. No dose–response relationship with breast cancer risk was evident with mg-months of oral conjugated oestrogen use. We computed relative risks according to daily dosage of oestrogen replacement therapy (data not shown), and similarly found no clear association.

We also studied women with no ovaries according to the risk factors identified *a priori*: age, age at last menstrual period, age at first full-term pregnancy, history of benign breast disease, and family history of breast cancer (Table 6); we compared oestrogen replacement therapy users with never-users in the same strata. Among oestrogen replacement therapy users, women aged 50–54 years old and women who reported a first-degree relative with a diagnosis of breast cancer appeared to have a twofold increased risk of breast cancer. The increased risk among the older women was statistically significant.

In Table 7, we compared women with no ovaries with women who reported natural menopause and who had never used oestrogen replacement therapy. The relative risk of breast cancer among women with no ovaries and no exposure to oestrogen replacement therapy was 0.8 with a 95% confidence interval (CI) of 0.6–1.1. However, when we compared women with no ovaries who had ever used oestrogen replacement therapy with the

Table 2 Relative risk of breast cancer by duration of oestrogen replacement therapy

Years of therapy	*Test for trend*	*Cases*	*Controls*	*Logistic regression RR* (95% CI)*
All women	$Z = 0.3$, $p = 0.7$			
never-users		942	1117	1.0 (referent)
ever-users		427	528	1.0 (0.9–1.2)†
< 1		81	105	1.0 (0.7–1.3)†
1–4		186	219	1.1 (0.8–1.3)†
5–9		104	123	1.1 (0.8–1.5)†
10–14		34	56	0.8 (0.5–1.3)†
15–19		15	19	1.3 (0.6–2.6)†
≥ 20		7	6	1.8 (0.6–5.8)†
Surgical menopause: no ovaries	$Z = 0.1$, $p = 0.9$			
never-users		85	133	1.0 (referent)
ever-users		210	268	1.3 (0.9–1.9)
< 1		31	34	1.6 (0.9–2.8)
1–4		88	105	1.3 (0.9–2.0)
5–9		56	79	1.1 (0.7–1.8)
10–14		23	32	1.5 (0.8–2.9)
≥ 15		12	18	1.7 (0.7–4.4)
Surgical menopause: 1–2 ovaries	$Z = 0.3$, $p = 0.7$			
never-users		417	488	1.0 (referent)
ever-users		147	164	1.1 (0.8–1.5)
< 1		33	45	0.9 (0.6–1.5)
1–4		57	63	1.1 (0.8–1.6)
5–9		37	28	1.6 (1.0–2.8)
10–14		10	21	0.6 (0.3–1.2)
≥ 15		10	7	2.0 (0.7–5.5)
Natural menopause	$Z = 0.4$, $p = 0.6$			
never-users		440	496	1.0 (referent)
ever-users		70	96	0.8 (0.6–1.1)
< 1		17	26	0.8 (0.4–1.4)
1–4		41	51	0.9 (0.6–1.3)
≥ 5		12	19	0.7 (0.3–1.4)

*Adjusted by age at last menstrual period, age at index date, age at first full-term pregnancy, history of benign breast disease, and family history of breast cancer; †also adjusted by menopausal status and number of ovaries; RR = relative risk

Table 3 Relative risk of breast cancer by latency of oestrogen replacement therapy

Years since first treatment	*Test for trend*	*Cases*	*Controls*	*Logistic regression RR* (95% CI)*
All women	$Z = 0.3$, $p = 0.8$			
never-users		942	1117	1.0 (referent)
ever-users				
< 1		22	31	0.9 (0.5–1.5)†
1–4		129	151	1.1 (0.8–1.4)†
5–9		162	192	1.1 (0.8–1.4)†
10–14		74	108	0.9 (0.7–1.3)†
15–19		24	31	1.1 (0.6–2.1)†
≥ 20		16	15	1.7 (0.8–3.7)†
Surgical menopause: no ovaries	$Z = 1.4$, $p = 0.2$			
never-users		85	133	1.0 (referent)
ever-users				
< 1		12	14	1.3 (0.5–3.1)
1–4		66	77	1.3 (0.8–2.1)
5–9		79	97	1.3 (0.8–2.0)
10–14		34	50	1.4 (0.8–2.5)
≥ 15		19	30	1.6 (0.7–3.8)
Surgical menopause: 1–2 ovaries	$Z = 0.5$, $p = 0.6$			
never-users		417	488	1.0 (referent)
ever-users				
< 1		6	11	0.8 (0.3–2.1)
1–4		39	32	1.5 (0.9–2.4)
5–9		51	60	1.1 (0.7–1.6)
10–14		30	45	0.8 (0.5–1.4)
≥ 15		21	16	1.6 (0.8–3.4)
Natural menopause	$Z = 0.3$, $p = 0.7$			
never-users		440	496	1.0 (referent)
ever-users				
< 5		28	48	0.6 (0.4–1.0)
5–9		32	35	1.0 (0.6–1.7)
≥ 10		10	13	0.9 (0.4–2.1)

*Adjusted by age at last menstrual period, age at index date, age at first full-term pregnancy, history of benign breast disease, and family history of breast cancer; †also adjusted by menopausal status and number of ovaries; **RR** = relative

Table 4 Relative risk of breast cancer by recency of oestrogen replacement therapy

Years since last treatment	*Test for trend*	*Cases*	*Controls*	*Logistic regression RR* (95% CI)*
All women	$Z = 0.5$, $p = 0.6$			
never-users		942	1117	1.0 (referent)
ever-users				
< 1		245	317	1.0 (0.8–1.2)†
1–4		97	105	1.2 (0.9–1.6)†
5–9		65	78	1.1 (0.8–1.6)†
≥ 10		20	28	1.0 (0.5–1.8)†
Surgical menopause: no ovaries	$Z = 1.6$, $p = 0.1$			
never-users		85	133	1.0 (referent)
ever-users				
< 1		141	184	1.3 (0.9–1.8)
1–4		40	48	1.4 (0.8–2.4)
5–9		24	28	1.6 (0.8–3.2)
≥ 10		5	8	1.9 (0.6–6.2)
Surgical menopause: 1–2 ovaries	$Z = 1.0$, $p = 0.3$			
never-users		417	488	1.0 (referent)
ever-users				
< 1		80	86	1.2 (0.8–1.6)
1–4		28	29	1.2 (0.7–2.0)
5–9		26	31	1.0 (0.6–1.8)
≥ 10		13	18	0.9 (0.4–1.9)
Natural menopause	$Z = 0.6$, $p = 0.5$			
never-users		440	496	1.0 (referent)
ever-users				
< 1		24	47	0.5 (0.3–0.9)
1–4		29	28	1.1 (0.7–2.0)
≥ 5		17	21	1.0 (0.5–1.9)

*Adjusted by age at last menstrual period, age at index date, age at first full-term pregnancy, history of benign breast disease, and family history of breast cancer; †also adjusted by menopausal status and number of ovaries; RR = relative risk

Table 5 Relative risk of breast cancer by mg-months of oral conjugated oestrogen use

	Test for trend	*Cases*	*Controls*	*Logistic regression RR* (95% CI)*
All women	$Z = 1.0$, $p = 0.3$			
never-users		942	1117	1.0 (referent)
ever-users				
< 25		119	138	1.1 (0.8–1.5)†
25–49.9		70	69	1.3 (0.9–1.9)†
50–74.9		33	42	1.1 (0.7–1.8)†
75–99.9		32	24	1.9 (1.1–3.3)†
≥ 100.0		52	86	0.8 (0.6–1.2)†
Surgical menopause: no ovaries	$Z = 0.2$, $p = 0.8$			
never-users		85	133	1.0 (referent)
ever-users				
< 25		46	62	1.2 (0.7–2.0)
25–49.9		41	34	1.9 (1.1–3.4)
50–74.9		17	28	1.1 (0.6–2.2)
75–99.9		21	14	2.4 (1.1–5.2)
≥ 100.0		32	62	0.9 (0.5–1.5)
Surgical menopause: 1–2 ovaries	$Z = 0.5$, $p = 0.6$			
never-users		417	488	1.0 (referent)
ever-users				
< 25		49	43	1.5 (1.0–2.3)
25–49.9		16	23	0.8 (0.4–1.6)
50–74.9		12	9	1.8 (0.7–4.4)
75–99.9		10	8	1.7 (0.7–4.5)
≥ 100.0		20	19	1.3 (0.6–2.5)
Natural menopause				
never-users		440	496	1.0 (referent)
ever-users				
< 25		24	33	0.7 (0.4–1.3)
≥ 25		18	24	0.8 (0.4–1.5)

*Adjusted by age at last menstrual period, age at index date, age at first full-term pregnancy, history of benign breast disease, and family history of breast cancer. Twenty-three cases and 21 controls with unknown dosage of conjugated oestrogen used or unknown dates of use are excluded; †also adjusted by menopausal status and number of ovaries; RR = relative risk

Table 6 Relative risk of breast cancer among women with no ovaries, by selected characteristics and oestrogen replacement therapy

	Cases		*Controls*		
Characteristic	*n*	*Oestrogen replacement therapy users (%)*	*n*	*Oestrogen replacement therapy users (%)*	*Logistic regression RR* (95% CI)*
Age (years)					
< 40	19	84.2	26	73.1	1.4 (0.3–6.7)
40–44	27	63.0	48	75.0	0.6 (0.1–1.9)
45–49	84	64.3	146	66.4	0.9 (0.5–1.6)
50–54	165	74.6	181	64.1	2.0 (1.2–3.2)
Age at last menstrual period (years)					
< 40	98	69.4	179	71.0	0.9 (0.5–1.5)
40–44	83	80.7	112	70.5	1.6 (0.8–3.4)
≥ 45	114	65.8	110	56.4	1.7 (1.0–3.1)
Age at first full-term pregnancy† (years)					
< 20	61	62.3	109	59.6	1.0 (0.5–2.0)
20–29	163	71.8	215	71.6	1.3 (0.8–2.1)
≥ 30	10	60.0	19	47.4	1.9 (0.4–9.7)
nulliparous	52	78.9	44	72.7	1.6 (0.6–4.5)
Benign breast disease					
yes	71	66.2	48	66.7	1.0 (0.4–2.2)
no	224	72.8	353	66.9	1.4 (1.0–2.1)
Family history of breast cancer					
none	96	77.1	180	70.0	1.5 (0.8–2.7)
first degree	48	66.7	21	47.6	2.2 (0.7–6.3)
second degree	51	66.7	41	75.6	0.8 (0.3–2.1)
unknown	100	70.0	159	63.5	1.2 (0.7–2.2)

*Referent is never-users of oestrogen replacement therapy in the same group. Adjusted by age at last menstrual period, age at index date, age at first full-term pregnancy, history of benign breast disease, and family history of breast cancer; †nine cases and 14 controls with unknown age at first full-term pregnancy are deleted; RR = relative risk

Table 7 Relative risk of breast cancer by duration of oestrogen replacement therapy: women with no ovaries vs. naturally menopausal women who had never used oestrogen replacement therapy

Years of therapy	*Cases*	*Controls*	*Logistic regression RR** *(95% confidence interval)*
Naturally menopausal women who have never used oestrogen replacement therapy	440	496	1.0 (referent)
Women with no ovaries			
never-use	85	133	0.8 (0.5–1.1)
ever-use	210	268	1.2 (0.9–1.6)
< 1	31	34	1.3 (0.8–2.3)
1–4	88	105	1.2 (0.8–1.7)
5–9	56	79	1.1 (0.7–1.7)
10–14	23	32	1.2 (0.6–2.3)
≥ 15	12	18	1.6 (0.6–4.1)

*Adjusted by age of last menstrual period, age at index date, age at first full-term pregnancy, history of benign breast disease, and family history of breast cancer

naturally menopausal never-users, the relative risk of breast cancer increased to 1.2 with a 95% CI of 0.9–1.6. The relative risks for the oophorectomized users appeared to be approximately constant for all durations of use, and stratification by time since oophorectomy did not produce different relative risks.

COMMENT

In this analysis, we were unable to demonstrate that oestrogen replacement therapy, in general, appreciably increases a woman's risk of breast cancer. When we consider the data for specific subgroups of women, however, the findings are more difficult to interpret. In particular, women with no ovaries appear to have consistently elevated risks according to all measures of exposure: duration, latency, recency, and mg-months of use. Those women appear to have a twofold increased risk if they are 50–54 years old or have a first-degree relative with a diagnosis of breast cancer.

Selection bias in the choice of our cases and controls seems unlikely to account for these findings. All histologically confirmed cases of breast cancer from the geographically defined regions were eligible for the study; controls were selected randomly from the general population of the same areas as the cases.

Our results are not likely to be attributable to errors in the diagnosis of breast cancer. A previous study indicated that the review by a committee of expert pathologists found that less than 3% of breast cancer diagnoses by community pathologists were inaccurate[19]. Because diagnostic errors are uncommon and breast cancer is well diagnosed by community pathologists, we accepted the diagnoses of breast cancer made by the community pathologists.

We excluded postmenopausal women who had used oestrogen replacement therapy during their reproductive years because we wished to focus on the risks of hormone replacement therapy for treating symptoms of menopause. Premenopausal oestrogen replacement therapy was uncommon and might have been related to hormonal conditions associated with the risk of breast cancer. Approximately 6% of the postmenopausal cases and controls used oestrogens before their last menstrual period or age 40 years; including these women in the analysis did not appreciably change the results.

Inaccurate reporting of oestrogen replacement therapy use or recall bias has probably been reduced by use of memory aids. To help respondents more accurately recall their use of oestrogen replacement therapy, we used four aids: first, a hand card listing possible reasons for using hormones, such as to alleviate hot flushes or sweats, to prevent bone thinning, to reduce discomfort during intercourse because of a dry vagina, or to replace hormones after ovaries have been removed; second, another hand card listing the major brand names of non-contraceptive hormones marketed in the United States since the 1940s; third, a colour photograph book of non-contraceptive oestrogen preparations; and fourth, a month-by-year calendar to relate the timing of hormone use to reproductive and other life events. Coulter and colleagues[20] reported that using a calendar improves the accuracy of historical contraceptive data collected during personal interviews.

Finally, it is unlikely that confounding variables account for our results. We used both logistic regression and Mantel–Haenszel methods to control for potentially confounding variables. The two approaches produced similar results; the relative risk estimates were neither appreciably different from each other nor from the unadjusted estimates.

Although our study is the largest case–control series to consider comprehensively the relationship between breast cancer and oestrogen replacement therapy, it can only address the association between breast cancer and oestrogen replacement therapy in postmenopausal women younger than 55 years of age. In our study, women who used oestrogen replacement therapy and who were 50–54 years old at diagnosis or interview had a relative risk of 1.2 with a 95% CI of 0.9–1.4, compared with women of the same ages who did not use it. However, among women who had undergone bilateral oophorectomy, 50- to 54-year-old users were twice as likely to develop breast cancer as similarly aged women who were not users (Table 6). This study provides no information on whether oestrogen replacement therapy use is associated with an increased risk of breast cancer among women older than 54 years.

Six previous studies, like ours, found no overall increased risk of breast cancer among women who had ever used oestrogen replacement therapy[4–9]. Three studies reported slightly elevated relative risks of borderline statistical significance: 1.4, 1.2, and 1.3, respectively[10–12]. One study used numbers of prescriptions noted in medical records instead of duration of use as reported by the respondent to estimate relative risks[10], and another study reported relative risks computed from US national cancer incidence data to derive the expected incidence of disease for women under the care of one physician[11]. Both studies, therefore, require cautious interpretation.

We did not find, overall, a trend of increasing risk with increasing duration of use or time since first use, not even for durations (Table 2) and latencies (Table 3) of 20 years or longer. Our failure to demonstrate statistically significant trends in duration of use and latency was consistent with three studies[4–6] but inconsistent with three others[10–12]. Hoover and colleagues reported statistically significant trends of increasing risk with increasing numbers of prescriptions[10] and length of follow-up[11]. For the latter study, the relative risk for 15 or more years of follow-up was 2.0 with a 95% CI of 1.1–3.4. Brinton and colleagues[12] found a statistically significant trend for duration of oestrogen replacement therapy use; however, the relative risk estimates for all strata were approximately 1.2.

Analyses of oestrogen replacement therapy use and breast cancer risk in naturally and surgically menopausal women are more difficult to resolve. We studied this issue by stratifying our data according to type of menopause:

(1) Surgical menopause, zero ovaries;

(2) Surgical menopause, one or two ovaries; and

(3) Natural menopause.

We found that oophorectomized women consistently had slightly higher but not significantly different ($p > 0.05$) estimates of risk than women with intact ovaries. Additionally, there appeared to be possible, but not statistically significant, trends of increasing risk with increasing time since first use and increasing time since last use among oophorectomized women. Brinton and colleagues reported trends of increasing risk with increasing duration of use among women whose ovaries had been removed[12] and suggested that oestrogen replacement therapy after surgery may obliterate the protective effect normally seen after oophorectomy[21]. Our data in Table 7 appear to support this hypothesis.

Table 8 summarizes relative risks of breast cancer from seven studies according to ovarian status and various dosage measurements of oestrogen replacement therapy. When we consider all studies together, there are no consistent patterns of increased or decreased risk. Whether ovaries are removed or intact, the risk of breast cancer does not appear to increase with either increasing duration of oestrogen replacement therapy or higher dosages. If a positive association between breast cancer and oestrogen replacement therapy does exist, we believe the increase in risk is slight. Two results from this analysis suggest an increased risk: firstly, most estimates of relative risk are greater than 1.0 and secondly, the protective effect of bilateral oophorectomy against breast cancer is reversed among women who have used oestrogen replacement therapy. In contrast, the absence of a duration effect and the biologic implausibility of an increased risk among women using oestrogen replacement therapy for less than 1 year argue against an increased risk. Clearly, certain aspects of the possible association between breast cancer and oestrogen replacement therapy deserve further study. Particular attention should be given to two factors: assessing whether long-term or high-dosage use has different effects on naturally and surgically menopausal women and identifying subgroups of women, possibly older women and women who report a family history of breast cancer, who may

Table 8 Relative risk of breast cancer, according to dosage measurements of oestrogen replacement therapy and ovarian status

Dosage measurement	*Authors*	*Number of cases/ controls*	*Ages of cases and controls* (years)	*Dosage* (mg)	*Relative risks* *Ovaries removed*	*Relative risks* *Ovaries intact*
Duration of use (years)	Wingo *et al.* (present study)	805/993	25–54	< 1	1.6	0.8*
				1–4	1.3	0.9
				5–9	1.1	0.7†
				10–14	1.5	
				≥ 15	1.7	
	Kaufman *et al.*[6]	671/762	< 70	< 1	0.4	0.9*
				1–4	0.8	0.9
				5–9	1.1	0.7
				≥ 10	0.5	1.3
	Brinton *et al.*[12]	802/781	35–74	< 5	1.4	1.2*‡
				5–9	1.6	1.2
				≥ 10	1.7	1.1
	Hulka *et al.*[14]	152/618	cases: mean, 65 controls: mean, 63	0.5–3	—	2.1*/**
				4–9	—	1.5
				≥ 10	—	1.7
	Brinton *et al.*[21]	155/425	35–74	< 5	—	0.9*/**
				5–9	—	1.8
				10–14	—	0.6
				≥ 15	—	0.5
Mg-months of use	Wingo *et al.* (present study)	724/886	25–54	< 25	1.2	0.7*
				25–49.9	1.9	0.8†
				50–74.9	1.1	
				75–99.9	2.4	
				≥ 100.0	0.9	
	Kelsey *et al.*[5]	327/1308	45–74	< 50	0.7	0.9**††
				≥ 50	1.0	0.6

continued

Table 8 (*continued*)

Dosage measurement	*Authors*	*Number of cases/ controls*	*Ages of cases and controls* (years)	*Dosage* (mg)	*Relative risks* *Ovaries removed*	*Relative risks* *Ovaries intact*
Daily dose (mg)	Wingo *et al.* (present study)	788/960	25–54	< 0.625	2.0	0.6*
				0.625	1.2	0.8
				1.25	1.3	0.8
				≥ 2.5	2.6	0.7
	Kaufman *et al.*[6]	587/619	< 70	< 1.25	2.0	1.2*
				≥ 1.25	0.5	0.7
	Brinton *et al.*[12]	672/664	35–74	0.3	0.9	0.8*‡
				0.6	2.1	1.2
				1.25	1.5	1.1
				2.5	1.2	2.5
	Hulka *et al.*[14]	133/585	cases: mean, 65	⩽ 0.625	—	1.9*/**
			controls: mean, 63	> 0.625	—	1.0
	Ross *et al.*[8]	123/247	50–74	⩽ 0.625	0.3	0.9**‡‡
				≥ 1.25	1.1	2.3

*Includes women who have undergone a natural menopause; †includes use greater than upper bound of last category; ‡includes women who have had a hysterectomy; **uncertain if women who have had a hysterectomy are included; ††includes premenopausal, perimenopausal, and postmenopausal women; ‡‡includes postmenopausal women with intact ovaries be at increased risk of breast cancer if they use oestrogen replacement therapy.

In conclusion, postmenopausal women and their physicians must balance the potential risks and benefits of oestrogen replacement therapy. A recent review suggested that the protective influence of oestrogens on cardiovascular disease and osteoporosis in all likelihood outweighs their harmful influence on endometrial and, possibly, breast cancer[1]. We agree with that assessment and anticipate that many postmenopausal women might use oestrogens to reduce their risk of cardiovascular disease and osteoporosis.

ACKNOWLEDGEMENTS

This investigation was supported in part by interagency agreement 3-Y01-HD-8-1037 between the Centers for Disease Control and the National Institute of Child Health and Human Development, with additional support from the National Cancer Institute.

The participants in this study included the following: principal investigator: George L. Rubin, MBBS, FRACP; project director: Phyllis A. Wingo, MS; project associates: Nancy C. Lee, MD, Michele G. Mandel, Herbert B. Peterson, MD; data collection centers principal investigators: Raymond Greenberg, MD, Atlanta; J. Wister Meigs, MD, W. Douglas Thompson, PhD, Connecticut; G. Marie Swanson, PhD, Detroit; Elaine Smith, PhD, Iowa; Dorothy Pathak, PhD, Charles Key, MD, New Mexico; Donald Austin, San Francisco; David Thomas, MD, Seattle; Joseph Lyon, MD, Dee West, PhD, Utah; pathology review principal investigators: Fred Gorstein, MD, Robert McDivitt, MD, Stanley J. Robboy, MD; project consultants: Lonnie Burnett, MD, Robert Hoover, MD, Peter M. Layde, MD, MSc, Howard W. Ory, MD, MSc, James J. Schlesselman, PhD, David Schottenfeld, MD, Bruce Stadel, MD, Linda A. Webster, MSPH, Colin White, MBBS; pathology consultants: Walter Bauer, MD, William Christopherson, MD, Deborah Gersell, MD, Robert Kurman, MD, Allen Paris, MD, Frank Vellios, MD.

REFERENCES

1. Bush, T.L., Barrett-Connor, E. (1985). Noncontraceptive estrogen use and cardiovascular disease. *Epidemiol. Rev.*, **7**, 80–104
2. Kennedy, D., Baum, C. and Forbes, M. (1985). Noncontraceptive estrogens and progestins: Use patterns over time. *Obstet. Gynecol.*, **65**, 441–6
3. Silverberg, E. and Lubera, J. (1986). Cancer statistics, 1986. *CA*, **36**, 9–25
4. Sartwell, P.E., Arthes, F.G. and Tonascia, J.A. (1977). Exogenous hormones, reproductive history and breast cancer. *J. Natl. Cancer Inst.*, **59**, 1589–92
5. Kelsey, J.L., Fischer, D.B., Holford, T.R., Livolsi, V.A., Mostow, E.D., Goldenberg, I.S. and White, C. (1981). Exogenous estrogens and other factors in the epidemiology of breast cancer. *J. Natl. Cancer Inst.*, **67**, 327–33
6. Kaufman, D.W., Miller, D.R., Rosenberg, L., Helmrich, S.P., Stolley, P., Schottenfeld, D. and Shapiro, S. (1984). Noncontraceptive estrogen use and the risk of breast cancer. *J. Am. Med. Assoc.*, **252**, 63–7

7. Jick, H., Walker, A.M., Watkins, R.N., D'Ewart, C.C., Hunter, J.R., Danford, A., Masden, S., Dinan, B.J. and Rothman, K.J. (1980). Replacement estrogen and breast cancer. *Am. J. Epidemiol.*, **112**, 586–94
8. Ross, R.K., Paganini-Hill, A. and Gerkins, V.R. (1980). A case–control study of menopausal estrogen therapy and breast cancer. *J. Am. Med. Assoc.*, **243**, 1635–9
9. Hulka, B. (1980). Effect of exogenous estrogen on postmenopausal women: the epidemiologic evidence. *Obstet. Gynecol. Surv.*, **35**, 389–99
10. Hoover, R., Glass, A., Finkle, W.D., Azevedo, D. and Milne, K. (1981). Conjugated estrogens and breast cancer risk in women. *J. Natl. Cancer Inst.*, **67**, 815–20
11. Hoover, R., Gray, L., Cole, P. and MacMahon, B. (1976). Menopausal estrogens and breast cancer. *N. Engl. J. Med.*, **295**, 401–5
12. Brinton, L.A., Hoover, R.N., Szklo, M. and Fraumeni, J.F. (1981). Menopausal estrogen use and risk of breast cancer. *Cancer*, **47**, 2517–22
13. Thomas, D.B. (1984). Do hormones cause breast cancer? *Cancer*, **53**, 595–604
14. Hulka, B., Chambless, L.E., Deubner, D.C. and Wilkinson, W.E. (1982). Breast cancer and estrogen replacement therapy. *Am. J. Obstet. Gynecol.*, **143**, 638–44
15. Centers for Disease Control Cancer and Steroid Hormone Study. (1983). Long-term oral contraceptive use and the risk of breast cancer. *J. Am. Med. Assoc.*, **249**, 1591–5
16. Waksberg, J. (1978). Sampling methods for random digit dialing. *J. Am. Stat. Assoc.*, **73**, 40–6
17. Schlesselman, J. (1982). *Case–Control Studies.* (New York: Oxford University Press Inc.)
18. Mantel, N. and Haenszel, W. (1959). Statistical aspects of the analysis of data from retrospective studies of disease. *J. Natl. Cancer Inst.*, **22**, 719–48
19. Thomas, L.B., Ackerman, L.V., McDivitt, R.W. *et al.* (1977). Report of NCI ad hoc pathology working group to review gross and microscopic findings of breast cancer cases in the HIP study. *J. Natl. Cancer Inst.*, **59**, 497–541
20. Coulter, A., Vessey, M. and McPherson, K. (1986). The ability of women to recall their oral contraceptive histories. *Contraception*, **33**, 127–38
21. Brinton, L.A., Williams, R.R., Hoover, R.M., Stegens, N.L., Feinelib, M. and Fraumeni, J.F., Jr (1979). Breast cancer risk factors among screening program participants. *J. Natl. Cancer Inst.*, **62**, 37–44

18

Case–control studies of exogenous sex hormones in relation to breast cancer in women conducted in western Washington

N.S. Weiss, J.L. Stanford and L.F. Voigt

As part of a programme of studies concerning the effects of exogenous sex hormones on the health of postmenopausal women, epidemiologists at the Fred Hutchinson Cancer Research Center and the University of Washington have conducted two case–control studies of breast cancer. The first identified and interviewed residents of King County, Washington, ages 50–74 years who were diagnosed during the period July, 1977–August, 1978 ($n = 189$). Controls ($n = 531$) were recruited through surveys of the King County female population during 1976, 1977, and 1979. Identical questions were asked of cases and controls; photographic displays of commonly used hormone preparations were shown to subjects to aid recall. The results of this study were published elsewhere[1]. A family history of breast cancer, as well as a late age at first birth and late age at menopause, were strongly associated with an increased risk. Postmenopausal oestrogens had been taken with slightly higher frequency by controls than cases, a difference that was well within the limits of chance. (The use of progestogens was exceedingly uncommon among the subjects, and so the influence of these hormones on breast cancer risk could not be studied.) Similarly, there was no appreciable case–control difference with regard to oestrogen use of long duration or long interval since first use. Neither was there any increased risk associated with oestrogen use in subgroups of women defined by oophorectomy status. While the results of this study suggested that, in King County, no important relationship had been present between the use of menopausal oestrogens and the occurrence of breast cancer, the fairly low level of response among cases (54% of those eligible) and the use of different interviewers for cases and controls argue for caution in interpreting the results.

Because of the increasing use of progestational hormones by postmenopausal women in western Washington during the 1980s, and because of concerns regarding the safety of these hormones, one decade later a second study was commenced. This study has sought to identify all 50–64 year-old female residents of King County diagnosed with breast cancer during

Table 1 Response status in women with breast cancer

	Number
Eligible	658
Deceased	22
Refusal	91
physician	37
patient	54
In process	131
Completed interview	414

January, 1988–June, 1990. As in the earlier study, identification of cases occurred with the assistance of the Cancer Surveillance System of Western Washington, a population-based cancer registry that has served western Washington since 1974. Excluded from participation in this study were women with a prior history of breast cancer, and a small number of non-white women and women who resided in households with no telephone.

A total of 658 potentially eligible women with breast cancer have been identified (Table 1). Of these, 22 died before an interview could be conducted, and 91 women or their physicians refused to take part in this study. As of mid-1991, 414 women completed a personal interview, and 131 were in process.

The personal interview sought detailed information concerning use of pre- and postmenopausal hormonal medications; recall was aided by colour displays of commonly used preparations. Additional information regarding menstrual, reproductive and menopausal history was obtained as well. An identical interview was sought with a sample of 50–64 year-old King County female residents identified via random digit dialling of telephone numbers. This method of control identification has been in use for several years at the University of Washington and the Fred Hutchinson Cancer Research Center. Table 2 summarizes our experience over the past 5 years with the household

Table 2 Control selection, including results of household screening for eligibility via random digit dialing in Western Washington, 1986–90, and results, as of February, 1991, of attempted interviews with women eligible to be controls

Status	%
Random digit dialling	
no answer (after 9 attempts)	8.7
telephone answered	
no household census provided	2.0
household census obtained	89.3
Attempted interviews	
refused interview	13.3
agreed to interview	
completed	77.0
in process	9.8

Table 3 Use of non-contraceptive hormones by women with breast cancer

	Number	%
Never	160	39.6
Ever	244	60.4
< 3 months	26	6.4
≥ 3 months	218	54.0
Unknown	10	—

Table 4 Use of non-contraceptive hormones (for more than 3 months) by type in women with breast cancer

	Number	%
Oestrogen only	139	61.0
Progestogen only	3	1.3
Oestrogen, + progestogen at some time	86	37.7
duration of progestogen use		
< 3 months	12	5.3
≥ 3 months	74	32.5
Hormone, type unknown	12	—

screening portion of this method. Among telephone numbers that potentially represent households (i.e. not non-working numbers or businesses), an answer has been obtained for 91.3% of numbers, although in some instances this has required up to nine attempts at calling. Only about 2% of individuals who do answer the telephone fail to provide a household census. Of the women potentially eligible to serve as a control subject in the present study, 13.3% have refused to provide an interview. However, an additional 9.8% of interviews are in process, and the percentage of non-response will almost certainly rise to some extent. Identification and interviewing of controls was to be completed in early 1992.

Even though a comparison of cases and controls cannot take place for some time, we have tabulated the use of oestrogens and progestogens among the 414 cases of breast cancer for whom interview data are complete. In doing so, we hope to get some idea as to the types of hormones and regimens that will be evaluable when the full analysis can be completed. In Table 3, it can be seen that of the 414 cases, 60.4% had used hormones of some type for purposes other than contraception. The large majority of these women had used them for 3 or more months, and will be the subject of most subsequent analyses. Only ten of the 414 women were unable to state whether or not they had used non-contraceptive hormones.

Among women who had used hormones for 3 or more months, 139 (61.0%) has used oestrogens alone, and 74 (32.5%) had for at least 3 months used both oestrogens and a progestogen (Table 4). Only three women had used a progestogen by itself. Among women who used oestrogens alone (Table 5), most had done so for more than 5 years, and the substantial majority were still taking these hormones at the time of diagnosis. Among the 98 current users of unopposed oestrogens who could specify the type (Table 6),

Table 5 Duration and recency of 'unopposed' use of oestrogens in women with breast cancer

	Number	%
Total*	139	100
Duration		
3 months–2.9 years	36	25.9
3–4.9 years	8	5.8
5–7.9 years	25	18.0
8–11.9 years	18	12.9
≥ 12 years	52	37.4
Recency		
current	101	72.7
former, with last use:		
< 5 years prior to diagnosis	10	7.2
≥ 5 years prior to diagnosis	28	20.1

*Excludes oestrogen users of < 3 months

Table 6 Type and dose of 'unopposed' oestrogens used by women with breast cancer

	Number	%
Total*	101	100
Type of oestrogen used at time of diagnosis		
conjugated	82	83.7
oestradiol cream or patch	6	6.1
other	10	10.2
unknown	3	—
Dose of conjugated oestrogens		
< 1.0 mg/day	52	65.0
≥ 1.0 mg/day	28	35.0
unknown	2	—

*Excludes former oestrogen users and users for < 3 months

82 (83.7%) were using conjugated oestrogens. Only six were using oestradiol creams or patches, and ten another form of oestrogen. Among the users of conjugated oestrogens, though most were using less than 1 mg per day, a substantial proportion (35%) were using a higher dose.

Use of a progestogen along with an oestrogen preparation for 3 or more months was reported by 74 women. The large majority of these women (83.8%) were still using the progestogen at the time of diagnosis (Table 7). Most progestogen users had been taking the drug for a total of less than 3 years, and only 23.6% had used them for 5 or more years. The majority (65.8%) were taking this hormone for 10 or more days per month, and 15.1% were taking it for more than 14 days per month. Nearly all current users were taking medroxyprogesterone acetate. Among current users of medroxyprogesterone acetate who could specify the amount they used, the majority (58.3%) took ≤ 50 mg per month (Table 8).

Most women with a history of bilateral oophorectomy had used hormones subsequently, and the large majority oestrogens alone (Table 9). Among

Table 7 Patterns of progestogen use in women with breast cancer

	Number	%
Progestogen use for ≥ 3 months*	74	100
Duration		
3 months–2.9 years	39	54.2
3–4.9 years	16	22.2
5–7.9 years	12	16.7
≥ 8 years	5	6.9
unknown	2	—
Recency		
current	62	83.8
former	12	16.2
Days used per cycle		
< 10	25	34.2
10–14	37	50.7
> 14	11	15.1
unknown	1	—

*Excludes three women who used a progestogen but no oestrogen

Table 8 Type and dose of progestogen used by women with breast cancer; excludes former progestogen users and users for < 3 months

	Number	%
Type of progestogen used at time of diagnosis		
medroxyprogesterone acetate	56	96.6
other	2	3.4
unknown	4	—
Average dose of medroxyprogesterone acetate per cycle (mg)		
< 20	10	20.8
20–50	18	37.5
51–100	15	31.3
> 100	5	10.4
unkown	8	—

women with at least one ovary intact, the proportions of users of opposed and unopposed oestrogen were more similar, with the latter being somewhat larger.

As can be seen from the foregoing data, in the Seattle area a sizeable proportion of postmenopausal women have taken hormone preparations, including approximately 18% who have been on opposed oestrogen therapy for a period of 3 or more months. Given this fairly high percentage, along with the relatively large number of cases and controls for whom we expect to have interview data, it would seem that this study would have reasonable power to identify any altered risk of breast cancer in women who have received hormonal replacement therapy. Nevertheless, several limitations in these data may well be present. Foremost among them is the relative recency of widespread progestogen use. Only a small fraction of all women (4.3%)

Table 9 Use of non-contraceptive hormones, by type and history of bilateral oophorectomy in women with breast cancer; excludes hormone users whose total duration of use was less than 3 months, women who used a progestogen alone, and women with unknown hormone type or unknown oophorectomy status

	Number	%
Women with at least one ovary present		
no hormones	178	53.8
oestrogen only	90	27.2
oestrogen plus progestogen*	63	19.0
total	331	100
Women with a bilateral oophorectomy		
no hormones	7	10.9
oestrogen only	47	73.4
oestrogen plus progestogen*	10	15.6
total	64	100

*Progestogen use for ≥ 3 months

have taken progestogens along with an oestrogen preparation for 5 or more years. Also, within this population there is little variability as to the type of oestrogen and progestogen used. Effectively, ours will be a study of the influence of recent use of conjugated oestrogen and medroxyprogesterone acetate on the risk of breast cancer in middle-aged women.

REFERENCE

1. McDonald, J.A., Weiss, N.S., Daling, J.R., Francis, A.M. and Polissar, L. (1986). Menopausal estrogen use and the risk of breast cancer. *Breast Cancer Res. Treatm.*, **7**., 193–9

19

Why can't we prove that hormone replacement therapy causes breast cancer? – Methodological and biological challenges

R.K. Ross and L. Bernstein

A large and compelling body of epidemiological and experimental data exist implicating oestrogens in the aetiology of human breast cancer[1]. Oestrogens, in addition to their important growth-stimulating effects on breast epithelium, increase dramatically the incidence of mammary tumours in rodents. Many studies have compared oestrogen fractions in breast cancer cases and controls and in populations at high and low risk of breast cancer, and the evidence is strong that oestrogen levels are elevated among the groups, as expected. Even the age – incidence curve for breast cancer, showing a rapid increase in incidence beginning several years after puberty and then slowing dramatically at menopause, suggests an extremely important role of ovarian activity, and most likely oestrogens, in breast cancer development[2]. Among the most consistently observed breast cancer risk factors, many are hormonal events involving alterations in oestrogen secretion and metabolism – age at menarche, age at menopause, age at first birth, parity, and postmenopausal weight[1].

While there has existed for many years a common clinical belief that progestogens may negate any oestrogen-related increase in breast cancer incidence, there is little biological rationale for such a belief. The simultaneous presence of progesterone, in fact, appears to enhance the rate of breast tissue epithelial cell proliferation associated with oestrogen alone; breast mitotic activity peaks during the later luteal phase of the menstrual cycle at the time of maximum progesterone levels[3]. There are data which strongly suggest that at least one type of progestogen can itself cause breast carcinomas in dogs[4]. While it has been argued that combination oral contraceptives may increase risk of breast cancer in a duration-related fashion, especially when taken early or late in reproductive life[5], there is no strong evidence to support the notion that oral contraceptives actually reduce risk of breast cancer. Not only do women who start menstruating at an early age have a higher risk of breast cancer than those starting later, but women who begin cycling regularly (and presumably ovulating regularly) very shortly after menarche have a substantially higher risk of breast cancer than women who take longer intervals to become regular, even for comparable ages at menarche[1].

All of these data have justifiably led to concerns that oestrogen replacement therapy will adversely affect breast cancer risk and that combination hormone replacement therapy might enhance this adverse effect. These concerns have been magnified by the popularity of these categories of medications. Hormone replacement therapy in the form of unopposed oestrogen therapy became widely popular in the United States in the 1960s and into the 1970s. By 1974, there were nearly 30 million prescriptions of oestrogen replacement therapy being filled annually in the United States and the most popular brand, the conjugated equine oestrogen, Premarin®, had become the fourth most frequently prescribed drug in the country[6]. Usage decreased dramatically in the mid-1970s after the initial reports showing that oestrogen replacement therapy caused endometrial cancer. As subsequent studies have demonstrated the enormous benefits from cardiovascular and cerebrovascular diseases and osteoporotic fractures to be derived from such treatment, the prevalence of use has begun to increase rapidly again. Concomitantly, use of progestogens has also been growing rapidly in popularity[6].

Results of more than 20 studies have been published in the past decade on the possible relationship between hormone replacement therapy and breast cancer. Various investigators have summarized this considerable literature, which mostly concerns the relationship between oestrogen replacement therapy and breast cancer, either by examining individual studies or as grouped data through a statistical approach known as meta-analysis. Persson and colleagues, for example, have summarized these studies by looking simultaneously at the point estimates of risk for hormone replacement therapy users overall and for 'long-term' users vs. non-users from each of these individual studies[7]. Among the 19 studies included in this analysis, five found a significant increase in breast cancer risk among hormone replacement therapy users compared to non-users, whereas the others found no significant overall alteration in risk. Although the definition of long-term use has varied across studies, results are somewhat more consistent with long-term use, with most studies finding at least a modest increased risk of breast cancer among those who have used hormone replacement therapy for extended periods.

Meta-analysis, a statistical technique for combining risk estimates from various studies into a single risk estimate, is an alternative approach to summarizing these data. Such an analysis has the disadvantage of not being able to weigh readily the methodological strengths and shortcomings of the individual studies. One such meta-analysis was conducted by investigators at the Centers for Disease Control in Atlanta[8]. This particular analysis concluded that, across all studies, there was some evidence of a duration-related increase in breast cancer risk associated with hormone replacement therapy use, but that this effect was of a relatively small magnitude, with about a 10% increase in risk among users for each 5 years of therapy, relative to non-users. Another meta-analysis concluded that this effect was even smaller[9].

Despite all the intense interest and the strong, albeit mainly indirect,

Table 1 Some methodological and biological issues related to studies of hormone replacement therapy and breast cancer

Power
Confounding
Study design: control selection
Incidence vs. mortality effects
Risks vs. benefits
Interactions
Validity
Latency

evidence supporting a cause and effect relationship between use of hormone replacement therapy and breast cancer, and despite the numerous studies which have now been conducted, it has clearly been surprisingly difficult up to now to prove that a real association exists. It is worthwhile to explore why this is true. The remainder of this paper examines several of the pertinent issues pertaining to this hypothesis, both epidemiological and biological in nature, which have complicated attempts to study, understand, and interpret fully the relationship between hormone replacement therapy and breast cancer (Table 1).

POWER

The statistical power of a study is a measure of its probability of detecting particular specified levels of risk with a certain degree of confidence. Statistical power depends on several factors: the relative risk of interest, the desired level of confidence, and the prevalence of the exposure of interest in the comparison population (Table 2). Based on empirical data, any association between hormone replacement therapy and breast cancer is likely to be of low magnitude. Statistical modelling of breast cancer incidence also supports

Table 2 Statistical power issues

Significance level (Type 1 error)
Conventionally, 0.05
Probability of concluding relative risk is different from 1.0 when it is not (with level set at 0.05, this error will occur less than 5% of time)
Sensitivity level (Type II error)
Conventionally, 0.20; power = 1 - 0.20 = 0.80
The probability of concluding relative risk is not different from 1.0 when it is, would be 0.20; this is equivalent to an 80% chance of finding a particular result and (correctly) labelling it significant
Relative risk
The higher the relative risk one wishes to detect, the smaller the sample size required
To detect small relative risks requires more subjects than needed to detect larger relative risks
Exposure rate
In general, the lower the prevalence of the exposure under study, the larger the required sample size

Table 3 Sample size requirements for case–control study with equal numbers of cases and controls; relative risk = 1.66; $\alpha = 0.05$; power = 80%

Exposure prevalence	*Sample size in each group*
0.05	1075
0.10	583
0.20	347
0.30	279
0.40	257
0.50	260

this notion. Pike and co-workers have developed and published one such model which is based, essentially, on the effects of endogenous oestrogen exposure on mitotic activity in breast tissue stem cells (hence, on breast cancer risk)[10]. This model incorporates all the major known hormonal breast cancer risk factors. Using this model one can predict the effects on breast cancer risk of various exogenous oestrogen preparations given in various doses for varying durations. Even after 15 years of use of the most commonly prescribed dose (0.625 mg) of conjugated equine oestrogen, this model predicts only a 66% increased risk of breast cancer.

Table 3 provides sample size requirements for a case–control study (given an equal number of cases and controls) to have an 80% chance of detecting a relative risk of 1.66 for breast cancer at a significance level of 0.05 (i.e. confidence level of 95%), for various possible prevalence rates of hormone replacement therapy exposure in the population. If the model of Pike and colleagues correctly predicts risk, a relative risk of 1.66 would be expected only after 15 years of therapy. Few of the published studies to date have had a sufficient number of such long-term users to detect confidently such low levels of risk.

CONFOUNDING

Confounding variables are variables related both to the exposure of interest (hormone replacement therapy) and to the disease in question (breast cancer), which can explain some or all of any observed association[11]. Obvious possible confounding variables in studies of the relationship between hormone replacement therapy and breast cancer include age, obesity, type of menopause and age at menopause; but more subtle confounding by other established breast cancer risk factors, by unknown ones, or by those less easily measured (such as social class) is probable, given the non-experimental nature of epidemiological research. Table 4 summarizes, for a few likely confounding variables, the probable 'direction' of the confounding effect; i.e. the probable impact of adjusting for the confounding variable on the magnitude of the relative risk estimate for hormone replacement therapy and breast cancer. For example, women with breast cancer would be

Table 4 Likely possible confounding variables in studies of hormone replacement therapy and breast cancer

Variable	*Expected effect of 'adjustment' on relative risk*
Age	↑↓
Weight	↑
Age at menopause	↑
Type of menopause	↑
Family history of breast cancer	↑
Benign breast disease history	↑
Social class	↓

expected, on average, to have a lower prevalence of artificial menopause including oophorectomy than 'control' women and will have a later average age at menopause. Both oophorectomy and early menopause are associated with a higher prevalence of use of hormone replacement therapy, so failure to adjust for these variables will overestimate the prevalence of such use in controls (relative to cases) and lead to an underestimation of the actual relative risk; as shown in Table 4, proper adjustment will correctly increase the relative risk estimate.

CONTROL SELECTION

Although a few cohort studies have evaluated the relationship between hormone replacement therapy and breast cancer, most studies exploring this association have been case–control in design. There is a common belief, especially among non-epidemiologists, that cohort studies are inherently better at determining exposure/outcome relationships. Such a belief is largely unfounded, at least for diseases that are relatively uncommon and for associations in which a reasonably long latent period is expected between the exposure and outcome of interest. Although the methodological challenges are somewhat different, well-conducted studies using either study design should provide similar results, in that a case–control study is essentially a cohort study conducted in 'reverse' order.

The most critical determinant of the quality of a case–control study is the appropriateness of the comparison group, i.e. how much it is truly representative of the source population from which the case group was drawn, in terms of the prevalence of the exposure of interest. Ideally the control group should provide an unbiased estimate of the prevalence of hormone replacement therapy use in the healthy 'source' population. Among recent case–control studies, there have been a wide variety of strategies used for selecting controls, but these strategies essentially fall into two general categories: those which have used hospitalized patients with conditions thought to be unrelated to hormone replacement therapy use; and those which have utilized healthy population controls. Overall, neither study type has provided any strong evidence that hormone replacement therapy users as a group have an increased risk of breast cancer (Table 5). None the less,

Table 5 Recent case–control studies of breast cancer after oestrogen replacement therapy

First author, year	*Number of cases*	*Controls exposed (%)*	*Relative risk, ever-use*	*Relative risk, long-term use*
Healthy controls				
Ross, 1981[12]	138	45	1.1	1.9
Hoover, 1981[13]	345	29	1.4	1.7
Hulka, 1982[14]	196	30	1.4	1.7
Hiatt, 1984[15]	119	90	0.7	1.8
Nomura, 1986[16]				
Japanese	183	50	1.1	1.9
Caucasian	161	62	0.9	1.3
Brinton, 1986[17]	1960	53	1.0	1.5
Wingo, 1987[18]	1369	31	1.0	1.7
Hospital controls				
Jick, 1980[19]	60	44	1.1*	—
	37	70	3.4†	—
Kelsey, 1981[20]	332	29	0.9	0.8
Hulka, 1982[14]	196	30	1.4	0.7
Sherman, 1983[21]	113	45	0.6	0.6
Kaufman, 1984[22]	1610	30	1.0	< 1.0
Nomura, 1986[16]				
Japanese	183	53	1.0	1.2
Caucasian	161	59	0.7	0.8
La Vecchia, 1986[23]	1108	4	1.8	—

*Natural menopause; †artificial menopause

there is a clear distinction between the results from the hospital-based studies and the studies using healthy controls, when examining effects of duration of use. The former group of studies provide no evidence of an increased risk even among long-term users, but the latter group of studies rather consistently show an elevated risk after long-term use.

The reason for this relatively clear distinction in the net results from these two general study design strategies is unknown, but the most likely explanation is that hospitalized patients are greater consumers of health care services than the population as a whole and, on that basis, are more likely to be prescribed elective drugs for lengthy periods. Such a bias would lead to an underestimate of the 'true' relative risk, when using hospitalized patients as a comparison group.

INCIDENCE VERSUS MORTALITY EFFECTS

Recently, some attention has been focused on the effects of hormone replacement therapy on breast cancer *mortality* as opposed to breast cancer incidence, both overall and after lengthy use. In the Swedish cohort study of Bergkvist and co-workers[24], women who were current hormone replacement therapy users when they developed breast cancer had a 5-year relative survival of 84%, compared to 74% for women who had discontinued such therapy prior to diagnosis[25]. While these investigators provided no specific data on breast cancer mortality rates in current oestrogen users vs. past users, these survival data clearly suggest that the mortality experience from breast cancer among hormone replacement therapy users may be more favourable than the morbidity experience.

We have utilized information provided in two separate reports from this cohort[24,25] to estimate the comparative mortality experience in these two groups of women. We have calculated that, for up to 6 years of hormone replacement therapy use, the mortality experience from breast cancer in hormone replacement therapy users compared to non-users is comparable, but thereafter becomes gradually less favourable for users[26]. By 8–10 years of use, we estimate an almost 40% excess mortality in the hormone replacement therapy users. It is noteworthy that several other groups have observed a reduction in mortality from breast cancer in oestrogen users overall[27,28], although no group has yet addressed the critical issue of mortality from breast cancer in long-duration users. Nevertheless, based on existing data, there appears to be some discrepancy between the observed increment in incidence from breast cancer in oestrogen users, as compared to mortality from breast cancer. One possible explanation for this anomaly, consistent with what has been proposed to explain a similar phenomenon which occurs with endometrial cancer[29], is that oestrogen users are diagnosed with breast (or endometrial) cancer at an earlier stage, on average, because as a group, such women are under closer medical surveillance than non-users. No published data exist on breast cancer screening rates (e.g. by mammography) in users compared to non-users of hormone replacement therapy, although one would predict higher screening rates in users. Importantly, no data exist to suggest that screening by mammography picks up tumours that would otherwise not come to medical attention, so detection bias *per se*, which has been suggested as the explanation for this phenomenon in endometrial cancer, is an unlikely explanation here. An alternative explanation is that there exists a fundamental difference in biological behaviour or the response to treatment of breast cancers diagnosed in women taking hormone replacement therapy.

RISK–BENEFIT ISSUES

As individual studies on the relationship between hormone replacement therapy and breast cancer have been published over the last few years, some suggesting a positive relationship and others no relationship, the level of interest in this possible relationship by the scientific community, the press, and the public has periodically waxed and waned. When those studies suggestive of a positive association have been published, the response of all interested parties has invariably been highly emotionally charged. It is especially important, therefore, that this purported association be kept in the appropriate context. We have developed a simple risk–benefit mortality model for hormone replacement therapy[30,31]. This model was developed by first determining the annual mortality rate from the five major disease categories thought to be affected by use of oestrogen replacement therapy and known to have substantial mortality associated with them. We utilized a summary estimate of the relative risks for each of these diseases associated with oestrogen replacement therapy, based on existing literature. We built in a very low case fatality rate for oestrogen-related endometrial cancer, but using a probable 'worst case' scenario we presumed that the incremental increased mortality from breast cancer associated with long-term hormone replacement therapy was comparable to the incremental increase in incidence. The net result of this analysis is that among 100 000 women using 0.625 mg of conjugated equine oestrogen for 10 years, 300 fewer deaths would be expected annually from these combined causes, relative to a comparable number of non-users (Figure 1), primarily because of the anticipated benefit in mortality from vascular diseases.

We have concluded from this analysis that, in terms of mortality, the overall risk–benefit equation balances strongly in favour of benefit. Moreover, despite the increase in endometrial cancer mortality, this benefit extends even to women with an intact uterus. This estimated reduction in mortality of approximately 300 deaths annually represents an approximately 17% annual overall reduction in mortality (i.e. from all causes). We have been following a cohort of 9000 elderly residents of a retirement community in Southern California since 1981. The median duration of oestrogen replacement therapy use among the 55% of women in this cohort who report having used oestrogen replacement therapy is 10 years. To date, this group of women has a 20% reduction in all-cause mortality[28], consistent with that predicted from the risk–benefit model. So, despite the adverse effects of oestrogen replacement therapy on endometrial and possibly breast cancer mortality, oestrogen replacement therapy, on balance, has enormous positive implications for women's health. We have done similar calculations for combination hormone replacement therapy, but many more assumptions

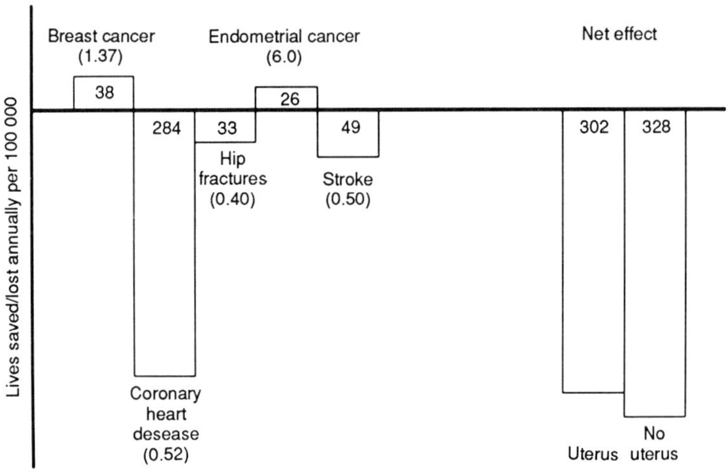

Figure 1 Estimated annual changes in mortality induced by oestrogen replacement therapy (0.625 mg conjugated equine oestrogen for 10 years). Figures in parentheses are relative risks

are required in such an analysis since few, if any, specific data currently exist on the association between combination hormone replacement therapy and any of the disease outcomes of interest.

OTHER ISSUES

There are many other important methodological issues in trying to establish a relationship between hormone replacement therapy and breast cancer development. If a duration-related increase in risk exists, it becomes crucial to establish whether there exist subgroups of women at particularly high risk or, for that matter, women at no increased risk at all. There have been some reports suggesting that only women with natural menopause have enhanced risk, but others have suggested the opposite (i.e. an increased risk limited to women with artificial menopause). There are reports that risk is enhanced especially among women with a history of benign breast disease, or among women with a family history of breast cancer, but others have not found these effects (for a summary, see reference 5). As described above, a principle issue in resolving these questions will be the design of studies with sufficient power to detect such interactions.

Evaluation of a 'dose–response' relationship between use of hormone replacement therapy and breast cancer would appear to be straightforward. In fact, establishing such a relationship is complicated because of marked changes over time in favoured doses, a tendency for women to use multiple doses over time (sometimes each for substantial periods of time), and the availability of many specific hormonal products with no bioassay to measure the relative potency of these individual products on breast tissue. For combination hormone replacement therapy, there is the added complication of evaluating the subset of women who have used both oestrogen replacement therapy *and* combination hormone replacement therapy at different times postmenopausally. Most studies of hormone replacement therapy and breast cancer to date have depended on self-reports to define exposure. In the United States, the oestrogen replacement therapy prescription market is largely controlled by a single brand (Premarin®), the dosages for which are readily distinguishable by pill colours. This fact has greatly simplified strategies for obtaining accurate data through these self-reports. In fact, we and others have established the validity of self-reports through use of pharmacy and clinic records[32]. To the extent that unbiased misclassification does occur, i.e. misclassification of a comparable degree in cases and controls, the effect will be to underestimate the 'true' relative risk.

There is a prevailing belief that oestrogens will act as 'promoters' and therefore that any effect on breast cancer risk will be apparent following a minimal latency period. There are some data which suggest that current hormone replacement therapy users have greater breast cancer risk for a constant duration of exposure than past users, lending some possible support to this hypothesis[33]. The consistently observed effects of duration of use on risk would argue against this phenomenon resulting simply from hormone replacement therapy leading to earlier detection of breast cancer.

ACKNOWLEDGEMENT

This work was supported by grant CA17054 from the National Institutes of Health.

REFERENCES

1. Henderson, B.E., Ross, R.K. and Bernstein, L. (1988). Estrogens as a cause of human cancer. The Richard and Hinda Rosenthal Foundation Award Lecture. *Cancer Res.*, **48**, 240
2. Pike, M.C., Ross, R.K., Lobo, R.A. and Key, K.J.A. (1989). LHRH agonists and the prevention of breast and ovarian cancer. *Br. J. Cancer*, **60**, 142–8
3. Ferguson, D.J.P. and Anderson, T.J. (1981). Morphological evaluation of cell turnover in the 'resting' human breast. *Br. J. Cancer*, **44**, 177–81
4. Finkel, M.C. and Berlinger, V.R. (1973). The extrapolation of experimental findings (animal to man): the dilemma of systematically administered contraceptives. *Bull. Soc. Pharmacol. Environ. Path.*, **4**, 13–18
5. Bernstein, L., Ross, R.K. and Henderson, B.E. (1992) The relationship of hormone use to cancer. *Natl. Cancer Inst. Monogr.* (in press)
6. Kennedy, D.L., Baum, C. and Forbes, M.F. (1985). Noncontraceptive estrogens and progestogens: use patterns over time. *Obstet. Gynecol.*, **65**, 441–6
7. Persson, I., Adami, H.O. and Bergkvist, L. (1990). Hormone replacement therapy and the risk of cancer in the breast and reproductive organs: a review of epidemiological data. In Drife, J.O. and Studd, J.W.W. (eds.) *HRT and Osteoporosis*, pp.165–75. (London: Springer-Verlag)
8. Steinberg, K.K., Thacker, S.B., Smith, S.J., Stroup, D.S., Zack, M.M., Handers, W.D. and Berkelman, R.L. (1991). A meta-analysis of the effect of estrogen replacement therapy on the risk of breast cancer. *J. Am. Med. Assoc.*, **265**, 1985
9. Dupont, W.D. and Page, D.L. (1991). Menopausal estrogen replacement therapy and breast cancer. *Arch. Intern. Med.*, **151**, 67
10. Pike, M.C., Krailo, M.D., Henderson, B.E. *et al.* (1983). 'Hormonal' risk factors, 'breast tissue age' and the age-incidence of breast cancer. *Nature* (*London*), **303**, 767–70
11. Smith, P.G. and Day, N.E. (1984). The design of case–control studies; the influence of confounding and interaction effects. *Int. J. Epidemiol.*, **13**, 356–65
12. Ross, R.K., Paganini-Hill, A., Gerkins, V.R., Hack, T.H., Pfeiffer, R., Arthur, M. and Henderson, B.E. (1980). A case–control study of menopausal estrogen therapy and breast cancer. *J. Am. Med. Assn.*, **243**, 1635–9
13. Hoover, R., Glass, A., Finkle, W.D., Azevedo, D. and Milne, K. (1981). Conjugated oestrogens and breast cancer risk in women. *J. Natl. Cancer Inst.*, **67**, 815–20
14. Hulka, B.S., Chambless, L.E., Deubner, D.C., Wilkinson, W.E. (1982). Breast cancer and estrogen replacement therapy. *Am. J. Obstet. Gynecol.*, **143**, 638–44
15. Hiatt, R.A., Bawol, R., Friedman, G.W. and Hoover, R. (1984). Exogenous estrogens and breast cancer after oophorectomy. *Cancer*, **54**, 139–44
16. Nomura, A.M.Y., Kolonel, L.N., Hirohata, T. and Lee, J. (1986). The association of replacement estrogens with breast cancer. *Int. J. Cancer*, **37**, 49–53
17. Brinton, L.A., Hoover, R., Fraumeni, J.F. (1986). Menopausal estrogens and breast cancer: an expanded case–control study. *Br. J. Cancer*, **54**, 825–32
18. Wingo, P.A., Layde, P.M., Lee, M.C., Rubin, G. and Ory, H.W. (1987). The risk of breast cancer in postmenopausal women who have used estrogen replacement therapy. *J. Am. Med. Assn.*, **257**, 209–15
19. Jick, H., Walker, A.M., Watkins, R.N., D'Ewart, D.C., Hunter, J.R., Danford, A., Madsen, S., Dinan, B.J. and Rothman, K.J. (1980). Replacement estrogens and breast cancer. *Am. J. Epidemiol.*, **112**, 586–94
20. Kelsey, J., Fischer, D.B., Holförd, T.R., LiVolsi, V.A., Mostow, E.D., Goldenberg, I.S. and White, C. (1981). Exogenous estrogens and other factors in the epidemiology of breast cancer. *J. Natl. Cancer Inst.*, **67**, 327–33
21. Sherman, B., Wallace, R. and Bean, J. (1983). Estrogen use and breast cancer. Interaction with body mass. *Cancer*, **51**, 1527–31

22. Kaufman, D.W., Miller, D.R., Rosenberg, L., Helmrich, S.P., Stolley, P., Schottenfeld, D. and Shapiro, S. (1984). Noncontraceptive estrogen use and the risk of breast cancer. *J. Am. Med. Assn.*, **252**, 63–7
23. La Vecchin, C., DiCarli, A., Parazzini, F., Gentile, A., Liberati, C. and Franceschi, S. (1986). Non-contraceptive oestrogens and the risk of breast cancer in women. *Int. J. Cancer*, **38**, 853–8
24. Bergkvist, L., Adami, H.O., Persson, I., Hoover, R., and Schairer, C. (1989). Risk of breast cancer after estrogen and estrogen–progestin replacement. *N. Engl. J. Med.*, **321**, 293–7
25. Bergkvist, L., Adami, H.O., Persson, I., Bergstroem, R. and Krusemo, U.B. (1989). Prognosis after breast cancer diagnosis in women exposed to estrogen and estrogen–progestogen replacement therapy. *Am. J. Epidemiol.*, **130**, 221–8
26. Pike, M.C., Bernstein, L. and Ross, R.K. (1990). Breast cancer and hormone replacement therapy. *Lancet*, **1**, 297
27. Hunt, K., Vessey, M., MacPherson, K. and Coleman, M. (1987). Long-term surveillance of mortality and cancer incidence in women receiving hormone replacement therapy. *Br. J. Obstet. Gynaecol.*, **94**, 620–35
28. Henderson, B.E., Paganini-Hill, A. and Ross, R.K. (1991). Decreased mortality in users of estrogen replacement therapy. *Arch. Intern. Med.*, **151**, 75–8
29. Chu, J., Schweid, A.I. and Weiss, N.S. (1982). Survival among women with endometrial cancer: a comparison of estrogen users and non-users. *Am. J. Obstet. Gynecol.*, **143**, 569–73
30. Henderson, B.E., Ross, R.K., Lobo, R.A., Pike, M.C. and Mack, T.M. (1988). Re-evaluating the role of progestogen therapy after the menopause. *Fertil. Steril.*, **49**, 9–15s
31. Ross, R.K., Pike, M.C., Henderson, B.E., Mack, T.M. and Lobo, R.M. (1989). Stroke prevention and oestrogen replacement therapy. *Lancet*, **1**, 505
32. Paganini-Hill, A. and Ross, R.K. (1982). Reliability of recall of drug usage and other health-related information. *Am. J. Epidemiol.*, **116**, 114–22
33. Colditz, G.A., Stampfer, M.J., Willett, W.C., Hennekens, C.H., Rosner, B. and Speizer, F.E. (1990). Prospective study of estrogen replacement therapy and risk of breast cancer in postmenopausal women. *J. Am. Med. Assoc.*, **264**, 2648–53

20

Oestrogen replacement therapy and breast cancer: results from the Slone Epidemiology Unit's Toronto Breast Cancer Study

L. Rosenberg, J.R. Palmer and S. Shapiro

INTRODUCTION

To evaluate whether the risk of breast cancer is influenced by alcohol consumption, we undertook a case–control study in Toronto, Canada in 1982[1]. We also collected information on many other potential risk factors, so that their influence could be evaluated as well. Non-contraceptive oestrogens were of particular interest: if endogenous oestrogens play a role in the aetiology of breast cancer[2,3], so too might exogenous oestrogens[4]. Whether the latter do indeed play a role is unclear, as the results of epidemiologic studies to date have been inconclusive[5–26]. Non-contraceptive oestrogens are very commonly used by menopausal women, at least in the United States and Canada; an increase in risk in users could have a substantial impact on the incidence of breast cancer.

We report here results from our Toronto Breast Cancer study on the relation of non-contraceptive oestrogen use to breast cancer risk.

MATERIALS AND METHODS

Data collection

Data collection was carried out from 1982 to 1986. Women were eligible to participate if they were under 70 years of age, lived in metropolitan Toronto, spoke English, and had no history of cancer other than non-melanotic carcinoma of the skin. Trained interviewers administered structured questionnaires in home interviews after the participants had given informed

Material used in this chapter has previously been published in Palmer, J.R. *et al.* (1991). *Am. J. Epidemiol.*, **134**, 1386–95 and is reproduced here with permission consent. The questionnaires elicited information about demographic factors, reproductive and medical histories, and medication use. For oestrogens and other female hormones, subjects were asked about the use of drugs for regulation of menstrual periods, menstrual problems, breast conditions, cessation of postpartum milk flow, maintenance of pregnancy, 'change of life', menopause, hot flashes and sexual difficulties. They were shown photographs of oestrogen pills marketed in Canada and the United States to aid recall. For each episode of use, the drug name, indication of use, frequency of use, time elapsed since first use, and duration of use were recorded.

Cases and controls

The cases, identified at the Princess Margaret Hospital, the major cancer treatment hospital in metropolitan Toronto, were women under age 70 with a histologically-confirmed primary carcinoma of the breast, diagnosed no more than 6 months before the interview. The physicians of 73 (9%) of 800 potential cases refused participation, and 97 (12%) women themselves refused. After exclusion of 23 (3%) cases for whom controls could not be found, the final case series consisted of 607 women. Oestrogen and progesterone receptor status were determined within 6 weeks of the diagnosis for 528 of the 607 cases[27].

Community controls, matched on neighbourhood and decade of age to the cases, were identified from Ontario tax assessment rolls. For each of the 607 cases, two controls were interviewed. Of 1874 eligible controls contacted, 1214 (65%) participated.

Of the total number of women (both cases and controls) 26% were 60–69 years of age, and 31% were 50–59; the remainder were less than 50. Most were White (cases, 85%; controls, 90%) and had been born in Canada (cases, 64%; controls, 63%). Fifty-one percent of cases and 47% of controls had at least 13 years of education. The cases tended more commonly than controls to have had a late menopause, a history of fibrocystic breast disease, a mother or sister with breast cancer, and to be Jewish or nulliparous[1]. Early age at menopause, leanness among the premenopausal women, and obesity among the postmenopausal women, were also associated weakly with an increased risk; late age at first birth was not associated with an increase[1].

Data analysis

We defined unopposed oestrogen replacement therapy as the use of oral or injectable oestrogens without progestogens during the year before the menopause, or after the menopause, for menstrual problems, 'change of life', menopause, hot flashes, or sexual difficulties. Oestrogen use for other purposes (cessation of lactation, breast conditions, and maintenance of pregnancy) was considered separately, and almost all such use occurred well before the menopause; we also included in this category the use of topical vaginal oestrogen cream (four women). Combination therapy (oestrogens taken together with a progestogen) was considered in a separate category.

Relative risks (odds ratios) for oestrogen use relative to never-use of a non-contraceptive oestrogen were estimated from conditional logistic regression analyses[28], which controlled for the matching factors, age and neighbourhood. Age at menopause was also controlled in all analyses, in the following categories: pre- or perimenopausal, menopause before age 45, menopause at age 45–49, menopause at age 50 or older, and unknown age at menopause because of a hysterectomy without bilateral oophorectomy. Multivariate relative risk estimates were obtained after allowance, in addition to the matching factors and age at menopause, for type of menopause, history of breast cancer in a mother or sister, age at menarche, age at first birth, parity, body mass index (weight/height^2), history of cystic breast disease, oral contraceptive use, alcohol consumption, years of education, and number of visits to a physician in the year previous to the year before interview. The multivariate estimates were similar to those adjusted only for the matching factors and age at menopause, and the latter estimates are given unless otherwise noted.

RESULTS

Replacement oestrogens unopposed by progestogens were taken by 15% of both the cases and controls (Table 1). Fewer women used unopposed oestrogens for reasons other than replacement (cases, 3.2%; controls 2.0%), or oestrogens opposed by progestogens (cases, 0.7%; controls, 1.2%).

With allowance for the matching factors and for age at menopause, the relative risk estimate for ever-use of unopposed oestrogens for replacement was 1.0 (95% confidence interval (CI), 0.7–1.3); for unopposed use for other reasons the estimate was 1.3 (95% CI, 0.7–2.6), and for use of oestrogens with progestogens it was 0.6 (95% CI, 0.2–2.0) (Table 2). The multivariate relative risk estimates were closely similar. Further attention is confined to use of unopposed oestrogens for replacement.

Among the 279 users of unopposed oestrogen for replacement (Table 3), 78% were able to name the oestrogen: among them, 93% had used conjugated oestrogens, and the remainder (7%) had taken other compounds. The relative risk estimate for ever-use of conjugated oestrogens was 0.8, while the estimates for other oestrogens, unknown oestrogens, and more than one type ranged

Table 1 Non-contraceptive oestrogen use in 607 breast cancer cases and 1214 neighbour controls

	Cases		*Controls*	
Non-contraceptive oestrogen use	*n*	(%)	*n*	(%)
Never used	493	(81.2)	991	(82.3)
Unopposed, for replacement	94	(15.5)	185	(15.2)
Unopposed, for other reasons	16	(3.2)	24	(2.0)
Opposed	4	(0.7)	14	(1.2)

Table 2 Relation of non-contraceptive oestrogen use to risk of breast cancer

Non-contraceptive oestrogen use	*Relative risk estimate* (95% confidence interval)*		*Multivariate relative risk estimate† (95% confidence interval)*	
Never used	1.0‡	—	1.0‡	—
Unopposed oestrogens, for replacement	1.0	(0.7–1.3)	1.0	(0.8–1.4)
Unopposed oestrogens, for other indications	1.3	(0.7–2.6)	1.4	(0.7–2.7)
Oestrogens taken with progestogens	0.6	(0.2–2.0)	0.6	(0.2–1.9)

*Adjusted for matching factors and age at menopause; †estimates from multivariate conditional logistic regression. Adjusted for the matching factors and the following factors: type of menopause, age at menopause, age at menarche, parity, age at first birth, family history of breast cancer, history of cystic breast disease, body mass index, education, alcohol consumption, oral contraceptive use, number of physician visits in previous year; ‡reference category

Table 3 Relation to unopposed oestrogen use for replacement to risk of breast cancer, by type of oestrogen

Type of oestrogen	*Cases*	*Controls*	*Relative risk estimate**	*95% confidence interval*
Total	94	185	1.0	0.7–1.3
Conjugated oestrogens only	60	144	0.8	0.6–1.1
Other oestrogens	8	7	2.2	0.8–6.3
Unknown oestrogens	21	31	1.4	0.8–2.6
More than one type	5	3	3.7	0.9–16

*Adjusted for matching factors and age at menopause; reference category is never-use of non-contraceptive oestrogens

Table 4 Relation of duration of use of unopposed oestrogens for replacement to risk of breast cancer

Duration of use of unopposed oestrogens for replacement (years)	*Cases*	*Controls*	*Relative risk estimate**	*95% confidence interval*
Never used	493	991	1.0†	—
< 1	29	42	1.3	0.8–2.2
1–4	62	70	0.7	0.4–1.1
5–9	17	34	1.0	0.5–1.8
10–14	7	17	0.9	0.4–2.3
15+	14	19	1.7	0.8–3.5

*Adjusted for matching factors and age at menopause; †reference category

from 1.4 to 3.7; none of the estimates differed significantly from 1.0.

When the duration of use of all types of unopposed replacement oestrogens together was considered (Table 4), the relative risk estimate for the shortest duration category, < 1 year of use, was 1.3; for all other duration categories except the longest, the estimates were less than 1.0; for the longest, 15+ years of use, the estimate was 1.7 (95% CI, 0.8–3.5). None of the estimates was statistically significant.

When conjugated oestrogens were considered separately (Table 5), the estimates according to categories of duration were similar to those for any type of oestrogen; in particular, the estimate was 1.4 (95% CI, 0.6–3.3) for 15+ years of use. When 15+ years of use was divided further into 15–19 and 20+ years, the estimates were 1.2 (4 exposed cases, 7 exposed controls), and 1.6 (5 exposed cases, 8 exposed controls), respectively. Virtually all of the conjugated oestrogen use was among postmenopausal women. When the analyses according to duration of conjugated oestrogen use were confined to postmenopausal women, the relative risk estimates for all duration categories were the same as those shown in Table 5.

The increased relative risk estimate for women who had used unopposed conjugated oestrogens for 15+ years was due to an excess of case users among women aged 60–69 (Table 6), for whom the relative risk estimate for 15 or more years of use was 2.6 (95% CI, 0.9–7.0). However, the estimate for the next longest duration category, 10–14 years, was 0.7 (95% CI, 0.2–2.8). In women under age 60, there was a deficit of long-term use in cases:

Table 5 Relation of duration of use of unopposed conjugated oestrogens for replacement to risk of breast cancer

Duration of use of unopposed conjugated oestrogens (years)	*Cases*	*Controls*	*Relative risk estimate**	*95% confidence interval*
Never used	493	991	1.0†	—
< 1	16	33	0.9	0.5–1.7
1–4	19	50	0.7	0.4–1.3
5–9	11	28	0.8	0.4–1.6
10–14	5	16	0.6	0.2–1.8
15+	9	15	1.4	0.6–3.3

*Adjusted for matching factors and age at menopause; †reference category

Table 6 Relation of duration of use of unopposed conjugated oestrogens for replacement to risk of breast cancer, according to age

Duration of use (years)	*Cases*	*Controls*	*Relative risk estimate**	*95% confidence interval*
Age < 60				
Never used	385	770	1.0†	—
< 5	22	47	0.8	0.5–1.4
5–9	8	14	1.1	0.4–2.7
10–14	2	8	0.5 } 0.3	} 0.1–1.4
15+	0	6	0	
Age 60–69				
Never used	108	221	1.0†	—
< 5	13	36	0.8	0.4–1.6
5–9	3	14	0.4	0.1–1.5
10–14	3	8	0.7	0.2–2.8
15+	9	9	2.6	0.9–7.0

*Adjusted for matching factors and age at menopause; †reference category

relative risk estimates for 10–14 and 15+ years of use were 0.5 and 0, respectively; the estimate for the combined category, 10+ years of use, was 0.3 (95% CI, 0.1–1.4).

To evaluate whether recent use influences risk, or whether an increased risk becomes apparent after a long interval (latency), we estimated relative risks according to the time elapsed since last use of unopposed conjugated oestrogens (Table 7). The relative risk estimate was decreased, 0.4 (95% CI, 0.2–0.9) for use that ended within the year before interview, elevated, 5.2 (95% CI, 2.0–13), for use that ended 1–2 years before interview, and less than 1.0 for all longer time-interval categories. For the longest elapsed interval, 15+ years, the estimate was 1.0 (95% CI, 0.5–2.3).

We repeated the analysis according to recency of last use for women who had used conjugated oestrogens for 5 or more years (Table 8). The estimates were 0.7 (95% CI, 0.3–1.5) for use that ended in the year before interview, 2.0 (95% CI, 0.6–7.4) for use that ended 1–2 years before interview, and 1.2 (95% CI, 0.4–3.5) for use that ended at least 10 years before interview.

Relative risk estimates for 5 or more years of unopposed conjugated oestrogen use for women in various categories of breast cancer risk factors are given in Table 9. All relative risk estimates were compatible with 1.0. The largest relative risk estimate, 1.5, was among women whose first birth was before age 25, and the smallest, 0.4, was among those whose first birth occurred at age 25 or older.

Table 7 Relation of use of unopposed conjugated oestrogens for replacement to risk of breast cancer, according to elapsed time since last use

Time since last use (years)	*Cases*	*Controls*	*Relative risk estimate**	*95% confidence interval*
Never used	493	991	1.0†	—
< 1	10	47	0.4	0.2–0.9
1–2	17	6	5.2	2.0–13
3–4	5	9	1.0	0.3–3.1
5–9	6	27	0.4	0.2–1.1
10–14	9	27	0.6	0.3–1.4
15+	12	23	1.0	0.5–2.3

*Adjusted for matching factors and age at menopause; †reference category

Table 8 Relation of use of unopposed conjugated oestrogens for replacement for at least 5 years to risk of breast cancer, according to elapsed time since last use

Time since last use (years)	*Cases*	*Controls*	*Relative risk estimate**	*95% confidence interval*
Never used	493	991	1.0†	—
< 1	9	30	0.7	0.3–1.5
1–2	5	5	2.0	0.6–7.4
3–9	5	14	0.7	0.2–2.0
10+	6	9	1.2	0.4–3.5

*Adjusted for matching factors and age at menopause; †reference category

Table 9 Relation of use of unopposed conjugated oestrogens for at least 5 years for replacement to risk of breast cancer, according to selected factors

Factor	*Cases* *Used 5+ years/ never used*	*Controls* *Used 5+ years/ never used*	*Relative risk estimate**	*95% confidence interval*
Type of menopause				
natural	10/189	26/375	0.7	0.3–1.6
surgical, both ovaries removed	10/20	22/38	1.0	0.4–2.6
surgical, ≤ 1 ovary removed	5/51	11/87	0.7	0.2–2.4
Age at menopause (years)				
natural and bilateral oophorectomy only				
< 45	6/21	16/70	1.2	0.4–3.4
≥ 45	13/175	31/333	0.8	0.4–1.5
Age at menarche (years)				
< 12	8/97	10/172	1.3	0.5–3.6
≥ 12	17/393	49/814	0.7	0.4–1.3
Age at first birth (years)				
< 25	12/176	16/375	1.5	0.7–3.4
≥ 25	7/193	34/409	0.4	0.2–1.0
Parity				
0	6/124	9/206	1.2	0.4–3.4
1–2	7/213	25/438	0.6	0.3–1.5
≥ 3	12/156	25/346	1.1	0.5–2.2
History of cystic breast disease				
yes	4/75	3/54	0.9	0.2–4.5
no	21/418	56/937	0.9	0.5–1.6
Family history of breast cancer				
yes	4/60	4/62	0.9	0.2–4.3
no	21/433	55/929	0.9	0.5–1.5
Body mass index (weight/height^2)				
≤ 20	6/101	8/196	1.3	0.4–4.2
21–28	16/296	45/647	0.8	0.4–1.4
≥ 29	3/89	6/134	0.7	0.2–3.1
Oral contraceptive use				
yes	7/220	16/469	1.0	0.4–2.7
no	18/273	43/522	0.8	0.4–1.4

*Adjusted for the matching factors and age at menopause

Among the 528 cases whose oestrogen receptor status was determined, 351 were classified as oestrogen receptor-positive (an assay of ≥ 10 fmol/mg) and 177 as oestrogen receptor-negative. For oestrogen receptor-positive women the relative risk estimate for 5 or more years of unopposed conjugated oestrogen use was 1.0 (95% CI, 0.5–1.8); for oestrogen receptor-negative women the relative risk estimate was also 1.0 (95% CI, 0.4–2.6).

We were unable to evaluate dosage because less than half of the women who used conjugated oestrogens were able to specify the dose.

DISCUSSION

Evidence from the present study

In the present data, use of unopposed non-contraceptive oestrogens for replacement for durations of less than 15 years was not associated with an increased risk of breast cancer. For 15 or more years of use, the point estimate of relative risk was elevated, 1.7, but not statistically significant. Results were similar when attention was confined to the most commonly used non-contraceptive oestrogen, conjugated oestrogens: in the women with 15+ years of use, the relative risk estimate was 1.4. The increased relative risk among women with 15+ years of conjugated oestrogen use was concentrated among the oldest women, those aged 60–69, but the increase was compatible with a value of 1.0, and for the next longest duration category the relative risk estimate was 0.7. In addition, there was a deficit of long-term users among cases who were under 60 years of age. While not entirely reassuring, the data do not provide consistent evidence of an adverse effect of long-term conjugated oestrogen use.

Current use of conjugated oestrogens was not associated with an increased risk. A statistically significant relative risk, 5.2, was estimated for any use that ended 1–2 years before interview, but the corresponding estimate for 5 or more years of use was 2.0 and not significant. The estimates for use that ended 3 or more years before interview were close to 1.0. A single elevation in relative risk coupled with no pattern or trend according to the length of the elapsed interval suggests sampling variation more strongly than any other explanation.

When conjugated oestrogen use was examined among women at varying risks of breast cancer, there was no evidence of an increased risk in any particular subgroup.

There were insufficient data for detailed evaluation of the use of oestrogens other than conjugated oestrogens, or the use of oestrogens concomitantly with progestogens.

It is possible that cases remembered oestrogen use more completely than controls; if so, this would have led to overestimation of the risk. We believe that this bias is more likely to have occurred in the reporting of short-term use than long-term use. Indeed, in the present study, the relative risk estimate was slightly elevated, 1.3, for women who reported less than 1 year of unopposed oestrogen use for replacement. That this estimate could have been due to information bias is supported by data from a validation study of breast cancer cases and hospital and neighbourhood controls[29]: subjects who were misclassified as to ever-use of oestrogens had relatively short durations of use; among confirmed users, agreement on duration of use was as good among controls as cases. Several other validation studies[30–32] indicate good agreement between subjects' reports of oestrogen use and physicians' records, for both cases and controls.

A satisfactorily high percentage of potential cases agreed to participate, so that bias due to selective participation is unlikely. We believe that admission to the Princess Margaret Hospital conditional on oestrogen use was also unlikely, but we have no quantitative evidence to support that belief. The participation rate for controls was 65% and this could have allowed a selection bias. In some studies, agreement to participate has been higher among persons who were better educated[33,34]. If participation was also related to education in our study, the effect would have been to underestimate a positive association, because well-educated women are more likely to be oestrogen users.

The standard breast cancer risk factors were controlled in the analysis, and this had little effect on the relative risk estimates. In addition, the matching of cases with neighbour controls may have served to control, to some extent, for subtle socioeconomic and cultural factors on which we had no information.

Evidence from other studies

A number of relatively large studies published since 1984 on the relation of oestrogen use to breast cancer risk have suggested a small positive association with breast cancer risk; others have provided strong evidence against an association, however. Of four follow-up studies[17,20,22,25], three reported an increased risk of breast cancer associated with ever- or long-term use of oestrogen[17,20,25]. The fourth found a positive association for recent use which was not influenced by the duration of use[22]. Of six large case–control studies[6,16,17,19,23,24], four found an increased risk to be associated with ever- or long-duration use[16,17,19,24]. Two studies, based on data collected in our Case–Control Surveillance Study, found no evidence of an increase[6,23], with close statistical confidence; the results of the most recent study are described elsewhere (Chapter 14). The strongest positive associations were observed in studies of European women, who had commonly used oestrogens other than conjugated oestrogens[17,20,24].

The Nurses' Health Study raised the hypothesis that current use, regardless of duration, increases the risk[22]. That hypothesis is weakly supported by two other studies[17,25], both of which did not clearly distinguish current from past use; strong evidence against the hypothesis is provided by data from the Cancer and Steroid Hormone study[18]. As noted, the present data provide little support for the hypothesis.

We conclude that there is reason for concern about an adverse effect of long-term oestrogen use on the risk of breast cancer, but that such an effect has not been established.

Future research

It is important to clarify whether very long-term use of non-contraceptive oestrogens increases the risk of breast cancer, because women are now taking oestrogens for increasingly longer durations with the hope of preventing osteoporosis and coronary heart disease. Previous studies have had limited statistical power to assess this question. As durations of use increase with the passage of time, future studies will have greater power to assess the effects of very long-term use of these drugs.

Combination oestrogen–progestin regimens are increasingly being used, because oestrogens taken with progestogens are thought to present less of a risk of endometrial cancer than unopposed oestrogens. Evidence on the effect of this regimen on breast cancer risk is sparse. Two studies suggest a possible protective effect[35,36], but two others suggest an increased risk[20,24]. More data on the effects of this regimen are needed, particularly as the durations of use increase.

Finally, it is possible that some types of oestrogen may increase the risk and that others may not. Once again based on sparse data, there is some evidence to suggest that oestrogens other than conjugated oestrogens may adversely influence risk[17,20,24]. Possible differences between oestrogens have not been adequately studied.

ACKNOWLEDGEMENTS

This work was supported by the Alcoholic Beverage Medical Research Foundation, Baltimore, MD; the US Food and Drug Administration (co-operative agreements U01 FD01222 and FD-U-000082); Hoffmann-LaRoche, Inc., Nutley, NJ; CIBA–GEIGY Corporation, Summit, NJ; Hoechst AG, Frankfurt, West Germany; McNeil Pharmaceutical, Spring House, PA; Merrell Dow Pharmaceuticals, Inc., Cincinnati, OH.

The authors are indebted to Dr E. Aileen Clarke, our collaborator in Toronto; to the attending physicians at Princess Margaret Hospital for their collaboration; to the interviewers who collected the data, Anne Allen, Rosemary Chepa, Suzanne Gale, Kathleen Gillespie, Lindsay Hall, Linda Harrel, Virginia Hunter, Beverly Linden, Muriel Relton, Shirley Rothery, Irene Servos, Ann Skene-Melvin, Linda West; to Verna Cundari and Phyllis Disenhouse for co-ordination of data collection; and to Leonard Gaetano and Marguerite Angeloni for data management.

REFERENCES

1. Rosenberg, L., Palmer, J.R., Miller, D.R., Clarke, E.A. and Shapiro, S. (1990). A case–control study of alcoholic beverage consumption and breast cancer. *Am. J. Epidemiol.*, **131**, 6–14
2. Henderson, B.E., Ross, R.K., Pike, M.C. and Casagrande, J.T. (1982). Endogenous hormones as a major factor in human cancer. *Cancer Res.*, **42**, 3232–9
3. Kelsey, J.L. and Berkowitz, G.S. (1988). Breast cancer epidemiology. *Cancer Res.*, **48**, 5615–23
4. International Agency for Research on Cancer. (1979). Sex hormones (II). *IARC Monograph on the evaluation of the carcinogenic risk of chemicals to humans*, **21**, 5–583
5. Kelsey, J.L., Fischer, D.B., Holford, T.R., LiVolsi, V.A., Mostow, E.D., Goldenberg, I.S. and White, C. (1981). Exogenous estrogens and other factors in the epidemiology of breast cancer. *J. Natl. Cancer Inst.*, **67**, 327–33
6. Kaufman, D.W., Miller, D.R., Rosenberg, L., Helmrich, M.S., Stolley, P., Schottenfeld, D. and Shapiro, S. (1984). Noncontraceptive estrogen use and the risk of breast cancer. *J. Am. Med. Assoc.*, **252**, 63–7

7. McDonald, J.A., Weiss, N.S., Daling, J.R., Francis, A.M. and Polissar, L. (1986). Menopausal estrogen use and the risk of breast cancer. *Breast Cancer Res. Treat.*, **7**, 193–9
8. Casagrande, J., Gerkins, V., Henderson, B.E., Mack, T. and Pike, M.C. (1976). Brief communication: Exogenous estrogens and breast cancer in women with natural menopause. *J. Natl. Cancer Inst.*, **56**, 839–41
9. Sartwell, P.E., Arthes, F.G. and Tonascia, J.A. (1977). Exogenous hormones, reproductive history, and breast cancer. *J. Natl. Cancer Inst.*, **59**, 1589–92
10. Hoover, R., Gray, L.A., Sr, Cole, P. and MacMahon, B. (1976). Menopausal estrogens and breast cancer. *N. Engl. J. Med.*, **295**, 401–5
11. Ross, R.K., Paganini-Hill, A., Gerkins, V.R., Mack, T.M., Pfeffer, R., Arthur, M. and Henderson, B.E. (1980). A case–control study of menopausal estrogen therapy and breast cancer. *J. Am. Med. Assoc.*, **243**, 1635–9
12. Hulka, B.S., Chambless, L.E., Deubner, D.C. and Wilkinson, W.E. (1982). Breast cancer and estrogen replacement therapy. *Am. J. Obstet. Gynecol.*, **143**, 638–44
13. Jick, H., Walker, A.M., Watkins, R.N., D'Ewart, D.C., Hunter, J.R., Danford, A., Madsen, S., Dinan, J. and Rothman, K.J. (1980). Replacement estrogens and breast cancer. *Am. J. Epidemiol.*, **112**, 586–94
14. Hoover, R., Glass, A., Finkle, W.D., Azevedo, D. and Milne, K. (1981). Conjugated estrogens and breast cancer risk in women. *J. Natl. Cancer Inst.*, **67**, 815–20
15. Hiatt, R.A., Bawol, R., Friedman, G.D. and Hoover, R. (1984). Exogenous estrogen and breast cancer after bilateral oophorectomy. *Cancer*, **54**, 139–44
16. Brinton, L.A., Hoover, R. and Fraumeni, J.R., Jr (1986). Menopausal oestrogens and breast cancer risk: an expanded case–control study. *Br. J. Cancer*, **54**, 825–32
17. Hunt, K., Vessey, M., McPherson, K. and Coleman, M. (1987). Long-term surveillance of mortality and cancer incidence in women receiving hormone replacement therapy. *Br. J. Obstet. Gynaecol.*, **94**, 620–35
18. Wingo, P.A., Layde, P.M., Lee, N.C., Rubin, G. and Ory, H.W. (1987). The risk of breast cancer in postmenopausal women who have used estrogen replacement therapy. *J. Am. Med. Assoc.*, **257**, 209–15
19. La Vecchia, C., Decarli, A., Parazzini, F., Gentile, A., Liberati, C. and Franceschi, S. (1986). Non-contraceptive oestrogens and the risk of breast cancer in women. *Int. J. Cancer*, **38**, 853–8
20. Bergkvist, L., Adami, H.-O., Persson, I., Hoover, R. and Schairer, C. (1989). The risk of breast cancer after estrogen and estrogen–progestin replacement. *N. Engl. J. Med.*, **321**, 293–7
21. Nomura, A.M.Y., Kolonel, L.N., Hirohata, T. and Lee, J. (1986). The association of replacement estrogens with breast cancer. *Int. J. Cancer*, **37**, 49–53
22. Colditz, G.A., Stampfer, M.J., Willett, W.C., Hennekens, C.H., Rosner, B. and Speizer, F.E. (1990). Prospective study of estrogen replacement therapy and risk of breast cancer in postmenopausal women. *J. Am. Med. Assoc.*, **264**, 2648–53
23. Kaufman, D., Palmer, J.R., Rosenberg, L., deMouzon, J., Stolley, P.D., Warshauer, E., Zauber, A.G. and Shapiro, S. (1991). Estrogen replacement therapy and the risk of breast cancer. *Am. J. Epidemiol.*, **13**, 86–95
24. Ewertz, M. (1988). Influence of non-contraceptive exogenous and endogenous sex hormones on breast cancer risk in Denmark. *Int. J. Cancer*, **42**, 832–8
25. Mills, P.K., Beeson, W.L., Phillips, R.L. and Fraser, G.E. (1989). Prospective study of exogenous hormone use and breast cancer in Seventh-day Adventists. *Cancer*, **64**, 591–7
26. Rohan, T.E. and McMichael, A.J. (1988). Non-contraceptive exogenous oestrogen therapy and breast cancer. *Med. J. Aust.*, **148**, 217–21
27. Ryan, E.D., Clark, A.F., Mobbs, B.G., Ooi, T.C., Sutherland, D.A. and Tustanoff, E.R. (1985). Inter-laboratory quality control of estrogen and progesterone receptor assays in breast cancer tissue using lyophilised cytosols. *Clin. Biochem.*, **18**, 20–6
28. Breslow, N.E., Day, N.E., Halvorsen, K.T., Prentice, R.L. and Sabai, C. (1978). Estimation of multiple relative risk functions in matched case–control studies. *Am. J. Epidemiol.*, **108**, 299–307
29. Goodman, M.T., Nomura, A.M.Y., Wilkens, L.R. and Kolonel, L.N. (1990). Agreement between interview information and physician records on history of menopausal estrogen use. *Am. J. Epidemiol.*, **131**, 815–25

30. Spengler, R.F., Clarke, E.A., Woolever, C.A., Newman, A.M. and Osborn, R.W. (1981). Exogenous estrogens and endometrial cancer: a case–control study and assessment of potential biases. *Am. J. Epidemiol.*, **114**, 497–506
31. Paganini-Hill, A. and Ross, R.K. (1982). Reliability of recall of drug usage and other health-related information. *Am. J. Epidemiol.*, **116**, 114–22
32. Persson, I., Bergkvist, L. and Adami, H.-O. (1987). Reliability of women's histories of climacteric oestrogen treatment assessed by prescription forms. *Int. J. Epidemiol.*, **16**, 222–8
33. McTiernan, A., Weiss, N.S. and Daling, J.R. (1986). Bias resulting from using the card-back system to contact patients in an epidemiologic study. *Am. J. Pub. Health*, **76**, 71–3
34. Marcus, A.C. and Crane, L.A. (1986). *The Validity and Value of Health Survey Research by Telephone*, pp. 49–55. (New York: The Commonwealth Fund)
35. Nachtigall, L.E., Nachtigall, R.H., Nachtigall, R.D. and Beckman, E.M. (1979). Estrogen replacement therapy. II. A prospective study in the relationship to carcinoma and cardiovascular and metabolic problems. *Obstet. Gynecol.*, **54**, 74–9
36. Gambrell, R.D., Jr, Maier, R.C. and Sanders, B.I. (1983). Decreased incidence of breast cancer in postmenopausal estrogen–progestogen users. *Obstet. Gynecol.*, **62**, 435–43

21

Hormone replacement therapy in the menopause: an analysis of benefits, risks and costs

E. Daly, M. Roche, D. Barlow, A. Gray, K. McPherson and M.P. Vessey

INTRODUCTION

The use of hormone replacement therapy by postmenopausal women has been recommended for many years for the relief of menopausal symptoms and the prevention of osteoporosis. More recently, there has been good evidence that hormone replacement therapy has a role in the prevention of coronary heart disease and possibly in the prevention of stroke. Weighing against these benefits is the possibility that the long-term use of hormone replacement therapy may increase a woman's risk of developing breast cancer. There is evidence that for non-hysterectomized users the increased risk of endometrial cancer associated with oestrogen therapy can be eliminated by the addition of a progestogen[1]. The opinion in North America, however, has been that the cardio-protective effect of oestrogen will be attenuated or reversed with the addition of progestogen[2], although in current British practice, the use of low doses of the androgenic progestogens[3] and certain newer non-androgenic progestogens, may avoid this effect[4].

For many women, drawbacks to combined therapy include withdrawal bleeding, and to a lesser extent progestogenic side-effects similar to premenstrual tension, which are likely to hinder compliance with therapy[5,6]. Attempts are now being made to develop preparations which do not induce uterine bleeding; this may be possible with the use of continuous combined preparations which successfully produce endometrial atrophy[7]. Also, it is possible that for many users of combined therapy, no adverse progestogen-associated symptoms will be experienced with certain forms of progestogen[8].

Unlike the United States, where hormone replacement therapy is used by many postmenopausal women, often for long periods of time, much lower

This article was previously published in the *British Medical Bulletin* (1992). **48**, 368–400 and is reprinted here with the kind permission of the publishers levels of use prevail in the UK, with very little long-term use[9,10]. A recent community survey of perimenopausal women in the UK revealed that while most respondents believed hormone replacement therapy could benefit hot flushes and osteoporosis, only about 10% felt it could reduce the risk of a stroke or myocardial infarction[11]. Given the role of hormone replacement therapy in preventing osteoporosis and perhaps cardiovascular disease, an assessment of its usefulness in the British context is timely. Decisions about treatment at the individual level must involve a careful weighing-up of all associated benefits and risks[12], while for a hard-pressed health service the economic repercussions of recommending hormone replacement therapy to postmenopausal women must be evaluated.

Two American studies have looked at the cost-effectiveness of hormone replacement therapy[13,14]. Weinstein and Schiff concluded that overall, oestrogen–progestogen therapy appeared to be cost-effective relative to oestrogen only therapy, except in women who considered the adverse effects of continued menstruation to offset the relief of menopausal symptoms[14]. However, this study included no asssumptions about the effect of hormone replacement therapy on cardiovascular disease. More recently, a British study published by members of our group found that, in terms of reduced mortality, the benefits of hormone replacement therapy outweigh the risks, especially for hysterectomized users[15]. The current analysis was undertaken to present a more complete assessment of the benefits, risks and costs of hormone replacement therapy by performing a cost-effectiveness analysis. However, as a consequence of the lack of published data on many aspects of hormone replacement therapy use, especially the long-term effects of combined therapy, it has been necessary to make assumptions about treatment effects. Such assumptions are derived from a review of the epidemiological literature and represent the authors' best estimates. In these situations we have taken a cautious view which may please neither the optimists nor the pessimists. However, for each assumption made, sensitivity analyses have been performed to evaluate its impact on the final results. In the face of conflicting evidence about the effects of hormone replacement therapy, this analysis attempts to highlight those factors which will have greatest influence on the final cost-effectiveness equation.

METHODS

Structure of the model

A cost-effectiveness framework in the form of a computer model was set up to study the impact of long-term hormone replacement therapy use in hypothetical cohorts compared with untreated control groups. Cost-effectiveness was defined as the ratio of the net increase in health care costs to the net effectiveness in terms of increased life expectancy and quality of life[16]. Three consequences of treatment were considered including mortality and morbidity induced or prevented by hormone replacement therapy, and health care costs associated with treatment.

For each of the diseases we wished to consider, age-specific mortality and morbidity rates (in 5-year age bands) were applied to a hypothetical control population. This enabled the numbers of deaths, hospital admissions and general practitioner consultations occurring each year from age 50 until the end of follow-up to be calculated. Corresponding numbers occurring in a hypothetical treatment cohort were calculated using mortality and morbidity rates to which appropriate relative risk estimates had been applied. For each disease of interest, age-specific hospital admission costs were applied to the annual difference in admissions between the two groups. Similarly, the cost of an average general practitioner consultation was applied to the annual difference in general practitioner consultations. Annual costs and savings thus calculated were appropriately discounted. Costs to the National Health Service of providing health care during the extended lifetime of women on hormone replacement therapy were estimated using age-specific annual health care costs per capita. Combining the above costs and savings with drug and monitoring costs enabled a treatment cost per user to be calculated. The cost per life year gained is given by dividing the discounted treatment cost per user by the discounted life years gained per user.

Treatment and monitoring options

Three main treatment strategies are considered throughout this analysis:

(1) Treating hysterectomized women with oestrogen only therapy;

(2) Treating non-hysterectomized women with oestrogen therapy with added progestogen; and

(3) Treating non-hysterectomized women with oestrogen replacement therapy.

The third strategy, although not currently recommended, may be suitable in certain cases where close supervision can be provided[17], and is considered here for comparative purposes. In our standard analysis, women are assumed to receive treatment for 10 years starting at age 50, and full compliance is assumed unless otherwise stated. For each treatment strategy considered, treatment and control groups are assumed to be identical with respect to uterine status.

For costing purposes it is assumed that oestrogen replacement therapy is taken in the form of 0.625 mg conjugated oestrogen daily (since most of the epidemiological evidence relates to the use of this preparation) and that combination hormone replacement therapy is taken as 0.625 mg conjugated oestrogen daily in combination with 0.075 mg levonorgestrel for 12 days each cycle. However, safer forms of progestogen which have less detrimental effects on serum lipid profiles are now available[4] – these are beginning to supersede the more androgenic progestogens in newer combined formulations.

It is assumed that current users see their general practitioner on two extra occasions each year for monitoring. In addition, because of the increased risk of endometrial cancer, non-hysterectomized women taking oestrogen replacement therapy are assumed to have an endometrial biopsy once every 2 years.

Health effects

Disease end-points considered in this analysis include (International Classification of Diseases (ICD9) 3-digit codes in brackets): endometrial cancer (179, 182), breast cancer (174), fractured neck of femur (820, 821), fractured wrist (814), fractured vertebrae (805), ischaemic heart disease (410–414) and cerebrovascular disease (430–438). In addition, the impact of treatment on a woman's risk of undergoing a hysterectomy (OPCS operation codes 690–694 or 696) or dilatation and curettage (Office of Population Censuses and Surveys (OPCS) codes 703, 704) is considered. Mortality and morbidity rates for all other causes are assumed to be identical in the treatment and control groups.

Data sources

For the untreated control group, current population mortality and morbidity rates are assumed to apply; this seems a reasonable assumption, given the very low levels of long-term use of hormone replacement therapy in this country[9,10]. Mortality rates used are taken from national mortality figures for 1988[18]. However, since national statistics are thought to underestimate the true mortality (and morbidity) associated with fractured neck of femur, we used an overall case–fatality rate of 25% applied to incidence rates for this disease. However, since this rate represents an overestimation for women under the age of 75 and an underestimation for older age-groups, we have performed some sensitivity analyses using different sets of published case–fatality rates.

For most of the diseases of interest, hospital admission rates, taken from the most recent Hospital Inpatient Enquiry[19], were regarded as a good proxy for morbidity. However, for the three types of fracture considered, different sources of data have been used. Incidence rates published by Boyce and Vessey[20] have been used as a measure of hip fracture morbidity, although average length of hospital stay data from the Hospital Inpatient Enquiry were used in our costing calculations for this disease. Fractured wrist incidence rates have been taken from a community survey by Donaldson and co-workers[21]. For the purpose of this study, management of wrist fractures is assumed to consist of initial treatment within an Accident and Emergency department followed by two outpatient visits. Since hospital admission data are unhelpful in estimating morbidity associated with vertebral fractures, incidence rates have been derived from the results of a survey by Melton and colleagues[22]. Based on informed clinical judgement regarding the outpatient and inpatient treatment of vertebral fractures, we have derived a cost per case for use in our analysis. General practice attendance rates for all the diseases of interest were obtained from the Third National General Practice Morbidity Survey[23].

Assumptions about disease risk

Our standard assumptions about disease risk following 10 years of treatment are summarized in Table 1 and are expressed in terms of relative risks.

Endometrial cancer

The evidence connecting oestrogen replacement therapy with an increased risk of endometrial cancer is compelling. A review of the topic[24] cited 20 case–control studies, all but one of which showed an increased risk. Most studies confirm that the risk appears to be related to duration of use, with roughly a 4–8-fold increase in risk after 5 years of use. Clinical research on the effect of progestogen on the endometrium shows that it reverses the action of unopposed oestrogen. In addition, a recent Swedish cohort study[1] supports the contention that the addition of a progestogen eliminates the increased risk of endometrial cancer.

For the purpose of this study, it is assumed that for women with uteri taking oestrogen replacement therapy, the relative risk of endometrial cancer increases sixfold following 5 years of treatment and returns to normal 5 years after treatment is discontinued. We have assumed that combination hormone replacement therapy users are at no increased risk of developing endometrial cancer. Although in our analysis we have assumed that the relative risk of dying from a disease approximates to the relative risk of incidence, this is probably incorrect in the case of endometrial cancer. Since this is a slow-growing disease with a good prognosis in the early stages, and since women on unopposed therapy are likely to be monitored closely, it is likely that oestrogen replacement therapy-associated endometrial cancers would have a lower case–fatality rate than that seen in the general population. Consequently, the results we present for non-hysterectomized oestrogen replacement therapy users probably underestimate the potential health benefits of this treatment strategy to a small extent.

Table 1 Standard assumptions about disease risk following treatment of 50-year-old women for 10 years with hormone replacement therapy. Standard assumptions about disease risk are expressed in terms of relative risks; ORT = oestrogen replacement therapy; CRT = combination hormone replacement therapy

		Age of women in cohort (years)				
		50–54	55–59	60–64	65–69	70+
Breast cancer	ORT/CRT	1	1	1.3	1.3	1
Endometrial cancer	ORT	2	6	2	1	1
Ischaemic heart disease	ORT	1	0.75	0.5	0.75	1
	CRT	1	0.88	0.75	0.88	1
Cerebrovascular disease	ORT	1	0.88	0.75	0.88	1
	CRT	1	0.94	0.88	0.94	1
Fracture	ORT/CRT	0.8	0.4	0.4	0.8	1
Hysterectomy/dilatation and curettage	ORT	2	2	1	1	1
	CRT	1.25	1.25	1	1	1

Breast cancer

The evidence on the effect of oestrogen replacement therapy on breast cancer risk remains inconclusive. While there is little evidence of an increase in risk with short-term use, there is accumulating evidence of a modest increase in risk with long-term use of 10 years or more. A review article by Henderson and co-workers[25] quotes eight case–control studies, all but one of which showed an increased risk of breast cancer with long-term oestrogen use (with relative risks ranging from 1.3–2.0). Such an effect is consistent with the known effect of a delayed natural menopause.

Since 1985 at least four cohort studies have been published on the effect of oestrogen replacement therapy on breast cancer risk[26–29], all of which showed a duration effect. More recently, updated results have been reported from two of these studies[26,27]. An updated analysis of the UK study conducted by Hunt and colleagues shows a temporal rise in breast cancer mortality (mortality ratio increased from 0.55 to 1.0) among hormone replacement therapy users, which is consistent with an adverse effect that has taken some time to manifest itself in a basically low-risk population[30]. This provides some evidence against the suggestion that oestrogen replacement therapy-induced cancers might have lower case–fatality rates[26,29,31] – the validity of this suggestion has indeed been questioned[32].

The Nurses' Health Study published in 1987[27] showed no evidence of any increased risk with up to 5 years of use of oestrogen replacement therapy, and no association was seen with current use. However, results from a longer follow-up of the same cohort[33] show a significant elevation of risk among current users (relative risk (RR), 1.36; 95% confidence interval (CI), 1.11–1.67), with a stronger relationship being observed with increasing age but not with increasing duration of use.

Two meta-analyses have been published recently on the effect of oestrogen replacement therapy on breast cancer risk[34,35], although these only considered studies published up to 1989. Dupont and Page[35] found no increased risk overall among those who had used low-dose conjugated oestrogens (< 0.625 mg), while women who took higher dose conjugated oestrogens had a relative risk of 2 or less. However, the variation in observed risks at this higher dosage was significant, indicating that other risk factors varied among these studies. Steinberg and co-workers[34] found a 30% increase in risk following 15 years of use (RR, 1.3, CI 1.2–1.6), the increase being largely due to studies that included premenopausal women or women using oestradiol (with or without progestogen). The corresponding relative risk for such studies was 2.2 (CI, 1.4–3.4). With regard to progestogen, speculations about its possible effects on breast cancer risk have been conflicting[36,37].

For the purpose of this analysis, it is assumed that 5 years of use of either oestrogen replacement therapy or combination hormone replacement therapy is associated with no increased risk of breast cancer. Risk is assumed to increase by 30% following 10 years of use (of either oestrogen replacement therapy or combination hormone replacement therapy) and 50% following 15 years of use, the risk remaining elevated after discontinuation of treatment for a period equal to the period of treatment.

Osteoporotic fractures of hip, wrist and spine

There is convincing evidence that oestrogen replacement therapy is effective in preventing the development of osteoporosis[38,39] and reducing the risk of associated fractures of the hip and wrist[40,41]. Weiss and colleagues[40] suggested a reduction of about 50–60% after 5 years use of oestrogen replacement therapy. A similar reduction in risk was reported recently by Swedish researchers[42], although this was found to be concentrated in women who received potent oestrogens before the age of 60. Furthermore, among this group of women, 41% of oestrogen use was opposed by a progestogen, a finding which corroborates clinical observations that combined regimens are effective in preserving bone mineral content[43]. What remains uncertain is the duration of effect after treatment is stopped.

In our analysis we have assumed a 20% reduction in fracture risk during the first 5 years of use of oestrogen replacement therapy or combination hormone replacement therapy, followed by a 60% reduction where treatment is continued. After discontinuation of treatment, this reduction in risk is assumed to persist for a period equal to the period of treatment.

Ischaemic heart disease

The mounting evidence for a protective effect of unopposed oestrogen on coronary heart disease is biologically plausible. It has been suggested that this protective effect is mediated partly through beneficial changes in high-density and low-density lipoprotein levels, and partly through other, non-lipid mechanisms[44]. A recent quantitative overview of the epidemiological literature yielded a relative risk of 0.56 (CI, 0.50–0.61) associated with oestrogen use[45]. This included 16 prospective studies, 15 of which showed decreased relative risks, in most instances statistically significant. One of the largest of these[46] showed a 50% reduction in the risk of both fatal and non-fatal heart disease in women who had ever used oestrogen replacement therapy. A recently published updated analysis of this study reports a 40% reduction in the risk of both major coronary disease and fatal cardiovascular disease for current oestrogen users[47]. A corresponding reduction of 20% is shown for former oestrogen users. However, evidence on the duration of effect after cessation of treatment is still inconclusive.

There is a noticeable lack of data on the effects of combination hormone replacement therapy in relation to coronary heart disease. Since progestogens have been shown to adversely affect serum lipid profiles, it has been suggested that the cardioprotective effect of oestrogen will be attenuated with concurrent use of progestogen. However, this may not be the case where low doses of the androgenic progestogens and certain newer non-androgenic progestogens are used in combined formulations[3,4].

In this study, we have assumed heart disease risk to decrease by 25% following 5 years use of oestrogen replacement therapy and 50% following 10 years of use, with risk remaining reduced after discontinuation of treatment for a period equal to the period of treatment. For combination hormone replacement therapy, we have assumed a halving of the cardioprotective effect. However, where appropriate, we have also presented results assuming full cardiovascular benefit with combination hormone replacement therapy.

Cerebrovascular disease

Studies looking at hormone replacement therapy and cerebrovascular disease have been scarce. Results from the British cohort study published in 1987 show a non-significant 30% reduction in the risk of death from stroke[26]. In the updated analysis of this study, the relative risk of death from cerebrovascular disease is estimated to be 0.54 (95% CI, 0.24–0.84)[30]. Another cohort study by Paganini-Hill and co-workers likewise shows a statistically significant 50% reduction in stroke mortality[48]. However, more recently, results published from the Nurses' Health Study suggest that current or former use of oestrogen is not associated with any change in the risk of stroke[47]. On the basis of this limited evidence, we have assumed a 25% reduction in the risk of stroke following the use of oestrogen replacement therapy and a 12% reduction following the use of combination hormone replacement therapy. Clearly, these assumptions are less well founded than those made for ischaemic heart disease; however, sensitivity analyses have been performed using a range of risk assumptions.

Hysterectomy and dilatation and curettage

Since any unexpected bleeding in a woman on hormone replacement therapy (oestrogen replacement or combination hormone replacement therapy) is likely to be thoroughly investigated, there are grounds for supposing there are increased gynaecological intervention rates among women undergoing treatment. One study by Ettinger and colleagues has demonstrated a marked increase in both hysterectomy and dilatation and curettage rates in oestrogen replacement therapy users[49]. We could find no studies in the literature looking at the effect of combination hormone replacement therapy on gynaecological intervention rates. In this analysis we have assumed a twofold increase in the risk of undergoing a hysterectomy or dilatation and curettage in oestrogen replacement therapy users and a 25% increase in women receiving combination hormone replacement therapy. The effect is assumed to last only during the period of treatment.

Health care costs

In the health sector, the cost-effectiveness of a particular intervention can be defined as the ratio of the net change in costs to the net change in health outcomes. In principle, cost-effectiveness analysis embraces all costs borne by society as a whole, including those borne by patients, their families, the private sector, and areas of government expenditure in addition to the health service. However, the availability of data and resources for research usually dictate that particular emphasis is placed on direct health care costs borne by the National Health Service, and this study follows this course.

It is the current convention to discount future costs and benefits to present values in order to ensure that comparisons are valid[16]. Discounting is used widely in economic analysis, and is based on the following reasoning: when given a choice between meeting a cost (or obtaining a benefit) now or some time in the future, individuals typically take the view that the further into the future a cost or benefit occurs, the less it matters to them. There are two basic reasons for this: first, people simply prefer the present to the future because they are impatient or view the future as holding risks and uncertainties; second, £1 now could be invested with the expectation that its future value will increase, say to £1.05 (allowing for any inflation) after 1 year. Therefore, £1 now is preferable to £1 in a year. To illustrate the actual net impact of treatment on mortality, regardless of when these effects occur, we have chosen to present undiscounted life years gained in this report. However, the cost per discounted life year gained results, presented alongside, encompass all health benefits and costs incurred, weighted for their occurrence in time. We have used the current UK Treasury-advised discount rate of 6% in our analysis, although we have performed sensitivity analyses using a range of alternative rates.

Costs used in the analysis

Direct costs to the National Health Service accounted for in this analysis include:

(1) An annual cost of £12 per woman treated with oestrogen replacement therapy (Premarin® 0.625 mg)[50] and £48 per woman treated with combination hormone replacement therapy (Prempak-C® 0.625 mg);

(2) The cost of two extra general practitioner consultations per year per user (costed at £6.70); and

(3) The cost of an outpatient endometrial biopsy once every 2 years for non-hysterectomized oestrogen replacement therapy users (costed as an outpatient visit at £36.89).

We estimated that at 1989/90 prices, the cost of an average general practitioner consultation was £16.86, and excluding any drugs prescribed, £6.70. The average cost per outpatient attendance in acute non-teaching hospitals given by the Department of Health is £36.89 (uprated to 1989/90 prices using the health specific inflation index[51]).

Indirect costs to the National Health Service incurred or averted as a result of treatment include the costs of treating side-effects and cost savings from reduced morbidity. Savings from wrist fractures prevented were estimated based on the assumption that management of such a fracture would include, on average, three outpatient attendances. For estimating savings associated with vertebral fractures, age-specific average costs per vertebral fracture case were calculated based on informed clinical judgement. In estimating hospital admission costs for each of the other diseases of interest, we have assumed that age–sex specific inpatient lengths of stay[19] multiplied by an average cost per inpatient day for acute non-teaching hospitals[52] of £135 (uprated to 1989/90 prices) will be sufficiently accurate.

However, we acknowledge the limitations of such an approach, given that costs incurred following discharge, such as those of long-term drug therapy and radiotherapy, are likely to contribute substantially to the overall cost per case. Also, the costs associated with an admission for acute myocardial infarction or unstable angina have risen over the last 10 years despite falling lengths of stay. Therefore, it is likely that we have underestimated the costs to the National Health Service associated with hormone replacement therapy-induced cancers, while on the other hand underestimating savings associated with a reduction in cardiovascular disease events.

If the net consequence of a health care intervention such as hormone replacement therapy is to extend a person's life expectancy, it is desirable in a cost-effectiveness study to take account of treating that person during their extra lifetime. One way of approaching this is to calculate the average annual age-specific per capita health care expenditure. The Department of Health programme budget gives age-specific annual per capita costs of providing all hospital and community health services. These costs range from £213 (age 45–64) to £1924 (age 85+) in 1989/90 terms. The Department of Health programme budget does not cover expenditure on the Family Health Service Authority (FHSA) services. However, since 70% of this expenditure is accounted for by general practitioner services, we have estimated age-specific per capita costs of providing FHSA services based on the age-distribution of expenditure on the general practitioner services. Using the General Household Survey data on average general practitioner consultations by different age/sex groups we have simply apportioned total FHSA expenditure to each age-group on the basis of the percentage of total annual general practitioner consultations attributable to that age-group. The resulting per capita expenditure on FHSA services ranges from £154 (age 45–64) to £191 (age 85+) in 1989/90 terms. Summing the age-specific costs per capita for all hospital and community health and FHSA services gives costs ranging from £367 (age 45–64) to £2115 (age 85+) in 1989/90 terms. Thus, if a 50-year-old person's life expectancy is increased by 1 year from 35 to 36 years as a result of treatment, we assume an additional National Health Service cost of £2115, discounted to present values.

Sensitivity analyses

Because of the uncertainty about many of the key assumptions used in this study, a large number of sensitivity analyses have been performed in an attempt to assess the impact of different assumptions on the final cost-effectiveness equation. Some of the variables considered include: the period of treatment, assumptions about disease risk, drug costs, monitoring arrangements and the discount rate used. Our standard assumptions provide a framework on which to perform sensitivity analyses. Unless otherwise stated, we have varied only one assumption at any one time (looking one by one at a range of possible values), while other assumptions remain as standard.

Quality of life adjustments

Life years gained is not an adequate measure of outcome if a health care programme makes an important impact on morbidity, or extends life expectancy at less than full health. The quality-adjusted life year is an attempt to address this problem. This approach involves attaching utilities or weights (between zero and one) to years of life in different health states. One of the methods used widely in the United States for the valuation of health states is the direct 'time trade-off' method which is based on an approach developed by Torrance and co-workers[53].

We have adopted an approach similar to that used by Weinstein (1980) in his study examining oestrogen use in postmenopausal women[13]. His quality adjustments were based on a time trade-off approach but made no use of survey data from patients or other groups, instead using his own judgements based on a reading of available literature. In this study, two different assumptions are made, based on informed clinical judgement, about the reduced quality of life experienced by women with menopausal symptoms. A preference value of 0.95 is assumed for severe symptoms, and a value of 0.99 for mild symptoms, the preference value for full health being 1. We are planning to undertake some fieldwork in the near future to obtain some empirical data on quality of life changes in the menopause. In addition, we intend to introduce into our analysis utility weights for each of the disease states of interest.

RESULTS

Standard assumptions about period of treatment and disease risk

Table 2 summarizes the estimated numbers of deaths induced or prevented (to age 69) per 1000 women treated for 10 years. Since with our standard assumptions, all relative risks of disease return to 1 at the age of 70 (see

Table 2 Deaths induced (+) and prevented (−) by cause (to age 69) per 1000 women treated with hormone replacement therapy for 10 years, using standard assumptions (see Table 1) about disease risk. ORT = oestrogen replacement therapy; CRT = combination hormone replacement therapy; n/a = not applicable

	Without uterus		*With uterus*		
	Control	*ORT*	*Control*	*ORT*	*CRT*
Endometrial cancer	n/a	n/a	2	+3	0
Breast cancer	18	+3	18	+3	+3
Fractured hip	4	−2	4	−2	−2
Ischaemic heart disease	39	−12	39	−12	−6
Cerebrovascular disease	14	−2	14	−2	−1
Other causes	99	+1	103	0	0
Total	175	−12	180	−9	−5
Average LYG per user*		0.25		0.19	0.11

*LYG: life years gained to extinction; 1 week = 0.02 year; 1 month = 0.08 year

Table 3 Hospital admissions induced (+) and prevented (−) by cause (to age 69) per 1000 women treated with hormone replacement therapy for 10 years, using standard assumptions (see Table 1) about disease risk. ORT = oestrogen replacement therapy; CRT = combination hormone replacement therapy; n/a = not applicable

	Without uterus		*With uterus*		
	Control	*ORT*	*Control*	*ORT*	*CRT*
Endometrial cancer	n/a	n/a	20	+33	0
Breast cancer	72	+11	72	+11	+11
Fractured hip	19	−7	19	−7	−7
Ischaemic heart disease	91	−26	91	−26	−12
Cerebrovascular disease	50	−7	49	−7	−4
Hysterectomy	n/a	n/a	54	+33	+9
Dilatation and curettage	n/a	n/a	136	+79	+21
Other causes	1671	+7	1634	+5	+4
Total	1903	−21	2075	+121	+22

Table 1), the difference in the number of deaths in the two groups (treated and untreated) peaks at age 69. However, when estimating the number of life years gained or lost as a result of treatment, we have followed the cohorts to extinction. All treatment strategies show an overall decrease in deaths, with a reduction of 7% among hysterectomized women, 5% among non-hysterectomized oestrogen replacement therapy users, and only 3% among women receiving combination hormone replacement therapy. Similarly, in terms of life years gained, greatest benefit is seen in the hysterectomized cohort treated with oestrogen replacement therapy, with an average of 0.25 life years gained per woman.

Hospital admissions (to age 69) induced or prevented per 1000 women treated for 10 years are detailed in Table 3. An overall reduction of 21 is seen per 1000 hysterectomized women treated with oestrogen replacement therapy, representing a reduction of about 1% on the baseline figure. For the other two treatment groups an overall increase is seen, accounted for by the extra admissions for endometrial cancer, hysterectomy and dilatation and curettage. Overall, the percentage increase in hospital admissions (to age 69) for non-hysterectomized women treated with oestrogen replacement therapy is 6%, but is only 1% with combination hormone replacement therapy. In all three groups, however, a total of 103 hip, wrist and vertebral fractures are preventable per 1000 women (to age 69), representing an overall reduction of 40% on the baseline figure of 259.

In Table 4, average discounted treatment costs per woman are shown for each of three different treatment strategies. For the combination hormone replacement therapy strategy, two treatment costs are shown, corresponding to assumptions about a full and reduced cardioprotective effect of oestrogen in combined regimens. An average treatment cost of £201 is seen for the hysterectomized oestrogen replacement therapy group, while a cost of £492 is estimated per combination hormone replacement therapy user when a full cardioprotective effect is assumed. For the latter, although greater savings are obtained in relation to cardiovascular disease (compared with the assumption of reduced benefit), the cost of keeping women alive during their

Table 4 Average cost/(saving) (£) to the health service per woman treated with hormone replacement therapy for 10 years, using standard assumptions (Table 1) about disease risk. ORT = oestrogen replacement therapy; CRT = combination hormone replacement therapy

	No uterus	*With uterus*		
	ORT	*ORT*	*CRT*	*CRT**
Drug	92	92	368	368
Monitoring	103	244	103	103
Endometrial cancer	—	23	—	—
Breast cancer	7	7	7	7
Fractured hip	(10)	(10)	(11)	(10)
Ischaemic heart disease	(15)	(16)	(8)	(15)
Cerebrovascular disease	(13)	(14)	(7)	(13)
Hysterectomy	—	43	10	10
Dilatation and curettage	—	20	5	5
Fractured wrist	(2)	(2)	(2)	(2)
Fractured vertebra	(4)	(4)	(4)	(4)
Net general practitioner cost/(saving)	(3)	0	(1)	(3)
Other items†	46	35	21	45
Total cost per user	201	420	482	492

*Assuming no change in the cardioprotective effect of oestrogen with combined replacement therapy; †additional health care costs incurred during added life expectancy

extended lifetime is higher (£45 compared with £21). The cost per discounted life year gained figures (Table 5) suggest that it is marginally more cost-effective to treat non-hysterectomized women with combination hormone replacement therapy than oestrogen replacement therapy if the addition of progestogen does not reverse the cardiovascular benefits of oestrogen.

Programme costs and the effect of reduced compliance

The annual steady-state programme costs of treating different populations of size 279 000 for 10 years, were estimated using our standard assumptions about disease risk (Table 6). Based on an estimated prevalence of hysterectomy of 18% amongst women aged 50–59, it is assumed in Scenario A that 18% of women receive oestrogen replacement therapy, the remainder receiving

Table 5 Average cost and life years gained per user and cost per life year gained for 10-year treatment period. ORT = oestrogen replacement therapy; CRT = combination hormone replacement therapy; LYG = life years gained; DLYG = discounted LYG; 1 week = 0.02 year; 1 month = 0.08 year

	No uterus	*With uterus*		
	ORT	*ORT*	*CRT*	*CRT**
Total cost per user (£)	201	420	482	492
Average LYG per user	0.25	0.19	0.11	0.24
Cost/DLYG (£)	2900	8300	14400	7000

*Assuming no change in the cardioprotective effect of oestrogen with combined replacement therapy

Table 6 Estimated annual steady-state programme costs (based on mid-year (1988) population of 50-year-old females in England and Wales) using different assumptions about compliance. Scenario A: 18% of women receive oestrogen replacement therapy, 82% receive combination hormone replacement therapy; Scenario B: as for A, but assuming no change in the cardioprotective effect of oestrogen with combination therapy; Scenario C: all women receive oestrogen replacement therapy. These scenarios are based on an estimated prevalence of hysterectomy of 18% amongst women aged 50–59; DLYG = discounted life years gained

	Treatment Scenario: cost (£ × 10^3)		
	A	*B*	*C*
Full compliance	121 000	123 000	106 000
Cost/DLYG	10.8	6.3	7.0
Reduced* compliance	66 000	67 000	59 000
Cost/DLYG	12.6	7.7	9.8

*Oestrogen replacement therapy: 100% compliance in first 5 years, falling to 50%; combination hormone replacement therapy: 67% compliance in first 5 years, falling to 33%

combination hormone replacement therapy. The same assumptions are made in Scenario B except that full beneficial effect on cardiovascular disease is assumed with combination hormone replacement therapy. In Scenario C, it is assumed that all women receive oestrogen replacement therapy. Programme costs associated with the latter strategy are lowest, reflecting the lower drug costs involved. In terms of cost-effectiveness, Scenarios B and C give comparable results, when full compliance with treatment is assumed. However, with reduced compliance, if a full cardioprotective effect is assumed with combination hormone replacement therapy, it appears to be more cost-effective to treat the non-hysterectomized subgroup with combination hormone replacement therapy (Scenario B) than with oestrogen replacement therapy (Scenario C). One explanation for this is that with shorter periods of use (resulting from lower compliance) of oestrogen replacement therapy by non-hysterectomized women, deaths from endometrial cancer are occurring in the early stages while the cardiovascular benefits are not so great. However, this is entirely dependent on the assumptions we have used about disease risk in this analysis.

Effect of different assumptions about period of treatment

The results for 5-, 10- and 15-year treatment periods are summarized in Table 7. Five years of treatment has relatively little impact on mortality in any of the treatment groups, whereas 15 years of treatment leads to a benefit in terms of life years gained exceeding that seen for 10 years of treatment. A reduction of approximately 30% is seen in the cost per life year gained when the period of treatment is increased from 10 to 15 years, suggesting that it is more cost-effective to treat women for longer periods of time.

Table 7 Average life years gained (LYG) per user and cost per discounted LYG for different treatment periods. ORT = oestrogen replacement therapy; CRT = combination hormone replacement therapy; 1 week = 0.02 year; 1 month = 0.08 year

Treatment period (years)	*No uterus*		*With uterus*		*With uterus*	
	ORT		*ORT*		*CRT*	
	LYG	£	*LYG*	£	*LYG*	£
5	0.04	7200	0.00	—	0.03	31 400
10	0.25	2900	0.19	8300	0.11	14 400
15	0.57	2100	0.45	5900	0.25	10 400

Effect of different assumptions about disease risk

The effects of varying assumptions about the risk of developing each of the diseases of interest are summarized in Tables 8–16.

Endometrial cancer

Table 8 details the results obtained when assumptions about endometrial cancer risk among non-hysterectomized oestrogen replacement therapy users are varied. The two factors considered include the magnitude of the increased risk, and the duration of effect after treatment is stopped. For the worst assumption made (EC2) there is a substantial reduction in life years gained per woman treated and a corresponding increase in cost per life year gained, compared with standard results (EC1).

Breast cancer

The effect of varying assumptions about breast cancer risk following treatment is shown in Tables 9 and 10. We have performed a large number of sensitivity analyses, varying both the magnitude of increased risk and the duration of effect, but have shown only a selection of results here. A twofold increase in breast cancer risk prevailing for 10 years (BC1) would substantially reduce the net life years gained per user, and for the combination hormone replacement therapy cohort, excess mortality from breast cancer would wipe

Table 8 Average life years gained (LYG) per user and cost per discounted life year gained following 10 years use of oestrogen replacement therapy by non-hysterectomized women, for a range of assumptions about endometrial cancer risk. Standard risk assumptions are used for other diseases of interest; figures given are relative risks; 1 week = 0.02 year; 1 month = 0.08 year

	Age group						
	50–54	55–59	60–64	65–69	70+	*LYG*	£
EC1*	2	6	2	1	1	0.19	8300
EC2	2	6	6	6	1	0.09	17 600
EC3	1.5	1.8	1.5	1	1	0.23	6300
EC4	1.5	1.8	1.8	1.8	1	0.22	6600

*EC1 = standard assumption about endometrial cancer risk

Table 9 Assumptions about relative risk of breast cancer (BC)

	Age-group				
	50–54	55–59	60–64	65–69	70+
BC1	1	1	2	2	1
BC2	1	1	2	2	2
BC3*	1	1	1.3	1.3	1
BC4	1	1	1.3	1.3	1.3
BC5	1	1	1	1	1

*BC3 = standard assumption about endometrial cancer risk

Table 10 Average life years gained (LYG) per user and cost per discounted life year gained, following 10 years use of hormone replacement therapy for a range of assumptions about breast cancer (BC) risk. ORT = oestrogen replacement therapy; CRT = combination hormone replacement therapy; figures in brackets represent life years lost. Standard risk assumptions are used for other diseases of interest. 1 week = 0.02 year; 1 month = 0.08 year

	ORT no uterus		*ORT with uterus*		*CRT with uterus*	
	LYG	£	*LYG*	£	*LYG*	£
BC1	0.12	5100	0.06	23 700	(0.01)	—
BC2	(0.08)	21 000	(0.13)	—	(0.20)	—
BC3*	0.25	2900	0.19	8300	0.11	14 400
BC4	0.19	3200	0.13	9900	0.06	19 100
BC5	0.30	2400	0.24	6500	0.17	10 200

*BC3 = standard assumption about breast cancer risk

out all benefits in relation to cardiovascular disease and hip fracture mortality. If this relative risk of 2 is assumed to last indefinitely (BC2), then for all three treatment strategies considered, a net loss of life years (undiscounted) per woman treated is predicted. However, when health benefits are discounted, a net life years gained figure is predicted for the hysterectomized cohort, with a corresponding cost per discounted life year gained of £21 000.

Similarly, assumptions BC3 and BC4 compare the effects of a 30% increase in breast cancer risk prevailing for a period of 10 years or indefinitely. For the combination hormone replacement therapy cohort, comparing results from BC3 and BC4 reveals a 50% reduction in net life years gained; for the other two treatment groups less variation is seen in the estimated life years gained and cost per discounted life year gained figures. For the hysterectomized woman, assuming no increased risk of breast cancer (BC5) reduces the cost per discounted life year gained by about 25%. In addition, the effect of an increased relative risk of 4.4 for combination hormone replacement therapy users (based on results published by Bergkvist and colleagues[29]), was considered. Assuming this increased risk prevails for a period of 10 years (immediately following cessation of treatment), a loss of life equivalent to about 5 months per woman (0.44 years) treated for 10 years is predicted by our model.

Fractures

Three sets of assumptions were made about the impact of hormone replacement therapy on the risk of developing osteoporotic fractures (Table 11). The factor varied was the duration of benefit following treatment. Per 1000 women treated for 10 years, a lasting reduction in fracture risk might prevent as many as 95 hip fractures, 80 Colles' fractures and 262 vertebral fractures. This represents a reduction of just over 40% on the baseline number of fractures. The relatively small difference in results obtained using assumptions F1 and F2 reflects the unimportant role of fractured neck of femur as a cause of morbidity among women under the age of 70. Similarly, in terms of life years gained, assuming a reduced risk of fracture until death has most impact on results (Table 12).

The effects of using different case-fatality rates for fractured neck of femur are detailed in Table 13. Shown are numbers of hip-fracture deaths prevented per 1000 users for different assumptions about fracture risk. It is only with assumption F3 (permanent benefit on fracture risk) that differences between the different case-fatality rates become marked. Even using a case-fatality rate of 25%, which is an overestimation for the younger age-groups in question, the number of preventable deaths (to age 69) per 1000 women

Table 11 Fractures prevented per 1000 women treated for 10 years for a range of assumptions about fracture risk. Standard risk assumptions are used for other diseases of interest; F2 = standard assumption about fracture risk; numbers given are fractures prevented to age when relative risk returns to baseline; baseline numbers of fractures are shown in brackets

	Age-group					
	50–54	55–59	60–64	65–69	70–74	75+
F1	0.8	0.4	1	1	1	1
F2	0.8	0.4	0.4	0.8	1	1
F3	0.8	0.4	0.4	0.4	0.4	0.4
	Hip		*Wrist*		*Vertebra*	
F1	3	(5)	14	(29)	26	(61)
F2	7	(19)	30	(72)	66	(168)
F3	95	(164)	80	(141)	262	(462)

Table 12 Average life years gained (LYG) per user and cost per discounted LYG, following 10 years use for a range of assumptions about fracture risk. ORT = oestrogen replacement therapy; CRT = combination hormone replacement therapy

	ORT no uterus		*ORT with uterus*		*CRT with uterus*	
	LYG	£	*LYG*	£	*LYG*	£
F1	0.23	3200	0.17	9400	0.09	17 300
F2*	0.25	2900	0.19	8300	0.11	14 400
F3	0.42	1800	0.36	5300	0.28	8000

*Standard risk assumptions are used for other diseases of interest; F2 = standard assumption about fracture risk; 1 week = 0.02 year; 1 month = 0.08 year

Table 13 Hip fracture deaths prevented per 1000 women treated for 10 years, using different case-fatality rates with varying assumptions about fracture risk. Numbers given are hip fracture deaths prevented up to age when relative risk returns to baseline; baseline numbers of hip fracture deaths are shown in brackets; case-fatality rate of 25% = standard assumption

Case-fatality rate	*F1*	*F2**	*F3*
25% overall	1 (1)	2 (4)	24 (41)
Boyce[54]	0 (0)	0 (1)	23 (40)
Evans *et al.*[55]	0 (0)	1 (2)	41 (72)

*Standard risk assumptions are used for other diseases of interest; F2 = standard assumption about fracture risk

Table 14 Assumptions about relative risk of ischaemic heart disease (IHD) and cerebrovascular disease (CVD). ORT = oestrogen replacement therapy; CRT = combination hormone replacement therapy

		Age-group				
		50–54	55–59	60–64	65–69	70+
	IHD1	0.75	0.5	1	1	1
Standard, ORT	IHD2	1	0.75	0.5	0.75	1
	IHD3	1	0.75	0.5	0.5	0.5
Standard, CRT	IHD4	1	0.88	0.75	0.88	1
	IHD5	1	1	1	1	1
	CVD1	0.75	0.5	1	1	1
	CVD2	1	0.75	0.5	0.75	1
	CVD3	1	0.75	0.5	0.5	0.5
Standard, ORT	CVD4	1	0.88	0.75	0.88	1
Standard, CRT	CVD5	1	0.94	0.88	0.94	1
	CVD6	1	1	1	1	1

treated for 10 years using assumption F2 is less than 2, reflecting the small impact of treatment on mortality in this age-group.

Ischaemic heart disease and cerebrovascular disease

Tables 14 and 15 show the effect of varying assumptions about cardiovascular disease risk. Note that assumptions about ischaemic heart disease and cerebrovascular disease are varied independently of each other. For the two groups on oestrogen replacement therapy, several possibilities are considered, including a beneficial effect confined to the period of treatment, a beneficial effect lasting after treatment is stopped for as long as treatment was given, a permanent beneficial effect and no effect. We deemed it relevant to consider the same possibilities for the combination hormone replacement therapy cohort, in the light of recent evidence on newer progestogens which do not appear to reverse the beneficial effects of oestrogen on serum lipid profiles[4].

It appears that altering assumptions about the duration of effect has a marked impact on life years gained for all treatment groups, although this effect is less marked for cerebrovascular disease than for ischaemic heart

Table 15 Average life years gained (LYG) per user and cost per discounted LYG, following 10 years use of hormone replacement therapy for a range of assumptions about ischaemic heart disease (IHD) risk and cerebrovascular disease (CVD) risk. ORT = oestrogen replacement therapy; CRT = combination hormone replacement therapy; standard risk assumptions are used for other diseases of interest; assumptions about IHD risk and CVD risk are varied independently of each other

	ORT no uterus		*ORT with uterus*		*CRT with uterus*	
	LYG	£	*LYG*	£	*LYG*	£
Ischaemic heart disease						
IHD1	0.10	4700	0.05	22 100	0.08	14 900
IHD2	0.25	2900	0.19	8300	0.22	7700
IHD3	1.17	1800	1.10	3100	1.14	3300
IHD4	—	—	—	—	0.11	14 400
IHD5	0.02	20 800	(0.03)	—	0.00	—
Cerebrovascular disease						
CVD1	0.24	2900	0.18	8300	0.13	12 100
CVD2	0.29	2400	0.23	6700	0.17	9400
CVD3	0.85	800	0.78	2600	0.72	3300
CVD4	0.25	2900	0.19	8300	0.13	12 300
CVD5	0.23	3200	0.17	9400	0.11	14 400
CVD6	0.21	3600	0.15	10 800	0.09	17 400

disease (Table 15). Varying assumptions about ischaemic heart disease risk yields a range from 0.02 to 1.17 life years gained per hysterectomized oestrogen replacement therapy user. Note that using assumption IHD3 for the combination hormone replacement therapy cohort gives a saving comparable to that obtained for the hysterectomized cohort (1.14 compared with 1.17 life years gained), the difference being entirely due to the standard assumptions used about cerebrovascular disease risk in the two groups (since all other disease risk assumptions are the same). However, the corresponding costs per discounted life year gained still differ quite considerably, reflecting the higher treatment costs associated with combined therapy. Similarly, when the risk of cerebrovascular disease is varied, any difference between life years gained figures for the hysterectomized and combination hormone replacement therapy cohorts reflects our standard assumptions about ischaemic heart disease.

Assuming no beneficial effect on ischaemic heart disease risk with combination hormone replacement therapy predicts no saving of life whereas when no beneficial effect on cerebrovascular disease risk is assumed some saving of life, albeit modest, is still predicted (0.09 life years gained), at a cost of £17 400 per discounted life year gained. This illustrates the greater importance of a reduction in ischaemic heart disease risk in terms of reducing mortality.

With regard to treatment costs per woman, an increase is seen when the beneficial effect on heart disease risk is assumed to increase – for the hysterectomized cohort, treatment costs obtained from using IHD5 (no benefit), IHD1, IHD2 and IHD3 (lasting benefit) are £170, £175, £201 and

£360, respectively. The likely explanation for this effect is the increasing cost associated with the provision of health care as the life expectancy of the treated cohort increases. Compared with ischaemic heart disease risk, assuming a lasting 50% reduction in the risk of stroke appears to have relatively more impact on cost per discounted life year gained figures than on life years gained alone, especially for the hysterectomized cohort. This is reflected in the corresponding changes seen in the average treatment costs per woman. For example, for the hysterectomized cohort, treatment costs obtained from using assumptions CVD6 (no beneficial effect), CVD1, CVD2 and CVD3 (lasting beneficial effect) are £211, £207, £191 and £129, respectively, which is not surprising given the gradient of benefit. Here, the increasing savings associated with a reduced rate of hospital admission for stroke outweigh any increase in the cost of health care provision as life expectancy increases.

Hysterectomy and dilatation and curettage

Table 16 illustrates the effect of using different assumptions about the risk of undergoing a hysterectomy or dilatation and curettage. Note that assumptions about hysterectomy and dilatation and curettage are varied independently of each other. For each assumption made, cost per discounted life year gained figures are shown along with expected numbers of excess hysterectomies or dilatations and curettages per 1000 users. Varying assumptions about hysterectomy yield average treatment costs ranging from £378 (relative risk of 1) to £573 (relative risk of 6) per woman treated with oestrogen replacement therapy. A smaller range of risk assumptions was

Table 16 Numbers of excess hysterectomies and dilatations and curettages induced per 1000 women treated for 10 years, for a range of risk assumptions, and corresponding cost per discounted life year gained. ORT = oestrogen replacement therapy; CRT = combination hormone replacement therapy; RR = relative risk. RR remains elevated during treatment period only and returns to baseline at age 60. Numbers shown are excess hysterectomies or dilatations and curettages to age 59; baseline numbers occurring in control group are shown in brackets; assumptions about hysterectomy and dilatation and curettage are varied independently of each other.

	Hysterectomy		*Dilatation and curettage*	
	Rate	£	*Rate*	£
ORT, with uterus				
RR = 1	0 (36)	7600	0 (85)	7900
RR = 2*	34 (36)	8300	81 (85)	8300
RR = 6	161 (36)	10 500	412 (85)	10 000
CRT, with uterus				
RR = 1	0 (36)	14 100	0 (85)	14 200
RR = 1.25*	9 (36)	14 400	21 (85)	14 400
RR = 2	34 (36)	15 300	84 (85)	14 900

*Standard risk assumptions are used for other diseases of interest

used for combination hormone replacement therapy which yielded average treatment costs between £472 (relative risk of 1) and £511 (relative risk of 2).

Using standard assumptions for hysterectomy while varying those for dilatation and curettage shows a substantial increase in the number of surgical procedures performed per 1000 women. However, less variation is seen in the cost per discounted life year gained than seen with hysterectomy, reflecting the lower costs associated with a hospital admission for dilatation and curettage. Assuming a relative risk of 6 of undergoing a dilatation and curettage, our results suggest that among 1000 women treated for 10 years with oestrogen replacement therapy, an extra 412 dilatations and curettages would be performed.

Effect of different assumptions about drug costs, monitoring and discount rates

Varying the drug costs used in our analysis has a large impact on both average treatment cost and cost per discounted life year gained. An assumed increase of 50% in the annual cost of combination hormone replacement therapy (from £48 to £72) would increase cost per discounted life year gained from £14 000 to £19 900, whereas a decrease of 50% (to £24) would yield a cost per discounted life year gained of £8900. Similarly, for the hysterectomized cohort on oestrogen replacement therapy, cost per discounted life year gained would increase from £2900 to £3500 for a 50% increase in drug costs (from £12 to £18), and would fall to £2200 for a 50% reduction. The annual cost of Premarin®, as given in the British National Formulary[50] ranges from £12 (0.625 mg dose) to £26 (2.5 mg dose). Using an annual drug cost of £26 for oestrogen replacement therapy yields total drug and treatment costs of £200 and £309, respectively. Note that in the latter, drug costs alone account for two-thirds of the average cost per woman treated.

Altering assumptions about the monitoring arrangements for the non-hysterectomized oestrogen replacement therapy group also has a large impact on cost per discounted life year gained. If an endometrial biopsy is performed annually, rather than every second year, the cost per discounted life year gained increases from £8300 to £11 100. In practice, the minimum recommended frequency of endometrial monitoring is every 2 years[17], although the more cautious recommend that biopsies be performed annually or whenever bleeding occurs[56].

Altering the discount rate applied to both life years gained figures and costs shows substantial variation in the cost per discounted life year gained figures. For the combination hormone replacement therapy cohort, cost per discounted life year gained figures of £10 900 and £18 700 were obtained when discount rates of 4 and 8%, respectively, were used. These figures represent a change of about 25% in the cost per discounted life year gained obtained from using a discount rate of 6%. For the non-hysterectomized oestrogen replacement therapy group, the corresponding costs per discounted life year gained were £6100 and £11 200.

Table 17 Average life years gained (LYG) per user, quality-adjusted for different assumptions about menopausal symptom relief (QALY), and cost per discounted quality adjusted life year (DQALY) (£) following 10 years of use, with standard assumptions about disease risk. ORT = oestrogen replacement therapy; CRT = combination hormone replacement therapy; Q1: severe symptoms (utility = 0.95) for 5 years; Q2: mild symptoms (utility = 0.99) for 5 years

	ORT no uterus		*ORT with uterus*		*CRT with uterus*	
	QALY	*Cost/DQALY* (£)	*QALY*	*Cost/DQALY* (£)	*QALY*	*Cost/DQALY* (£)
Q1	0.50	700	0.44	1500	0.36	1900
Q2	0.30	1700	0.24	4400	0.16	6200
Unadjusted LYG and cost per discounted LYG						
	0.25	2900	0.19	8300	0.11	14400

Measuring quality of life benefits derived from symptom relief following treatment

In Table 17 life years gained figures are shown adjusted for menopausal symptom relief yielding quality-adjusted life years. Unadjusted life years gained and cost per discounted life year gained are shown also for comparison. It is noticeable that even for a fairly modest assumption about symptom relief following hormone replacement therapy (Q2), the cost per discounted quality-adjusted life year for each of the three treatment strategies is substantially reduced, compared with the unadjusted figures. For women with severe menopausal symptoms, the figures look even more encouraging, with costs per discounted quality-adjusted life year ranging from £700 for hysterectomized women, to £1900 for women on combination hormone replacement therapy.

DISCUSSION

The results presented above consistently underline the substantial benefits of oestrogen replacement therapy for hysterectomized users, particularly in relation to a reduction in cardiovascular disease. For non-hysterectomized women, the gynaecological consequences of long-term treatment must be considered. Although progestogen supplements will eliminate the increased risk of endometrial cancer, it is not clear whether the full cardioprotective effect of oestrogen will be maintained. In addition, studies on compliance with treatment have shown that it is the progestogen element that causes most problems[6]. However, with good management and tailoring of treatment to suit the individual woman, satisfactory levels of compliance should be attainable[57–59].

Given that, by the age of 50, up to 20% of the female population of England will have had a hysterectomy[60], a strategy aimed at this group alone would have major public health implications. On the basis of our results, offering treatment to both hysterectomized women and to those with severe menopausal symptoms might be a relatively cost-effective way of treating a substantial proportion of perimenopausal women. It has been reported that at least 82% of menopausal women experience acute oestrogen deficiency-related symptoms for more than 1 year[61], and that in 25% of women these symptoms last for more than 5 years. Of those women who experience symptoms, 51% suffer severely[62].

What is clear from our results is the life-saving potential of a reduction in cardiovascular disease risk following treatment. Our model predicts an increase in life expectancy of almost 2 years when a lasting 50% reduction in risk is assumed. For the hysterectomized cohort, assuming a permanently reduced relative risk of 0.5 for both ischaemic heart disease and cerebrovascular disease yields a life years gained figure of 1.9 years (cost per discounted life year gained is £1000). The corresponding results for the combination hormone replacement therapy cohort are 1.9 life years gained per user at a cost of £2000 per discounted life year gained. Assuming, additionally, permanent benefit with respect to fracture risk increases this figure marginally to 2.1 years. Hillner and colleagues, in their analysis of the benefits and risks of oestrogen use, also showed an overwhelming impact of oestrogen on cardiovascular mortality which overshadowed all other effects[63]. If a 50% reduction in ischaemic heart disease risk but only a 25% reduction in cerebrovascular disease risk is assumed to persist indefinitely following treatment, our model predicts an average saving of 1.5 years per hysterectomized woman, at a cost of £1300 per discounted life year gained.

The small increase in breast cancer risk which may be associated with long-term use is unlikely to overwhelm the benefits of treatment. Our results show that the excess mortality associated with a 30% increase in breast cancer risk would be more than offset by reduced mortality from cardiovascular disease, even when this increased risk is assumed to last indefinitely. Nevertheless, this potential side-effect of treatment may heavily influence the overall balance of benefits and risks as perceived by women. It is important for individual women and their doctors to have conclusive evidence relating to hormone replacement therapy and its effect on breast cancer risk.

Recent studies have consistently shown lower mortality from cardiovascular disease among hormone replacement therapy users[30,47,64,65]. Sullivan and co-workers concluded that oestrogen replacement therapy after the menopause prolongs survival when coronary artery disease is present, but that it has less effect in the absence of coronary artery disease[65]. Indeed, in the United States, the recommendations for treatment now appear to be shifting to women at high risk of heart disease[44,66]. A recent study by Persson and colleagues[67] showed a slightly increased survival among women over 60 receiving oestrogen replacement therapy, 10% of which was opposed with progestogen. However, in women under 60, 45% of whom received combined therapy, survival seemed to be unaffected, which, suggest the authors, might be partly due to a reduced cardioprotective effect with combined regimens.

The most important unanswered question today is whether combined treatment will have less cardioprotective effect than that seen with unopposed oestrogen treatment. In presenting our results, we have chosen to assume a halving of the cardioprotective effect of oestrogen when progestogen is added, although what must be borne in mind is that this may be a pessimistic view. In the general analysis, assuming full cardiovascular benefit with the use of combination hormone replacement therapy will give a reduction in mortality almost identical to that obtained for the hysterectomized cohort treated with oestrogen replacement therapy. With this assumption, a life years gained figure of 0.24 is obtained per woman treated for 10 years with combination hormone replacement therapy, while the corresponding figure per hysterectomized oestrogen replacement therapy user is 0.25 life years gained (see Table 5). Therefore, our standard assumptions serve to illustrate the net reduction in life years gained which would be expected if progestogen halved the cardioprotective effect of oestrogen. It can be seen from Table 5 that cost per discounted life year gained still differs quite substantially for these two treatment scenarios, estimated at £7000 and £2900, respectively.

In the United States, the issue of whether women with an intact uterus might be given oestrogen replacement therapy has been raised, since the data suggest that this would prevent a much greater volume of cardiovascular morbidity and mortality than the endometrial cancer it might cause. This is a difficult clinical issue weighing an act of commission (causing endometrial cancer) against an act of omission (failing to prevent cardiovascular disease). It has been noticeable in the results of this study that long-term treatment of women with a uterus with oestrogen replacement therapy compares favourably with a combination hormone replacement therapy strategy (see Table 2), if one assumes only half the cardioprotective effect with combination therapy. However, increased rates of hospitalization for hysterectomy and dilatation and curettage in this group could have a substantial impact on morbidity (Table 3), and such surgical procedures carry their own inherent risks[68]. If the full cardioprotective effect of oestrogen can be maintained after the addition of a progestogen, then treating non-hysterectomized women with combination hormone replacement therapy would appear to be slightly more cost-effective than using oestrogen replacement therapy (Table 5). This results from the different life years gained figures estimated for these two groups (0.24 compared with 0.19 per user), which reflect the assumptions made about endometrial cancer. Similar conclusions were reached by Weinstein and Schiff[14], although no consideration was given to the effects of treatment on cardiovascular disease. However, we may have underestimated the beneficial effects on mortality associated with treating non-hysterectomized women with oestrogen only therapy since we have assumed that oestrogen replacement therapy-associated endometrial cancers have the same case-fatality rate as that seen in the general population. This may be a pessimistic view, given that women with a uterus treated with oestrogen replacement therapy are likely to be under close gynaecological surveillance.

In Britain, prescribing unopposed oestrogen for women with an intact uterus is only recommended for the small number of women who cannot tolerate progestogens. It may be that in the future, women on hormone replacement therapy who suffer from intolerable bleeding and progestogenic side-effects might be advised to undergo a prophylactic hysterectomy[17]. However, this would require a careful weighing up of the long-term benefits of oestrogen replacement therapy and the inherent risks associated with surgery.

From our results, it appears to be less cost-effective to treat women for short periods of time because the benefits derived in terms of life years gained and averted costs are not so great (see Table 7). A reduction of approximately 30% is seen in the cost per discounted life year gained when the period of treatment is increased from 10 to 15 years. The argument for long-term therapy of up to 20 years has already been made for those women in whom treatment is clearly beneficial and devoid of side-effects[69]. If the full benefits of hormone replacement therapy are to be reaped, we should perhaps be encouraging women (especially those at high risk of heart disease) to undergo long-term prophylactic treatment. The treatment period currently recommended in this country is 5–6 years as this is thought to be the minimum period for achieving bone protection[57]. However, our results suggest that a reduction in fracture risk following long-term hormone replacement therapy, even if permanent, would not have a substantial impact on mortality. It is possible that targeting women at high risk of osteoporosis would be more cost-effective than a universal treatment strategy; however, the specificity and sensitivity of screening procedures for osteoporosis have not been firmly established[70–73].

A comparison of our results with costs per quality-adjusted life year for other health care interventions (Table 18) gives an indication of the relative cost-effectiveness of hormone replacement therapy. On the basis of cost per quality-adjusted life year, it appears that the cost-effectiveness of treating hysterectomized women with severe menopausal symptoms is comparable to that of a general practitioner giving advice to stop smoking, and offers very good value for money. Long-term (15 years) prophylactic treatment of hysterectomized women, on the basis of our assumptions, also compares favourably with currently accepted health interventions, including screening for breast cancer. The annual cost of the breast screening programme in the United Kingdom (estimated at £25 million with a capital cost of £44 million[76]), falls well below our estimated costs for the universal treatment of

Table 18 Cost per quality-adjusted life year of different health interventions

Health intervention	*Cost* (£)*
Advice by general practitioner to stop smoking[74]	300
10 years oestrogen replacement therapy for hysterectomized women with severe menopausal symptoms	700
Coronary artery bypass grafting for severe angina with left main disease[75]	1500
10 years oestrogen replacement therapy for hysterectomized women with mild menopausal symptoms	1700
Prophylactic treatment of hysterectomized women (no menopausal symptoms) for 15 years with oestrogen replacement therapy	2100
Action by general practitioners to control hypertension[74]	2400
Coronary artery bypass grafting for moderate angina with three-vessel disease[75]	3500
Breast cancer screening programme[76]	4700
10 years' combination hormone replacement therapy for women with mild menopausal symptoms	6200
Heart transplantation[75]	7200

*Updated to 1989–90 prices using National Health Service price index (Social Services Committee memorandum)

50–59-year-olds in England and Wales with hormone replacement therapy. However, in terms of cost per life year gained, two of the programme strategies we considered (see Table 6) yielded results comparable to those for the breast screening programme. Indeed, our results would compare more favourably if we excluded the costs of providing health care during the extended lifetime of treated women, costs which were not included in the breast screening programme costs. The programme costs for Scenarios A, B and C (Table 6), when one excludes the costs of health care provision during the extended lifetime of those treated, fall to £113, £110 and £96 million respectively (assuming full compliance), with corresponding costs per discounted life year gained of £10 100, £5600 and £6400.

Results published recently from a study similar to ours indicate that possible net financial savings to the health service could be made[77]. On the contrary, our results suggest that treatment of women with hormone replacement therapy, even in the face of substantial benefits, will involve a net cost to the National Health Service, accounted for mainly by drug and monitoring costs. One explanation for these conflicting results is the different populations of women considered in these two studies. Whereas our analysis was based upon 10 years of treatment of women starting at age 50, the other study proposed treating a hypothetical group of women aged between 65 and 74 (at commencement of treatment) for a total of 10 years. Few data exist concerning the effects of treatment on women in this age-group. Indeed, most of the evidence suggests that the greatest benefit is obtained from treating women close to the menopause.

What must be borne in mind when interpreting the results of a cost-effectiveness analysis is that these are dependent on the assumptions used, must not be viewed in isolation, and should be seen as decision-aiding information rather than decision-taking yardsticks. Given the lack of consistent data about the effects of hormone replacement therapy, the results presented above seek merely to underline those factors which will have most impact in terms of health benefits and costs. Until better data become available, the overall balance of benefits and risks must ultimately be assessed on an individual level.

ACKNOWLEDGEMENTS

The authors acknowledge the financial support of the Department of Health, and thank Dr Ruairidh Milne for his useful critique of the manuscript.

REFERENCES

1. Persson, I., Adami, H.-O., Bergkvist, L., Lindgren, A., Petterson, B., Hoover, R. and Schairer, C. (1989). Risk of endometrial cancer after treatment with oestrogens alone or in conjunction with progestogens: results of a prospective study. *Br. Med. J.*, **298**, 147–51
2. Ross, R.K. (1989). Stroke prevention and oestrogen replacement therapy. *Lancet*, **1**, 505
3. Jensen, J. and Christiansen, C. (1987). Dose–response effects on serum lipids and lipoproteins following combined oestrogen–progestogen therapy in post-menopausal women. *Maturitas*, **9**, 259–66

4. Siddle, N.C., Jesinger, D.K., Whitehead, M.I., Turner, P., Lewis, B. and Prescott, P. (1990). Effect on plasma lipids and lipoproteins of postmenopausal oestrogen therapy with added dydrogesterone. *Br. J. Obstet. Gynaecol.*, **97**, 1093–1100
5. Hahn, R.G. (1989). Compliance considerations with estrogen replacement: withdrawal bleeding and other factors. *Am. J. Obstet. Gynecol.*, **161**, 1854–8
6. Randall, S. (1990). Problems encountered by long-term hormone replacement therapy users. *Br. J. Fam. Planning*, **16**, 101–5
7. Christiansen, C. and Riis, B.J. (1990). Five years with continuous combined oestrogen/progestogen therapy. Effects on calcium metabolism, lipoproteins, and bleeding pattern. *Br. J. Obstet. Gynaecol.*, **97**, 1087–92
8. Siddle, N.C., Fraser, D., Whitehead, M.I., Jesinger, D.K., Endacott, J., Prescott, P. and Pryse-Davies, J. (1990). Endometrial, physical and psychological effects of postmenopausal oestrogen therapy with added dydrogesterone. *Br. J. Obstet. Gynaecol.*, **97**, 1101–7
9. Spector, T.D. (1989). Use of oestrogen replacement therapy in high risk groups in the United Kingdom. *Br. Med. J.*, **299**, 1434–5
10. Barlow, D.H., Brockie, J.A. and Rees, C.M.P. (1991). Study of general practice consultations and menopausal problems. *Br. Med. J.*, **302**, 274–6
11. Kadri, A.Z. (1991). Hormone replacement therapy – a survey of perimenopausal women in a community setting. *Br. J. Gen. Pract.*, **41**, 109–12
12. Hunt, K. and Vessey, M. (1991). The risks and benefits of hormone replacement therapy: an updated review. *Curr. Obstet. Gynaecol.*, **1**, 21–7
13. Weinstein, M.C. (1980). Estrogen use in postmenopausal women – costs, risks and benefits. *N. Engl. J. Med.*, **303**, 308–16
14. Weinstein, M.C. and Schiff, I. (1983). Cost–effectiveness of hormone replacement therapy in the menopause. *Obstet. Gynecol. Surv.*, **38**, 445–55
15. Roche, M. and Vessey, M.P. (1990). Hormone replacement in the community: risks, benefits and costs. In Drife, J.O. and Studd, J.W.W. (eds.) *HRT and Osteoporosis*. (London: Springer–Verlag)
16. Weinstein, M.C. and Stason, W.B. (1977). Foundations of cost-effectiveness analysis for health and medical practices. *N. Engl. J. Med.*, **296**, 716–21
17. Leather, A.T. and Studd, J.W.W. (1990). Can the withdrawal bleed following oestrogen replacement therapy be avoided? *Br J. Obstet. Gynaecol.*, **97**, 1071–9 (commentary)
18. Office of Population Censuses and Surveys (1990). Mortality Statistics: cause 1988. (London: HMSO)
19. Department of Health and Social Security and Office of Population Censuses and Surveys (1987). Hospital Inpatient Enquiry 1985. (London: HMSO)
20. Boyce, W.J. and Vessey, M.P. (1985). Rising incidence of fracture of the proximal femur. *Lancet*, **1**, 150–1
21. Donaldson, L.J., Cook, A. and Thomson, R.G. (1990). Incidence of fractures in a geographically defined population. *J. Epidemiol. Commun. Health*, **44**, 241–5
22. Melton, L.J., Kan, S.H., Frye, M.A., Wahner, H.W., O'Fallon, W.M. and Riggs, B.L. (1989). Epidemiology of vertebral fractures in women. *Am. J. Epidemiol.*, **129**, 1000–11
23. Department of Health and Social Security and Office of Population Censuses and Surveys (1986). Morbidity Statistics from General Practice, Third National Study 1981–1982. (London: HMSO)
24. Hunt, K. and Vessey, M.P. (1987). Long-term effects of postmenopausal hormone therapy. *Br. J. Hosp. Med.*, **38**, 450–60
25. Henderson, B.E., Pike, M.C., Ross, R.K., Mack, T.M. and Lobo, R.A. (1988). Re-evaluating the role of progestogen therapy after the menopause. *Fertil. Steril.*, **49** (Suppl.), 9–15S
26. Hunt, K., Vessey, M., McPherson, K. and Coleman, M. (1987). Long-term surveillance of mortality and cancer incidence in women receiving hormone replacement therapy. *Br. J. Obstet. Gynaecol.*, **94**, 620–35
27. Buring, J.E., Hennekens, C.H., Lipnick, R.J., Willett, W., Stampfer, M.J., Rosner, B., Peto, R. and Speizer, F.E. (1987). A prospective cohort study of postmenopausal hormone use and risk of breast cancer in US women. *Am. J. Epidemiol.*, **125**, 939–47
28. Mills, P.K., Beeson, W.L., Phillips, R.L. and Fraser, G.E. (1989). Prospective study of exogenous hormone use and breast cancer in Seventh-Day Adventists. *Cancer*, **64**, 591–7
29. Bergkvist, L., Adami, H.-O., Persson, I., Hoover, R. and Schairer, C. (1989). The risk of

breast cancer after estrogen and estrogen–progestin replacement. *N. Engl. J. Med.*, **321**, 293–7
30. Hunt, K., Vessey, M. and McPherson, K. (1990). Mortality in a cohort of long-term users of hormone replacement therapy: an updated analysis. *Br. J. Obstet. Gynaecol.*, **97**, 1080–6
31. Brinton, L.A., Hoover, R. and Fraumeni, J.F., Jr (1986). Menopausal oestrogens and breast cancer risk: an expanded case–control study. *Br. J. Cancer*, **54**, 825–32
32. Pike, M.C., Bernstein, L. and Ross, R.K. (1990). Breast cancer and hormone replacement therapy. *Lancet*, **335**, 297 (letter)
33. Colditz, G.A., Stampfer, M.J., Willett, W.C., Hennekens, C.H., Rosner, B. and Speizer, F.E. (1990). Prospective study of oestrogen replacement therapy and risk of breast cancer in postmenopausal women. *J. Am. Med. Assoc.*, **264**, 2648–53
34. Steinberg, K.K., Thacker, S.B., Smith, S.J., Stroup, D.F., Zack, M.M., Flanders, W.D. and Berkelman, R.L. (1991). A meta-analysis of the effect of estrogen replacement therapy on the risk of breast cancer. *J. Am. Med. Assoc.*, **265**, 1985–90
35. Dupont, W.D. and Page, D.L. (1991). Menopausal estrogen replacement therapy and breast cancer. *Arch. Int. Med.*, **151**, 67–72
36. Key, T.J. and Pike, M.C. (1988). The role of oestrogens and progestogens in the epidemiology and prevention of breast cancer. *Eur. J. Cancer Clin. Oncol.*, **24**, 29–43
37. Gambrell, R.D., Jr (1984). Proposal to decrease the risk and improve the prognosis of breast cancer. *Am. J. Obstet. Gynecol.*, **150**, 119–32
38. Lindsay, R., Hart, D.M., Aitken, J.M., MacDonald, E.B., Anderson, J.B. and Clarke, A.C. (1976). Long-term prevention of postmenopausal osteoporosis by oestrogen: evidence for an increased bone mass after delayed onset of oestrogen treatment. *Lancet*, **1**, 1038–41
39. Horsman, A., Gallagher, J.C., Simpson, M. and Nordin, B.E.C. (1977). Prospective trial of oestrogen and calcium in postmenopausal women. *Br. Med. J.*, **2**, 789–92
40. Weiss, N.S., Ure, C.L., Ballard, J.H., Williams, A.R. and Daling, J.R. (1980). Decreased risk of fractures of the hip and lower forearm with postmenopausal use of oestrogen. *N. Engl. J. Med.*, **303**, 1195–8
41. Paganini-Hill, A., Ross, R.K., Gerkins, V.R., Henderson, B.E., Arthur, M. and Mack, T.M. (1981). A case–control study of menopausal estrogen therapy and hip fractures. *Ann. Int. Med.*, **95**, 28–31
42. Naessen, T., Persson, I., Adami, H.-O., Bergstrom, R. and Bergkvist, L. (1990). Hormone replacement therapy and the risk for first hip fracture – a prospective, population-based cohort study. *Ann. Int. Med.*, **113**, 95–103
43. Christiansen, C., Christensen, M.S. and Transbol, I. (1981). Bone mass in postmenopausal women after withdrawal of oestrogen/gestagen replacement therapy. *Lancet*, **1**, 459–61
44. Barrett-Connor, E. and Bush, T.L. (1991). Estrogen and coronary heart disease in women. *J. Am. Med. Assoc.*, **265**, 1861–7
45. Stampfer, M.J. and Colditz, G.A. (1991). Estrogen replacement therapy and coronary heart disease: a quantitative assesment of the epidemiologic evidence. *Prev. Med.*, **20**, 47–63
46. Stampfer, M.J., Willett, W.C., Colditz, G.A., Rosner, B., Speizer, F.E. and Hennekens, C.H. (1985). A prospective study of postmenopausal estrogen therapy and coronary heart disease. *N. Engl. J. Med.*, **313**, 1044–9
47. Stampfer, M.J., Colditz, G.A., Willett, W.C., Manson, J.E., Rosner, B., Speizer, F.E. and Hennekens, C.H. (1991). Postmenopausal estrogen therapy and cardiovascular disease: ten-year follow-up from the Nurses' Health Study. *N. Engl. J. Med.*, **325**, 756–62
48. Paganini-Hill, A., Ross, R.K. and Henderson, B.E. (1988). Postmenopausal oestrogen treatment and stroke: a prospective study. *Br. Med. J.*, **297**, 519–22
49. Ettinger, B., Golditch, I.M. and Friedman, G. (1988). Gynecologic consequences of long-term unopposed estrogen replacement therapy. *Maturitas*, **10**, 271–82
50. British National Formulary Number 19 (March, 1990). (London: British Medical Association and the Royal Pharmaceutical Society of Great Britain)
51. Social Services Select Committee, 8th report (1989). (HMSO)
52. Health and Personal Social Services Statistics (1989). (London: HMSO)
53. Torrance, G.W. (1986). Measurement of health state utilities for economic appraisal: a review. *J. Health Econ.*, **5**, 1–30
54. Boyce, W.J. (1987). Fracture of the proximal femur: studies of the distribution, risk factors, care and outcome in Oxford 1983–1985. *DM Thesis*, Oxford University

55. Evans, J.G., Prudham, D. and Wandless, I. (1979). A prospective study of fractured proximal femur: incidence and outcome. *Pub. Health*, **93**, 235–41
56. Managing the Menopause – a practical guide to HRT. (1991). (Oxted: Medical Communications Services)
57. Coope, J. (1991). Management of the menopause in the community. *Br. J. Fam. Planning*, **16** (Suppl.), 42–5
58. Siddle, N. (1990). Treatment strategies. In Page, M.L. (ed.) *Current Approaches – Hormone Replacement Therapy*, pp. 47–51 (Southampton: Duphar Medical Relations)
59. Ettinger, B. (1988). Optimal use of postmenopausal hormone replacement. *Obstet. Gynecol.*, **72** (Suppl.), 31–36S
60. Coulter, A., McPherson, K. and Vessey, M.P. (1988). Do British women undergo too many or too few hysterectomies. *Soc. Sci. Med.*, **27**, 987–94
61. McKinlay, S.M. and Jefferys, M. (1974). The menopausal syndrome. *Br. J. Prev. Soc. Med.*, **28**, 108–15
62. Samsioe, G., Bryman, I. and Ivansson, E. (1985). Some anthropological aspects of the climacteric syndrome. *Acta Obstet. Gynecol. Scand.*, **130** (Suppl.), 5–7
63. Hillner, B.E., Hollenberg, J.P. and Pauker, S.G. (1986). Postmenopausal estrogens in prevention of osteoporosis. Benefit virtually without risk if cardiovascular effects are considered. *Am. J. Med.*, **80**, 1115–27
64. Henderson, B.E., Paganini-Hill, A. and Ross, R.K. (1991). Decreased mortality in users of estrogen replacement therapy. *Arch. Int. Med.*, **151**, 75–8
65. Sullivan, J.M., Vander Zwaag, R., Hughes, J.P., Maddock, V., Kroetz, F.W., Ramanathan, K.B. and Mirvis, D.M. (1990). Estrogen replacement and coronary artery disease. Effect on survival in postmenopausal women. *Arch. Int. Med.*, **150**, 2557–62
66. Bush, T.L. (1990). The epidemiology of cardiovascular disease in postmenopausal women. *Ann. NY Acad. Sci.*, **592**, 263–71
67. Persson, I., Adami, H.-O., Bergstrom, R., Krusemo, U.B. and Hoover, R. (1990). Survival in women receiving hormone replacement therapy. A record-linkage study of a large population-based cohort. *J. Clin. Epidemiol.*, **43**, 677–85
68. Loft, A., Andersen, T.F., Bronnum-Hansen, H., Roepstorff, C. and Madsen, M. (1991). Early postoperative mortality following hysterectomy. A Danish population based study, 1977–1981. *Br. J. Obstet. Gynaecol.*, **98**, 147–54
69. Whitehead, M. and Studd, J. (1988). Selection of patients for treatment: which therapy and for how long? In Studd, J.W.W. and Whitehead, M.I. (eds.) *The Menopause*. (Oxford: Blackwell Scientific Publications)
70. Cummings, S.R., Browner, W.S., Grady, D. and Ettinger, B. (1990). Should prescription of postmenopausal hormone therapy be based on the results of bone densitometry? *Ann. Int. Med.*, **113**, 565–7 (editorial)
71. Tosteson, A.N.A., Rosenthal, D.I., Melton, L.J. and Weinstein, M.C. (1990). Cost–effectiveness of screening perimenopausal white women for osteoporosis: bone densitometry and hormone replacement therapy. *Ann. Int. Med.*, **113**, 594–603
72. Melton, L.J., Eddy, D.M. and Johnston, C.C. (1990). Screening for osteoporosis. *Ann. Int. Med.*, **112**, 516–28
73. Johnston, C.C., Slemenda, C.W. and Melton, L.J. (1991). Clinical use of bone densitometry. *N. Engl. J. Med.*, **324**, 1105–9 (review)
74. Williams, A. (1987). Screening for risk of CHD: is it a wise use of resources? In Oliver, M., Ashley-Miller, M. and Wood, D. (eds.) *Screening for Risk of Coronary Heart Disease*, pp. 97–105 (Chichester: Wiley)
75. Williams, A. (1985). Economics of coronary artery bypass grafting. *Br. Med. J.*, **291**, 326–9
76. Department of Health and Social Security (1986). Breast Cancer Screening. A report to the Health Ministers of England, Wales, Scotland and Northern Ireland by a working group chaired by Sir Patrick Forrest. (London: HMSO)
77. Goddard, M. (1990). The cost-effectiveness of hormone replacement therapy: a review. Discussion Paper No. 73. (University of York, Centre for Health Economics)

22

Hormone replacement therapy and breast cancer risk: summing up

C.E.D. Chilvers

I will begin by picking out in chronological order a few general issues that have been discussed before trying to summarize the main results. We started with Dr Mann and an informal overview of the studies that have been carried out to date. He posed a number of questions:

(1) What is the overall effect of hormone replacement therapy?

(2) What is the effect of long-term use?

(3) What is the effect of dose?

(4) What difference does adding a progestogen make to oestrogen replacement therapy?

Professor Jacobs then gave a very lucid account of the physiology of the menopause; one of the points he made is particularly important: the very small proportion of women who are being studied of all those prescribed replacement hormones. If we are to advance our knowledge, more (and larger) studies must be carried out.

Mr Ellerington looked at specialist practice. I was particularly interested in the different methods by which oestrogens and progestogens can be given, and the present uncertainty that we have about these different methods in terms of both short- and long-term effects.

Dr Upsdell told us about general practice, reminding us of the very profound effect that menopausal symptoms have on women's lives, and how important this therapy is for many women to be able to continue to function effectively. I was also reminded of the recent Green Paper in the United Kingdom on the Health of the Nation; this highlights the necessity for the identification of health needs in the population. The debate that we have had over the last few days seemed pertinent; this is an area of need about which we do not know as much as we should.

Professor Smith's paper on osteoporosis highlighted the lack of information on its epidemiology, and the likely costs related to it in the future with our aging population. Osteoporosis is a major public health problem today, and the role of hormone replacement therapy in preventing bone loss will be increasingly important.

Mr Burn talked about clinical factors, and in particular about how hormone replacement therapy can be used more safely. There are a number of points that I think are important here. Firstly, who are the women at high risk of developing breast cancer? Family history (in a first-degree relative) is quoted widely, but it is important to take into account the age at which a mother or sister developed breast cancer. The increased risk is confined to women whose first-degree relative developed breast cancer before the menopause. Secondly, there is benign breast disease and this term covers a number of conditions. Proliferative disease, particularly atypical hyperplasia, is associated with an increased risk. There are, however, types of benign disease which do not fall into this category and do not confer an excess risk. Then there is the very difficult question of women who have already had a cancer, and what should be done for them in terms of hormone replacement therapy.

CASE–CONTROL STUDIES

Table 1 summarizes the data from case–control studies that have been presented at this meeting. The risks associated with ever-use are generally close to unity and few are greater than 1.2–1.3. As Professor Shapiro has argued very persuasively, there are real difficulties in interpreting risks as low as this because they could easily be explained by the sorts of bias to which this type of study is particularly subject.

Most of the studies summarized in Table 1 have found raised risks with long durations of use, but most of them show no evidence of any trend with duration of use. The latter is, of course, one of the most persuasive ways in which we can begin to distinguish causal relationships from chance associations.

What we have, then, are relative risks of no more than 1.2–1.3 for ever use, and some evidence from some studies of raised risks after long-term use. Dr Ross, in his paper on the methodological problems of studying the association between hormone replacement therapy and breast cancer risk, cites a number of factors that may help to explain the difficulty in reaching conclusions about this relationship; studies tend to have a rather low power to detect small relative risks (i.e. under 2). Failure to allow for confounding factors may, in this particular context, lead to underestimation of risk, and studies using population-based controls have consistently found elevated risks for long-term use, whereas studies with hospital controls have not.

COHORT STUDIES

Cohort studies (Table 2) are particularly problematic because of the possibility of selection bias. This arises where the cohort mortality or morbidity is compared with that in the general population. Selection bias is likely to arise

Table 1 Summary of case–control studies presented at the conference: overall results

Author	*Country*	*No. of cases*	*Type of therapy*	*Relative risk (95% CI)*	*Duration of use* (years)
Brinton	USA	881*	Oestrogen	1.24 (1.0–1.5)	Ever
		1960†	Oestrogen	1.0‡	Ever
La Vecchia	Italy	3037	Oestrogen	1.3 (1.0–1.8)	Ever
			Oestrogen	1.5 (0.9–2.6)‡	≥ 3
Hulka**	USA	152	Oestrogen	1.7 (1.1–2.6)	Ever
				1.5 (0.6–4.0)	≥ 10
Kaufman	USA	1686	Oestrogen	1.1 (0.9–1.4)	Ever
			Conjugated oestrogen	1.2 (1.0–1.6)	Ever
			Conjugated oestrogen	0.9 (0.4–1.9)	≥ 15
			Other oestrogen	1.2 (0.6–2.7)	Ever
			Oestrogen + progestogen	1.7 (0.9–3.6)	Ever
Rohan	Australia	281	All	0.82 (0.50–1.34)	Ever
			All	0.50 (0.15–1.63)	≥ 4
Rosenberg	Canada	607	Oestrogen	1.0 (0.8–1.4)	Ever
			Oestrogen	1.7 (0.8–3.5)	≥ 15
			Conjugated oestrogen	0.8 (0.6–1.1)	Ever
			Conjugated oestrogen	1.4 (0.6–3.3)	≥ 15
			Other oestrogen	2.2 (0.8–6.3)	Ever
			Oestrogen + progestogen	0.6 (0.2–1.9)	Ever
Wingo	USA	1369	Oestrogen	1.0 (0.9–1.2)	Ever
			Oestrogen	1.8 (0.6–5.8)	≥ 20
Adami††	Sweden	253	Oestrogen	2.3 (1.1–4.8)‡	> 9
Vessey††	UK	53	All	3.6 (0.9–15.0)	> 6

*1973–77; †1973–80; ‡Test for trend, $p < 0.05$; **results for natural menopause, community controls; ††case–control study within cohort

Table 2 Summary of cohort studies presented at the conference: overall results

Author	*Country*	*No. of cases*	*Type of therapy*	*Relative risk (95% CI)*	*Duration of use* (years)
Colditz	USA	1050	All	1.33 (1.12–1.57)	Current
			All	0.92 (0.79–1.09)	Past
			Conjugated oestrogen	1.42 (1.19–1.70)	Current
			Other oestrogen	1.14 (0.72–1.81)	Current
			Oestrogen + progestogen	1.54 (0.99–2.39)	Current
Adami	Sweden	253	Oestrogen	1.1 (1.0–1.3)	Ever
			Oestrogen	1.7 (1.1–2.7)*	> 9
			Oestrogen + progestogen	4.4 (0.9–22.4)	> 6
Gambrell	USA	6	Oestrogen + progestogen	0.22	Ever
Vessey	UK	12†‡	All	0.55 (0.28–0.96)	Ever
		19†**	All	1.0 (0.55–1.45)	Ever
		50	All	1.59 (1.18–2.10)	Ever

*Test for trend, $p < 0.05$; †mortality study – breast cancer deaths; ‡1978–June 1984; **July 1984–December 1988

because women prescribed hormone replacement therapy may be screened with respect to breast problems and thus, at least for short term follow-up, their breast cancer rates may be much lower than those expected in the general population.

Dr Adami and Dr Colditz both report raised risks, in contrast to Dr Gambrell and Professor Vessey (Table 2). Dr Gambrell's very low relative risk (0.22) based on 6 cases is likely to be due to selection bias, and Professor Vessey has explored this in some detail in his analyses. In terms of new cases of breast cancer, Professor Vessey reports a relative risk of 1.59 for ever-use, but a relative risk of 0.55 in his first mortality study. After further follow-up (by which time some of the selection effect may have worn off), the relative risk has increased to 1.0 and he speculates that with further follow-up the relative risk is likely to exceed unity.

TYPE AND DOSE OF REPLACEMENT THERAPY

In some studies, different types of hormone replacement therapy have been considered (see Table 1). In two studies (Colditz and Kaufman) there is no difference between risks associated with conjugated oestrogens or 'other' oestrogens. Dr Adami reports a risk of 1.8 for oestradiol relative to oestriol, and Dr Rosenberg a higher (but non-significant) risk associated with 'other' oestrogen relative to conjugated oestrogen. Dr Brinton also reported that she had found some evidence of a greater risk for non-conjugated, compared to conjugated, oestrogens.

In most studies there has been relatively little use of oestrogen opposed by a progestogen. Five studies have some relevant results; Dr Colditz and Professor Vessey report no difference, while Dr Adami and Dr Kaufman report higher odds ratios for opposed therapy and Dr Rosenberg a reduced odds ratio (Table 1). The data collected by Dr Ross in his as yet unpublished study will be of considerable relevance to the debate about the relative merits of opposed and unopposed therapy.

Results reported for different daily dosages of conjugated oestrogen are shown in Table 3. There is no evidence of a dose response. Wingo and colleagues also report results with doses categorized as mg-months of conjugated oestrogen use. There is no evidence of a trend in relative risks. Dr Brinton reported higher risks among 'high-dose' users in her first dataset, but not in the results updated to 1980.

Table 3 Dose of conjugated oestrogen

Author	*Dose* (mg)	*Relative risk* (95% *CI*)
Hulka*	≤ 0.625	1.8 (0.9–8.6)
	> 0.625	0.9 (0.4–2.0)
Kaufman	< 1.25	0.8 (0.4–1.5)
	1.25	1.2 (0.7–2.0)
Colditz	0.625	1.45 (1.16–1.83)
	1.25	1.44 (1.07–1.93)

*Natural menopause, community controls

SUBGROUP ANALYSES

A number of studies included extensive subgroup analyses, but generally without formal tests of interaction. Few of the studies have sufficient power for this type of analysis. Although most studies found at least one subgroup at apparently high risk from hormone replacement therapy, the lack of any consistency between the studies suggests that these are likely to be chance findings. There are two subgroupings that may be worth further investigation, in that for each of these, two of the studies reported do show some consistency: age at diagnosis, where the effect of hormone replacement therapy appears to be greater in older women, and body-mass index, where the effect appears to be greater in leaner women.

CONCLUSIONS

My final conclusions are as follows:

(1) Most of the studies presented at this meeting have been of unopposed oestrogens and mainly conjugated oestrogens.

(2) The relative risks for ever-use are certainly not in excess of 1.3.

(3) We have not been able to establish the safety of very long-term use (15 years or more). This may be the only type of use that is relevant in long-term protection against heart disease and osteoporosis.

(4) Overall, the risks associated with conjugated oestrogens may be lower than for 'other' oestrogens.

(5) We need much more information about combined treatment with oestrogen and progestogen.

(6) Few of the studies have found convincing dose–response relationships in terms of either duration of use or of daily dosage.

(7) There are many opportunities in these studies for bias and other methodological problems. It is unlikely that we will be able to distinguish causality from bias in further observational studies.

(8) We have been considering breast cancer in isolation; it is really only in the last paper from Dr Roche that the whole spectrum of effects of hormone replacement therapy has been looked at. We are very uncertain about the long-term effects on cardiovascular disease and osteoporosis: for how long hormones must be taken, and for how long after ceasing treatment the effect is likely to last. One of the questions I was considering was partially answered in Dr Roche's presentation: with current levels of knowledge of the effects of cardiovascular disease and osteoporosis, what level of breast cancer risk would still be consistent with overall benefit? I think that the relative risk would be about 2.

(9) There seems to be little information about short-term effects apart from

relief of symptoms. What happens when a woman stops taking hormone replacement therapy? Has she to go through all the vasomotor symptoms of the menopause at the age of 60 rather than at 50?

There seem to me to be a number of possible ways forward. There will soon be more epidemiological data on long-term use and on opposed oestrogens. These will need to be looked at very carefully. Much more work is needed on the epidemiology of osteoporosis in order to have firmer evidence on which to base a cost–benefit analysis. Account also needs to be taken of other possible ways of preventing osteoporosis and cardiovascular disease. The biphosphonates, for example, are being tried now for preserving bone mass. Exercise is another alternative which also has other benefits.

What about clinical trials? There will clearly be many difficulties in carrying out randomized controlled trials. In the United Kingdom, compliance is not very good, particularly in older women. There may be ways of manipulating the hormones so that bleeding, which seems to be the main barrier to compliance, is reduced. Finally, if we do opt for large randomized controlled trials, I think it would be a great mistake not to allow unopposed oestrogen as well as opposed oestrogen in women with an intact uterus.

General discussion V

(Chairman: Dr Ronald D. Mann)

Dr C.H. Hutton Can Prof. Weiss tell us whether, with the very high usage of HRT in Washington State, there has been any absolute change in the overall incidence of breast carcinoma?

Prof. N.S. Weiss In our State, as in most of the USA, the incidence of breast cancer has been rising steadily for at least the last 10 years. I do not know to what extent this increased incidence is more or less present in post- and premenopausal women. My impression is that it is rising in both groups, particularly in the former, so it is not clear whether the impact of oestrogens and the increasing incidence can be related.

Dr L. Rosenberg My impression is just the opposite to that of Prof. Weiss. I think the incidence in the USA is rising more rapidly in older women than in younger women. In fact, the Institute of Child Health and Human Development used this as evidence that the oral contraceptives could not be increasing the risk in younger women since there was this huge rise in older women.

Dr R.D. Gambrell I have a different impression. Certainly the incidence of breast cancer is increasing, for which I think there are two reasons in the USA: first, with our aging population, and the ever-increasing incidence by age, we are seeing more cancers because women are living longer. Secondly, 40% of women now have mammograms after the menopause (although only 20% have regular annual mammograms, as recommended by the American Cancer Society). With this increased use of mammography in the USA, we are certainly seeing an increase in earlier diagnosis, *in situ* lesions – and this has come out in several presentations at this meeting. These are the reasons why an increase is being seen.

Prof. Weiss When Dr Rosenberg and I described our perceptions of the incidence of breast cancer we referred to age-adjusted rates, not just total numbers – but I understand what you are saying.

Prof. R.K. Ross Breast cancer rates in Los Angeles have risen about 20% in the last 7 or 8 years – a big increase for a common disease. As has also been done in the San Francisco Bay area of northern California, we have looked at some of the demographic characteristics of this increase. The magnitude is certainly greater in older women than in younger women and, by and large, is restricted to higher social class women in the early stages of the disease. I think this is compatible with Dr Gambrell's hypothesis that the change has resulted from increased mammography, but it is certainly also compatible with an effect of hormone replacement therapy, and we know that this therapy is more commonly used in higher social class women. Women who use hormones, and are later diagnosed with breast cancer, might well tend to be diagnosed at an early stage of their disease.

Prof. W.D. Dupont The other part of this equation that needs to be pointed out is that, in spite of the alarming increase in the incidence of breast cancer with time in the USA, there is very little increase in breast cancer mortality; the curves are quite flat. We are left with a real dilemma regarding whether this increase in incidence represents a real change in disease (which somehow is being counterbalanced by earlier detection or better treatment) or whether it is truly an artefact of our new detection methods (and results from the fact that through mammography we are detecting far more benign disease which will either take its time before killing people or, conceivably, would never progress to the point of clinical presentation).

Mr I. Burn Some risk is probably acceptable if we can be sure of providing a useful protective effect – for example, on cardiovascular disease. But is it not a fact that the administration of HRT is as much for social reasons as for health? My impression, from the patients I see in my own clinic, is that there is a very big social use of this particular agent.

Prof. Weiss I cannot evaluate the 'social' reasons for use, either here or in the USA. I am prepared to ignore them when evaluating the overall risks and benefits, and simply concentrate on the actual health benefits and risks. I think it is probably best left at that.

Prof. J. Drife What is the difference between a social and a health indication? In gynaecology, we have learnt over the last 50 years that there is a very close correlation between social conditions and health problems. I do not believe that it is possible to separate the two categories of 'social' and 'health' usage. I would be interested to know what is wrong with having social indications for medication.

Mr Burn What concerns me is not the difference between social and medical indications. I am happy to go along with the wishes of women if they feel absolutely safe in taking these agents for whatever reason. When I use the word 'social', I mean 'cosmetic'; if you like, the effect of taking these agents produces a sense of well-being and also induce a sense of youthfulness. There is nothing wrong with that, but I do think that we should not pretend that these agents are being taken by the majority of women because they wish to avoid heart problems or osteoporosis. I am sure that these long-term indications are not in the minds of most women when they go to their doctor to ask for HRT.

Prof. Drife I would wish to emphasize that there is nothing immoral in making women feel happier. There is, I think, a rigorous kind of feeling that somehow we must weigh only medical indications and serious life-threatening diseases in the balance in deciding to prescribe, and this is, perhaps, an inappropriate point of view.

Mr M. Pugh I have a menopause clinic, and the most important thing is the quality of life. It is not only the women who benefit, but the men benefit too. It makes family life better and improves the quality of living of all concerned.

Dr P.E. Belchetz As a clinician I want to go on record as saying that I find some of these comments, regarding 'social' indications, both patronizing and offensive. To suggest that the treatment is simply social, when it is given because women want to be youthful, is putting at a very low level the motivation that they have to live the high quality life that Mr Pugh has just mentioned. We have no qualms about treating headache, depression or insomnia. These are very important symptoms. The absolute devastation that many women suffer at the menopause is of the highest medical priority. We should make no excuses and give no apologies for treating them. These are not 'social' indications.

Mr Burn It was not my intention to be in any way offensive. I must just reiterate, though, that my role in life is dealing, as a surgeon, with breast cancer, and I have a real concern about it.

Prof. C.E.D. Chilvers I would like to thank Dr Belchetz. The bottom line is that women must be given the facts. We are well able to make up our own minds as to how we want to live and what we want... (*applause*)

Dr U. Lachnit-Fixon Should we differentiate between women on high- and low-fat diets, thus taking into account the fact that diet might be a confounding factor?

Prof. Weiss In our study we have not attempted to undertake the fairly arduous task of validly ascertaining dietary information.

Prof. R.E. Mansel Prof. Weiss addressed the difference between English and USA practice: in the USA some women with a uterus would receive opposed, but some would receive unopposed oestrogen; in the UK all such women would receive opposed oestrogen. Could he make a statement about the relative cost – not the drug cost alone, but the fact that it could perhaps be argued that women on unopposed therapy need more attention, in order to pick up those endometrial cancers? Can we be told whether one of the two regimens would cost the country, or the system, more than the other?

Prof. Weiss It is my understanding that in the USA there is a variety of regimens for following women who receive unopposed oestrogens. These range from giving a simple caution to respond promptly and seek medical attention if there is any bleeding, to other regimens in which the physician would routinely, on a 6-month or annual basis, attempt to do an endometrial biopsy. Which regimen is ultimately the most cost-effective has, I think, not been studied.

Dr Lachnit-Fixon We should perhaps just note that vaginal sonography is an extremely useful tool now for determining the height of the endometrium, and is probably an extremely useful method for finding very early endometrial cancer.

Prof. J.A. Collins Can Prof. Ross tell us if there is a published reference for the 'Leisure World' mortality data?

Prof. Ross They were published in *Archives of Internal Medicine* earlier in 1991[1].

Prof. Mansel Prof. Ross said that in a screened population vs. a non-screened population there would be the same detection bias in terms of mammography; i.e., that it is not possible to get a reference population. This may be a major problem in the USA because the non-screened population is still having a very high level of mammography. In Britain, there is very little mammography outside the screening programme, apart from certain special units, so that the background population may not be having a lot of mammography. We know the screening programme has shown a tenfold increase in the detection of *in situ* cancer, which may or may not be important.

Dr B. Santra Prof. Ross's statistics showed that cancer of the breast is very high (2.45%) in those women who use oestrogen and progesterone for 7 years or more. In some West German studies with unopposed oestrogen the findings were 123 cancers per 100 000, but with oestrogen and progesterone they were 105 per 100 000. What does this imply in terms of using opposed vs. unopposed oestrogens?

Prof. Ross There are virtually no data on combination therapy in relation to breast cancer – I think primarily because of the recency of this type of medication.

Dr A.H. Ross I have a slight concern about the case selection in Dr Rosenberg's series because the cases were selected from a cancer treatment hospital. The majority of cancers, or certainly early stage primary cancers, are treated in general hospitals, and the cancer treatment hospitals only have a referral population. Is it possible that the cases selected were systematically different, and is it therefore difficult to compare the findings to other series in which case selections were done differently?

Dr Rosenberg That concern is well taken, and it certainly is possible that they were different. I should say that the standard breast cancer risk factors were present in the case–control comparisons. The risk factors had the same strength as in other studies, except for age at first birth, which was not a risk factor, and which also seems to be absent in other Canadian studies.

Prof. Mansel Can Dr Roche please tell us the start point of treatment in her cost-effectiveness study? [*Dr M. Roche* 50] I tried to allude earlier to the fact that 10% of the work-load of breast clinics is now related to Hormone Replacement Therapy. No assumptions were made in Dr Roche's model regarding breast morbidity. If more mammograms are done, there is more cost, and more biopsies which would not have been done otherwise. I know that women at 50 are included in the screening programme, but women on HRT are being mammogrammed more frequently than 3-yearly, so the monitoring costs have been underestimated quite substantially.

Dr Roche We have underestimated them if we accept your assumption that these women would be screened more frequently than they would be under the national breast screening programme. Our assumption has been that as these women are all over the age of 50 they fall within the 50–64 age group who, as you say, will be screened 3-yearly as part of the national programme. I take your point, we have not included any extra costs.

Prof. Collins The presentation of Dr Roche was important and very informative. I agree entirely that the feelings of individual women are important and should be taken into account. When the quality-adjusted life years were estimated, was some factor for compliance built in? This may also be an important characteristic associated with the feelings of women.

Dr Roche The result I presented was based simply on some assumptions regarding informed clinical opinion, which basically means that some assumptions were made about what we thought might be the impact of menopausal symptoms on quality of life. We are now doing the fieldwork – asking menopausal women (women both from a specialist menopausal clinic and from a general practice setting) what they are thinking. We do not have the results yet. The women at the menopause clinic are, predominantly, users of HRT, but we are also looking for a more unselected population from general practice who will include both.

Dr G. Colditz I enjoyed Dr Roche's presentation, and wonder whether adding a sensitivity analysis that allowed for cardiovascular benefit far earlier than 5 years might be considered. I noticed that there is a 25% reduction at 5 years, and we have to wait 10 years before there is a 50% reduction. A lot of evidence would suggest that the effect on coagulation profiles is present well before 5 years.

Dr Roche That has not been done. It is interesting to get people's opinions about things that we should be doing with the model.

Dr K.H. Kimbel I liked the study very much and the possibilities of cost-savings, both for the community and for the insurance companies, but the patient who gets the benefit is not the same as the patient who gets the adverse effects. The woman with the lowest oestrogen and the most need for it gets the benefit, and the woman with an average or higher oestrogen level gets the risks. Therefore, it is astonishing that HRT is not titrated like other hormone replacement therapies, such as insulin.

Secondly, only oestriol and oestradiol are real replacement hormones. All the others are chemically distorted hormones, especially the progestogens. Is it really possible to talk about replacement therapy?

It is slightly disappointing for a clinical pharmacologist that our data on hormone treatment, on metabolism, on interactions (we know that progestogens interact with the oestrogen metabolism) are so poor, and that our statistical evidence has such a poor foundation that we have to rely on a standard dose for large and small women, and women from the USA, Asia and from Europe, regardless of their varying metabolizer status.

Dr C.W. Jones What happens when realistic estimates for compliance are entered into your model?

Dr Roche It obviously reduces the cost-effectiveness quite dramatically, although I do not have the figures readily available. Obviously, not 100% of women will take HRT for 10 years, and in the UK very few women take HRT for long periods at the moment. There is a significant effect of reducing cost-effectiveness, although as long as women are not having the prescription filled and then not taking the medication, there is a reduction both in drug and monitoring costs.

Dr E.C.G. Grant There are interesting figures from the oral contraceptive cohort studies for total death rates and the vascular and neoplasm death rates that are relevant to this subject. Prof. Vessey was one of the co-authors of the publication of the Oxford Family Planning Association (FPA) contraceptive study on the pill (mostly the combined pill) between 1968 and 1979, which showed that both the overall death rate and the circulatory disease death rates in this study were half of those for England and Wales. The Royal College of General Practitioners' (RCGP) study also had a lower overall death rate than the national figures, but a higher death rate for circulatory disease. The Walnut Creek figures matched the English figures for deaths due to neoplasms, accidents and violence better than either of the two British studies, but also had a low proportion of circulatory deaths. Does Prof. Vessey really agree that oral contraceptives reduce the death rate by half, and is this the sort of thing we are looking at here?

Prof. M. Vessey The main reason for seeing a reduced overall death rate in the Oxford FPA contraceptive study and in all the publications dealing with mortality – the last and most detailed one was in December, 1989 – is, unquestionably, selection. Fortunately, this selection affects the women in the different groups that are contrasted: pill, intrauterine device (IUD) and diaphragm users. All the women in the study were reasonably fit at entry; they had to be able to walk to a family planning clinic, and to have sufficient motivation to attend it. The only surprise was that this so-called 'healthy worker' effect persisted so long. It has to be due to selection, but this does not invalidate comparisons within the cohort between the different groups because this selection affects all the groups. The RCGP study also had some slight selection in it. I think their rates are much closer to the rates expected nationally. I may say, too, that both the RCGP and the Oxford FPA studies showed an increase in mortality from cardiovascular disease. I was unaware that the Walnut Creek figures were similar to the figures for England and Wales. If this is the case, it must be due to chance. This is all not directly relevant, as far as I can see, to the present discussion.

Dr B.M. Campbell-Brown A cost that I think has been omitted in the cost–benefit survey is the cost of comfort drugs given to women who have the menopause and who are not receiving oestrogens. These include propanolol, investigations for palpitations, and often expensive cardiological investigations. Such costs are very real and, I appreciate, very difficult to assess, but they should be borne in mind.

Dr Roche Yes, they would be difficult to quantify, but are important.

Dr T. Rohan As I understand it, only one assumption was varied at a time. Why were several not varied at the same time? I think it would be important to do something like this to produce a sort of upper and lower range of plausible estimates.

Dr Roche We have looked at best- and worst-case scenarios. Today, for simplicity (although it was not that simple) I have presented the results of varying only one assumption.

Dr Rosenberg We have been talking about quality of life issues. The woman who gets endometrial cancer or has to go for endometrial biopsy every 6 months or once a year while she is on oestrogens, is not having her quality of life increased. Here we are, from our platform, talking about the public health benefits, but for the individual woman it is not very pleasant to get endometrial cancer. I know the argument is made that it is usually not fatal – maybe not, but it is fatal for some small proportion of women, and the treatment is not very pleasant either. This needs to be remembered.

Prof. Ross The point is well taken. On the other hand I said earlier that, typically, adding a progestogen tends to make women feel worse rather than better. I think there is yet another factor in quality of life in adding progestogen.

Prof. H.S. Jacobs When outlining oestrogen replacement therapy to American postmenopausal women, do American physicians say: 'Here is unopposed oestrogen therapy; you do understand that it has a sixfold increased risk of cancer of the uterus?' – or what-fold increased risk of cancer of the uterus are American women informed about these days?

Dr R.D. Gambrell As a gynaecologist who has treated and seen many cases of endometrial cancer, with the type of lesion that occurs with unopposed oestrogen therapy, hysterectomy is usually curative and the morbidity is fairly low. If American women understood endometrial cancer as we do, using progestogens would be very difficult to sell to them because there are some side-effects. These can be managed by changing to a different progestogen, but it would be difficult to sell progestogens on this benefit alone. The gynaecologist does not tell the American woman that she has a choice between using unopposed therapy with biopsies or opposed oestrogen. The gynaecologist does not usually offer the patient the opportunity to use unopposed therapy because as soon as the word 'cancer' is mentioned, these women will not accept any type of therapy.

Dr R.D. Mann Are you saying that valid informed consent is not obtained from these women – they are not told that there are alternative lines of therapy?

Dr Gambrell We tell our patients that with unopposed oestrogen therapy, as they well know, there is a five- to eightfold increased risk of endometrial cancer. In our studies, adding progestogens decreases the risk to less than the natural incidence in untreated women. This is what American women accept. There are few physicians who recommend unopposed therapy, saying they will monitor the women with biopsies, but their patients do not comply and continue on that therapy.

Prof. Collins There are possibly two other reasons why the majority of women in North America use unopposed oestrogens. One is the extent of hysterectomy in their 50s and 60s. Secondly, very few gynaecologists in litigious North America would fail to inform women of risks. Even after that information, I think women are voting with their feet and taking unopposed oestrogens in low doses, accepting whatever the risks of endometrial cancer may be.

I would like to describe how one gynaecologist approaches this, because it allows me to introduce a fourth meta-analysis published in Canada[2]. (Dr Rohan referred to a third, which I think was published in the *Medical Journal of Australia* a couple of years ago.) This meta-analysis arose because Dr Bates was inundated by patients in August 1989 asking what to do about HRT and breast cancer. He is also a graduate student in epidemiology, so he did a meta-analysis and arrived at the same conclusion as the three previous meta-analyses. There is the single difference that the Steinberg meta-analysis is the only one to look at duration and to find any effect of duration. He uses this in his practice now, saying that according to all the published studies we are left with this uncertainty – that there is this possible, but unproven, 10% increase in breast cancer. He tells the 50+ woman in his office, who is asking the question, that her residual lifetime risk of breast cancer is probably about 9%, and therefore there is a possibility that her risk will increase to 10%. The majority of his patients' eyes glaze over with boredom by the time he gets to this point, and they make their decision based on the other issues that he has discussed. This might be one way in which we can understand and try to use the epidemiological evidence that we have been hearing.

Dr Rosenberg The relative risk of 5–8 that is quoted is, of course, an average based on all durations of use. There is a very strong duration–response curve for oestrogen, with a much higher risk for women who have been on oestrogens for long periods, so that women who have been on them for 10 or 20 years have a greater increase.

Dr Gambrell As a practising physician treating a large number of menopausal patients, I have this unique opportunity to interact with so many epidemiologists. The new studies – the more than 50 studies over the last 15 years – have failed to show any significant increased risk, with some slight increased risk over 15 years (quoting a figure of 30%) and others showing no increased risk over 20 years of therapy.

May I make a plea, as epidemiologists continue their studies on oestrogen therapy and publish them: whether or not there is a risk of breast cancer, please be very sure of the data. Every time a study is published, the impact when it gets into the press (in the USA, and probably the same is true in England) is tremendous. I overheard some English physicians talking about 'thieves' of HRT, referring to what happens when a study is publicized and gets into the press: women on HRT will stop their therapy, women considering it will not start, and women in the future will never take therapy because of something they read.

I do not like to single out an individual study, but the impact of the Swedish study, published in the *New England Journal of Medicine* (August 1989) was great. Because of the wide press coverage, many women throughout the USA went off their therapy and many others will never take therapy for this reason.

It seems as though in nearly 20 years, if there is an increased risk it would have been possible to show it. There is still some doubt among the epidemiologists about a reduction in cardiovascular disease or even osteoporosis. Perhaps they could direct their attention and energies there. But please be very careful when publishing data to be very sure about them, so that our women are not unnecessarily alarmed, because the impact upon their health, their future health and quality of life is great.

Mr Burn May I support Prof. Mansel's earlier comment about benign breast disorder induced by HRT. The cost factor is not just the question of screening, but the cost of attending clinics, the aspirations that go with this, and the therapy that is often necessary for reintroduction of breast symptoms.

Following Dr Gambrell's comments about publications, I would like to comment that these very elegant cost-effective studies can have an enormous impact. To give two examples in the UK: first, in my opinion, it was a very theoretical cost-effective study that postponed the introduction of breast screening in the UK for some 10 years. Likewise, about 5 years ago, the UK Department of Health commenced a series of theoretical cost-effective studies for hospital beds. This resulted in the closure of 2000 hospital beds in the North-West Thames Region, essentially based on cost-effective studies of very doubtful validity. I would make the plea that if publications are made on the sort of presentation we have heard from Dr Roche today, that it is made absolutely clear that these are extremely theoretical considerations and should not lead to any direct action.

Dr Roche I accept the point. When a cost-effective study is published we make very clear that a large number of assumptions have to be made, some of which are based on good evidence and some of which are not. This is certainly the case with this study. We could stand up in court with some of the assumptions, but with others there would be great dispute. This is why sensitivity analysis is done and a range of possible values presented. The real value is that because we have to be explicit about what has been assumed, the areas where more evidence is needed before a final answer can be given are highlighted.

Prof. Dupont In response to the troubling comments by Dr Gambrell and to take a specific example; I – and I believe most people here – found the recent study of Dr Colditz and colleagues very reassuring. Yet, in our local newspaper it made an enormous splash with 'Harvard professors found a 40% increase in breast cancer risk' – which was perceived to be a finding of very major concern to the general public. I have no idea what the answer is. It does not matter how carefully we write our papers or describe our results and their certainty (or lack of it); the lay press remains in the business of selling newspapers or television or whatever – and scaring people silly sells newspapers. It is the nature of our profession that we will never have simple answers; it is the nature of the newspaper business that they will strive to oversimplify and be provocative.

Prof. Ross Unfortunately, how the press deals with our publications is completely out of our hands. However cautious we may be in our own language, the press may be incautious in how they deal with our findings. It is no secret that I am a proponent of oestrogen replacement therapy – I think probably of routine use of ERT. I also believe that the Swedish paper got the right answer, that there is a duration-related increase in breast cancer risk association with ERT, and probably combination therapy adds a little to that risk. The press obviously finds breast cancer much more interesting to deal with than a reduction in heart disease and, as a result, the Swedish paper received much more publicity than probably all the papers on the reduction in heart disease risk combined. This is bad, in a sense, but it may parallel the way many women feel about the issue; that one breast cancer does not equate to one heart attack, but might equal 10 or even 100 heart attacks. For some women, the equation may never balance. For women, breast cancer is a much more emotional issue than heart disease, so they may deal with it personally in the same way as the press.

Dr H.P. McEwan To the gynaecologist, endometrial carcinoma is the cancer with the lowest risk; it would not concern us too greatly. The extremely interesting thing that is coming out of this meeting is whether we should now, in fact, advise opposed oestrogen therapy.

Prof. Jacobs I thought Prof. Ross gave a most persuasive account of why, on biological grounds, he thinks hormones cause breast cancer. If we think it likely, *a priori*, that hormones cause breast cancer, then – applying Popperian ideas of science – the obligation on the scientist is to try to flaw that hypothesis. Thus, it is not good enough to say that the epidemiologists have failed to prove that oestrogens cause breast cancer. It is their failure to produce negative results that we should be worrying about.

Dr Mann It is interesting, and perhaps worrying, that we are trying, both with the pill and with HRT, to establish safe conditions of use while a generation of women are using them.

Dr Santra If we suspect that oestrogen increases the risk of breast cancer perhaps we should ask if there is a role for calcitonin nasal spray – because calcitonin reduces reabsorption of bone – in the management of postmenopausal osteoporosis. Could we give calcitonin nasal spray and low oestrogen at the same time, in the hope of reducing the risk of breast cancer? There was a report from Belgium, in 1989, in which oestrogen therapy was not given to those women who needed replacement therapy for osteoporoses, but they were treated with a calcitonin nasal spray, and there was the same effect. Do we have an opinion on this? (*Prof. Ross indicated that he had no experience of the use of calcitonin*)

Dr Mann It is difficult – perhaps as difficult as looking at diet and exercise under double-blind conditions, yet we would not want to give long-term hormone therapy if diet and exercise are equally effective in preventing bone loss and cardiovascular disease.

Prof. S. Shapiro I must take issue with Prof. Ross regarding his certainty concerning the reduction in the risk of ischaemic heart disease.

None of the studies that have been done have taken life-style factors into account; they have failed to take into account the fact that oestrogen users are undoubtedly more health conscious than non-users, thus they engage in practices that have not been controlled in the studies. In my judgement, it is likely that oestrogens do reduce the risk of ischaemic heart disease, but to a much lesser extent than has been suggested in many of the studies.

If the reduction is low, and if it should turn out, in due course, that one or other of the hormonal preparations increases the risk of breast cancer, then we may have an entirely different perspective than we have now.

It worries me that we are currently recommending that women should use, for prophylaxis, and for 10, 15 or 20 years, a preparation about which uncertainties remain regarding the evidence of benefit and risk... (*applause*)

Prof. Mansel Am I correct in presuming that those people who are certain that hormone replacement therapy is safe, and has no effect on breast cancer, do no monitoring of the breast when they treat their patients?

Dr Gambrell We feel that it is safe. The same monitoring should be done for women on, and not on, replacement therapy. In the USA, this is recommended by the American Cancer Society. This involves a baseline mammogram between the ages of 35 and 40, every 1–2 years in women with breasts which are normal on palpation at ages between 40 and 50, and annually after age 50.

Mr Pugh With regard to the use of continuous oestrogen, we are doing a trial now of administering it for 3 months, and then giving progestogen for the fourth month. We have no figures because the work has not yet been completed. Clearly, we are still worried about endometrial cancer and want to know whether this regime might retain the safety that we have already.

Prof. Ross We are doing the same kind of trial at the University of Southern California, trying the intermittent use of progestogens. We do not yet have evidence of what this does in terms of endometrial hyperplasia, let alone the risk of endometrial cancer.

Mr H.H. Hamed We seem to discuss the issue in absolute terms. We know that during the postmenopausal period, the main symptomatic impact and the maximum bone loss occur during its early phase. From what we have heard today, it would seem that the risk of breast cancer is observed following a prolonged use of HRT, and if the protective effect of HRT lasts for 5–10 years after stopping it, why can't it be used, say, for 7–10 years after the menopause, thus achieving a prolonged protection without increasing the risk of breast cancer?

Dr Roche The problem is that we do not know whether the beneficial effect on fractures *does* last permanently after HRT is stopped. Given that hip fractures really only start being common in women when they are in their late 70s and 80s, it is important to know whether the effect of the medication lasts into the period of fracture risk – and we do not know that. If we did, your suggestion would be fine.

Dr Mann I must bring the discussion to a close. Clearly there are a number of alternative views on the use of HRT: let me ask each of you to indicate which of the following main alternatives you would choose:

(1) HRT is dreadful and you would never give it to a woman, whatever her opinion. (*One person*)

(2) You would use it primarily symptomatically for up to, say, 5 years. (*About half of those present*)

(3) You would also use it prophylactically for 10 or 20 years? (*The other half of the audience*)

We should not treat this result too seriously but it is interesting to note that of the 134 persons who voted in response to this question, 92 are British, 21 are American or Canadian, and 21 are from other countries. In terms of forms of medical practice the split is as follows: 36 pharmaceutical physicians; 33 physicians; 25 surgeons or gynaecologists; 23 non-medical scientists, epidemiologists or statisticians; nine family doctors; and eight lawyers, or members of non-medical professions.

REFERENCES

1. Henderson, B.E., Paganini-Hill, A. and Ross, R.K. (1991). Decreased mortality in users of oestrogen replacement therapy. *Arch. Int. Med.*, **151,** 75–8
2. Bates, S.K. (1991). Postmenopausal estrogen replacement therapy and breast cancer. *J. Soc. Obstet. Gynecol. Canada*, **12**, 9–13

Index